Historical Atlas of

Immunology

Historical Atlas of
Immunology

Julius M. Cruse BA BS DMedSc MD PhD Dr hc FAAM FRSH FRSM

Guyton Distinguished Professor
Professor of Pathology
Distinguished Professor of the History of Medicine
Director of Immunopathology and Transplantation Immunology
Director of Graduate Studies in Pathology
Department of Pathology
Associate Professor of Medicine and Associate Professor of Microbiology
University of Mississippi Medical Center
Historian of the American Association of Immunologists
Historian of the American Society for Histocompatibility and Immunogenetics
Investigator of the Wilson Research Foundation
Mississippi Methodist Rehabilitation Center
Jackson, Mississippi, USA

Robert E. Lewis BA MS PhD FRSH FRSM

Professor of Pathology
Director of Immunopathology and Transplantation Immunology
Department of Pathology
University of Mississippi Medical Center
Investigator of the Wilson Research Foundation
Mississippi Methodist Rehabilitation Center
Jackson, Mississippi, USA

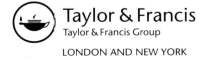

Taylor & Francis
Taylor & Francis Group
LONDON AND NEW YORK

© 2005 Taylor & Francis, an imprint of the Taylor & Francis Group

First published in the United Kingdom in 2005
by Taylor & Francis,
an imprint of the Taylor & Francis Group,
2 Park Square, Milton Park
Abingdon, Oxon OX14 4RN, UK

Tel.:   +44 (0) 20 7017 6000
Fax.:   +44 (0) 20 7017 6699
Website: www.tandf.co.uk

Although every effort has been made to ensure that all owners of copyright material have been acknowledged in this publication, we would be glad to acknowledge in subsequent reprints or editions any omissions brought to our attention.

British Library Cataloguing in Publication Data

Data available on application

Library of Congress Cataloging-in-Publication Data

Data available on application

ISBN 1-84214-217-8

Distributed in North and South America by

Taylor & Francis
2000 NW Corporate Blvd
Boca Raton, FL 33431, USA

Within Continental USA
Tel.: 800 272 7737; Fax.: 800 374 3401
Outside Continental USA
Tel.: 561 994 0555; Fax.: 561 361 6018
E-mail: orders@crcpress.com

Distributed in the rest of the world by
Thomson Publishing Services
Cheriton House
North Way
Andover, Hampshire SP10 5BE, UK
Tel.: +44 (0) 1264 332424
E-mail: salesorder.tandf@thomsonpublishingservices.co.uk

Composition by Parthenon Publishing
Printed and bound by T. G. Hostench S.A., Spain

Contents

Dedication   vii

Preface   ix

Foreword   x

The Authors   xi

Acknowledgments   xiii

Chapters

1. Origins of immunity in antiquity: Rhazes; variolation; Lady Mary Wortley Montagu; Edward Jenner and smallpox vaccination by cowpox inoculation   1

2. Germ theories and the advent of classical immunology   15

3. Immunochemistry (molecular immunology)   49

4. The complement system: chronology and mystique   93

5. Anaphylaxis   109

6. Allergy, atopy, Arthus and Shwartzman reactions   121

7. Cellular immunity and delayed-type hypersensitivity   137

8. Immunobiology, cellular immunology and tumor immunity   149

9. Autoimmunity   177

10. Immunohematology   207

11. Immunogenetics, immunologic tolerance, transfusion and transplantation   225

12. Immunization against infectious diseases; interferon; congenital immunodeficiences; AIDS   269

13. Immunological methods   289

14. Immunological societies   305

15. Landmarks in the history of immunology   313

Suggested further reading   320

Epilogue   321

Credits for illustrations   323

Index   329

In celebration of the 150th birthday of

Paul Ehrlich
(1854–1915)

whose magnificent and indomitable spirit will continue to inspire future generations of immunologists from all nations

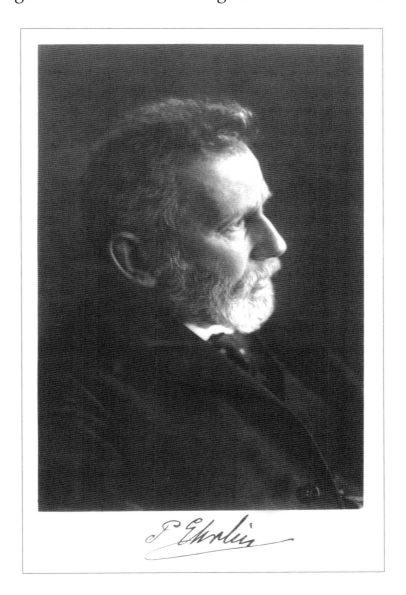

Geheimer Medicinalrat

Professor Dr. PAUL EHRLICH

Direktor des Instituts für experimentelle Therapie

FRANKFURT a. M.

hrlich, Paul, geboren zu Strehlen in Schlesien am 14. März 1854, studierte in Breslau, Freiburg, Straßburg und Leipzig Medicin. 1878 promoviert, trat er im selben Jahre als Assistent von Frerichs in die Berliner I. medicinische Klinik ein. Seit 1895 war er externer Assistent der II. medicinischen Klinik unter Gerhardt. Im Jahre 1887 habilitierte er sich als Privatdozent für innere Medicin und wurde im Jahre 1890 zum Professor extraordinarius ernannt. 1890 trat Ehrlich als Mitarbeiter Kochs in das neubegründete Institut für Infektionskrankheiten zu Berlin ein. 1896 wurde ihm die Direktion des eben errichteten kgl. Instituts für Serumforschung und Serumprüfung in Steglitz übertragen, welches unter Erweiterung seiner Aufgaben im Jahre 1899 als Institut für experimentelle Therapie nach Frankfurt am Main verlegt wurde. 1897 wurde ihm der Titel eines Geheimen Medicinalrats verliehen.

Ehrlichs zahlreiche histologische Arbeiten führten zur Begründung einer rationellen, auf chemischen Grundsätzen beruhenden Farbenanalyse der Gewebe und zur nutzbringenden Einführung der Anilinfarben in verschiedene Gebiete der mikroskopischen Technik. Durch seine Arbeiten über die normale und pathologische Histologie des Blutes, die im Jahre 1891 gesammelt als „Farbenanalytische Studien zur Histologie und Klinik des Blutes" erschienen, schuf er die grundlegenden Auffassungen für das Wesen der Bluterkrankungen. Die bisherigen Resultate der Forschung auf diesem Gebiete stellte Ehrlich gemeinsam mit Lazarus in einem 1899 erschienenen größeren Werk „Die Anämie" unter einheitlichen Gesichtspunkten dar. Im Zusammenhang mit Ehrlichs Blutstudien stehen zahlreiche klinische und klinisch-experimentelle Untersuchungen.

Von besonderer, praktischer Bedeutung ist die Auffindung der Diazo-Reaktion des Harns und die auf die Entdeckung der Säurefestigkeit der Tuberkelbazillen begründete differentielle Untersuchungen.

Von großer Wichtigkeit für die Biologie wurde Ehrlichs Entdeckung der Methylenblaureaktion der lebenden Nervensubstanz (1886). Auf rein biologisches Gebiet führt Ehrlichs Arbeit „Ueber das Sauerstoffbedürfnis des Organismus" (1885). Zahlreiche neuere Arbeiten Ehrlichs betreffen die Immunitätslehre. Hier sind zunächst die Immunisierungsversuche gegen die pflanzlichen Toxalbumine und die Studien über die Vererbung der Immunität anzuführen. Das Prinzip der quantitativen Betrachtung der Immunität und der systematischen Steigerung derselben, welche Ehrlich als erster eingeführt hat, bewährten sich bei der Uebertragung der Serumtherapie auf die Praxis. Gemeinsam mit Behring arbeitete Ehrlich jahrelang an der Ausgestaltung der Serumtherapie. Er begründete vor allem ein genaues, fast allgemein akzeptiertes Verfahren der Wertbestimmung des Diphtherieheilserums, das die Grundlage der zuerst in Deutschland eingeführten staatlichen Kontrolle bildete.

Diese Untersuchungen sind hauptsächlich in der Schrift: „Die Wertbestimmung des Diphtherieheilserums und ihre theoretischen Grundlagen" (1897) niedergelegt, wo Ehrlich zugleich seine theoretischen Anschauungen über den Wirkungsmodus der Toxine und die Entstehung der Immunität niederlegte. Ehrlichs bekannte „Seitenkettentheorie" der Immunität bringt die Erscheinungen der Immunität in Zusammenhang mit allgemeinen biologischen Gesetzen und hat sich als ein fruchtbares Prinzip der Forschung bewährt. In letzter Zeit beschäftigten Ehrlich hauptsächlich Studien über die durch Immunisierung erzeugten und die im normalen Serum vorkommenden Haemolysine. Gemeinsam mit seinem Assistenten, dem Japaner Hata, Entdeckung eines Mittels gegen Syphilis. Im Handel seit Dezember 1910 als „Salvarsan".

Von Auszeichnungen besitzt Ehrlich den preußischen Kronenorden III. Klasse, das Kommandeurkreuz II. Klasse des norwegischen Olaf-Ordens, das Kommandeurkreuz II. Klasse des Danebrog-Ordens. Er ist Mitglied der dänischen Akademie der Wissenschaften, Ehrenmitglied der Deutschen balneologischen Gesellschaft und korrespondierendes Mitglied der Société de Biologie. Der Zar zeichnete ihn durch den Armeeorden I. Klasse mit Brillanten, der König von Spanien durch das Großkreuz des Ordens Alfons XII und der König von Serbien durch den heiligen Savaorden I. Klasse aus. Er ist auswärtiges Mitglied der medicinischen Klasse der Akademie der Wissenschaften in Stockholm und Ehrenmitglied des Instituts für experimentelle Therapie in St. Petersburg. 1908 erhielt er den Nobelpreis.

Preface

The *Historical Atlas of Immunology* chronicles the metamorphosis of immunology with the aid of numerous photographs and illustrations that depict major persons and events responsible for pivotal advances in the development of the modern and eclectic science of immunology.

Following each historical account is a section in shaded boxes that presents the current status of knowledge on that topic for those unfamiliar with the field. It is our hope that this approach will make the publication attractive not only to immunologists, but to other scientists and lay-persons alike with an appreciation for the history of science and medicine.

Beginning with the origins of immunology in antiquity, the book is divided into chapters as shown in the Contents. The development of key concepts and theories

that stimulated an exponential increase in scientific research has culminated in a critical mass of data that intersect all aspects of biomedical science. Immunology has relevance for many other branches of medical science ranging from transplant surgery to molecular biology. To appreciate the current status of knowledge in the field, one needs to understand the pathfinders and events that led to an improved understanding of immunology, perhaps the most fascinating of all contemporary scientific research. Not only students, but researchers, physicians, investigators in related fields and even non-scientists should find the development of immunological concepts a scientific adventure worth reading. To appreciate the present, we must not forget the past. This book should fulfill that need for those interested in immunology today.

Foreword

Immunology is an eclectic science with foundations in clinical medicine, molecular biology and biophysical chemistry. It is that branch of biomedical science concerned with the response of the organism to immunogenic (antigenic) challenge, the recognition of self from non-self, all the biological (*in vivo*), serological (*in vitro*), physical and chemical aspects of immune phenomena and immunological tolerance.

The origins of immunology in antiquity include a mythological story which claimed that Mithridates, King of Pontus, protected himself against poisons by drinking the blood of ducks that had been treated with them. Pliny the Elder regarded the livers of mad dogs as a cure for rabies. Numerous African tribes practiced immunization against various venoms.

Although prophylactic inoculation against smallpox (variola) was practiced in China, India and Persia for many centuries before it was introduced into Europe, the practice of variolation was made popular in England in the 1720s, principally through the efforts of Lady Mary Wortley Montagu.

The first physician to vaccinate against smallpox with a non-virulent cowpox vaccine was Edward Jenner, who observed that milkmaids frequently remained resistant to smallpox as a consequence of prior infections on their hands by cowpox. It is remarkable that the principles of active immunization for protection against infectious disease established by Jenner's work were ignored for so many years.

Louis Pasteur and Robert Koch isolated bacterial agents of infectious diseases and grew them in pure culture. Pasteur developed an attenuated anthrax vaccine in 1881 and Koch's brilliant researches on tuberculosis formed the basis for understanding delayed-type hypersensitivity and cell-mediated immunity in disease.

The Authors

Julius M. Cruse, BA, BS, DMedSc, MD, PhD, Dr hc, is Guyton Distinguished Professor, Professor of Pathology, Director of Immunopathology and Transplantation Immunology, Director of Graduate Studies in Pathology, Associate Professor of Medicine, Associate Professor of Microbiology and Distinguished Professor of the History of Medicine at the University of Mississippi Medical Center in Jackson. Formerly, Dr Cruse was Professor of Immunology and of Biology in the University of Mississippi Graduate School. Dr Cruse graduated in 1958 receiving BA and BS degrees in Chemistry with honors from the University of Mississippi. He was a Fulbright Fellow at the University of Graz (Austria) Medical Faculty, where he wrote a thesis on Russian tickborne encephalitis virus and received the DMedSc degree *summa cum laude* in 1960. On his return to the United States, he entered the MD, PhD program at the University of Tennessee College of Medicine, Memphis, completing his MD degree in 1964 and PhD in Pathology (immunopathology) in 1966. Dr Cruse also trained in Pathology at the University of Tennessee Center for the Health Sciences, Memphis.

Dr Cruse is a member of numerous professional societies, including the American Association of Immunologists (Historian), the American Society for Investigative Pathology, the American Society for Histocompatibility and Immunogenetics (Historian; Member of Council, 1997–99; formerly Chairman, Publications Committee (1987–1995)), the Societé Française d'Immunologie, the Transplantation Society and the Society for Experimental Biology and Medicine, among many others. He is a Fellow of the American Academy of Microbiology, a Fellow of the Royal Society of Health (UK) and a Fellow of the Royal Society of Medicine (London). He received the Doctor of Divinity, *honoris causa* in 1999 from The General Theological Seminary of the Episcopal Church, New York City.

Dr Cruse's research has centered on transplantation and tumor immunology, autoimmunity, MHC genetics in the pathogenesis of AIDS, and neuroendocrine immune interactions. He has received many research grants during his career and is currently funded by the Wilson Research Foundation for neuroendocrine–immune system interactions in patients with spinal cord injuries. He is the author of more than 300 publications in scholarly journals and 45 books, and has directed dissertation and thesis research for more than 40 graduate students during his career. He is editor-in-chief of the international journals *Immunologic Research*, *Experimental and Molecular Pathology* and *Transgenics*. He was chief editor of the journal *Pathobiology* from 1982 to 1998 and was founder of *Immunologic Research*, *Transgenics* and *Pathobiology*.

Robert E. Lewis, BA, MS, PhD, is Professor of Pathology and Director of Immunopathology and Transplantation Immunology in the Department of Pathology at the University of Mississippi Center in Jackson. Dr Lewis received his BA and MS degrees in Microbiology from the University of Mississippi and earned his PhD in Pathology (Immunopathology) from the University of Mississippi Medical Center. Following specialty postdoctoral training at several medical institutions, Dr Lewis has risen through the academic ranks from Instructor to Professor at the University of Mississippi Medical Center.

Dr Lewis is a member of numerous professional societies, including the American Association of

Immunologists, the American Society for Investigative Pathology, the Society for Experimental Biology and Medicine, the American Society for Microbiology, the Canadian Society for Immunology and the American Society for Histocompatibility and Immunogenetics (Chairman, Publications Committee; Member, Board of Directors), among numerous others. He is a Fellow of the Royal Society of Health of Great Britain and a Fellow of the Royal Society of Medicine (UK). Dr Lewis has been the recipient of a number of research grants in his career and is currently funded by the Wilson Research Foundation for his research on neuroendocrine–immune system interactions in patients with spinal cord injuries.

Dr Lewis has authored or coauthored more than 120 papers, 150 abstracts and 35 books. He has made numerous scientific presentations at both national and international levels. In addition to neuroendocrine–immune interactions, his current research also includes immunogenetic aspects of AIDS progression. Dr Lewis is a founder, senior editor and deputy editor-in-chief of *Immunologic Research* and *Transgenics* and is senior editor and deputy editor-in-chief of *Experimental* and *Molecular Pathology*. He was senior editor and deputy editor-in-chief of *Pathobiology* from 1982 to 1998.

Acknowledgments

It is a great pleasure and privilege to thank Mrs Dorothy Whitcomb, formerly Historical Librarian and Curator of the Cruse Collection in Immunology at the Middleton Health Sciences Library at the University of Wisconsin, Madison. Much of her scholarly and indefatigable research into the history of immunology is reflected in the contents of this volume. We offer her our eternal gratitude.

The authors express genuine appreciation to Ms Julia Peteet, who transcribed the manuscript through numerous revisions, Mr G. W. (Bill) Armstrong, who prepared most of the photographs and illustrations for publication, and Mr William Buhner for computer graphics. We also thank Mr Michael Schenk and Mr Kyle Cunningham for art and scientific illustration. We are most grateful to the magnificent team at Taylor & Francis, especially Mr Nick Dunton, acquiring editor, Mrs Pam Lancaster, production editor, Ms Dinah Alam, developmental editor, and their staff.

Special thanks are expressed to Dr Daniel Jones, Dean of Medicine and Vice Chancellor for Health Affairs, University of Mississippi Medical Center, for his unstinting support of our research and academic endeavors. His wise and enthusiastic leadership has facilitated our task and made it enjoyable.

CHAPTER 1

Origins of immunity in antiquity:

Rhazes; variolation; Lady Mary Wortley Montagu; Edward Jenner and smallpox vaccination by cowpox inoculation

The metamorphosis of immunology from a curiosity of medicine associated with vaccination to a modern science focused at the center of basic research in molecular medicine is chronicled in the following pages. The people and events that led to this development are no less fascinating than the subject itself. A very great number of researchers in many diverse areas of medicine and science contributed to building the body of knowledge we now possess. It will be possible to name only a few, but we owe a debt to them all. We are standing on the shoulders of giants, and in remembering their achievements we come to understand better the richness of our inheritance.

Resistance against infectious disease agents was the principal concern of bacteriologists and pathologists who established the basis of classical immunology in the latter half of the 19th and early 20th centuries. Following the brilliant investigations by Pasteur on immunization against anthrax and rabies and Koch's studies on hypersensitivity in tuberculosis, their disciples continued research into the nature of immunity against infectious disease agents. Emil von Behring and Paul Ehrlich developed antitoxins, while Metchnikoff studied phagocytosis and cellular reactions in immunity. Buchner described complement and Bordet discovered complement fixation. With the studies of Landsteiner on immunochemical specificity, the discovery of immunological tolerance by Medawar, the announcement of Burnet's clonal selection theory of acquired immunity and the elucidation of immunoglobulin structure by Porter and Edelman, modern immunology emerged at the frontier of medical research.

This eclectic science, with foundations in clinical medicine, molecular biology and biophysical chemistry, has relevance today for essentially every biomedical discipline, ranging from molecular recognition to organ transplantation. For many years it was considered a part of what has come to be known as microbiology, and in some universities it is still taught in the same department. The discipline has acquired a number of subspecialties as knowledge about the action of the living body has been expanded, so that now research and teaching are progressing in molecular immunology (immunochemistry), immunobiology, immunogenetics, immunopathology, tumor immunology, transplantation, comparative immunology and the related fields of serology, virology and parasitology. The *New Oxford Dictionary* gives as the origin of the word immune, the Latin word *immunis*, from *im* plus *munis*, ready to be of service: hence the meaning of exemption from a service or obligation to certain duties or to taxation[1]. We still use this meaning when we speak of diplomatic immunity. The contemporary medical usage of the word is cited as being found in literature in England starting in 1879 with the meaning of freedom from infection, resistance to poison or to contagion.

Immunology, therefore, becomes the study of the biological mechanisms producing non-susceptibility to the invasive or pathogenic effects of foreign microorganisms or to the toxic effects of antigenic substances, or, more vividly phrased, the capacity to distinguish foreign material from self. The ability of the human body to resist infection and disease must have been recognized in very ancient civilizations. There are references to this recognition in early literature. Thucydides of Athens is quoted as observing that, during a plague epidemic in about 430 BC, those who recovered were used to tend the sick, 'as the same man was never attacked twice, never at least fatally'. Procopius is also quoted as recording during the plague of Justinian in AD 541 that those who recovered were not liable to a second attack[2].

King Mithridates of Pontus was a particularly blood-thirsty Middle Eastern ruler who systematically exterminated all whom he thought might usurp his throne and feared that he might be poisoned, so he protected himself with repeated small doses of poison[3]. His name survives in the modern dictionary as the noun 'Mithridatism' for the tolerance produced in the body as a result, or in the universal antidote 'theriac' of the medieval formularies.

SMALLPOX

This disease was known in India and China very early. Writings in the sacred canon of Hinduism describe inoculation with pus from the lesions of smallpox using thread soaked in the matter, which was introduced into small incisions in the skin, traditionally done by members of the priestly Brahmin caste. A different custom was reported from possibly the year AD 1000 or thereabouts, in China, where crusts from smallpox vesicles were wrapped in cotton or powdered and introduced into the nostrils of those who were to be protected, thereby producing a mild form of the disease[4].

Muhammed ibn Zakariya, Abu Bakr al-Razi, better known to the world as Rhazes, wrote the first modern description of smallpox, which he described as a mild childhood disease, caused by excess moisture in the blood, which fermented and escaped from the body through the pustules[5] (Figures 1 and 2). Smallpox probably spread in Europe between the sixth and ninth centuries, and certainly had become widespread by the Crusades. It was introduced into the Americas by the Spaniards. Epidemics were of frequent occurrence thereafter. Probably fewer than 20% of the population escaped infection. At best, it was disfiguring and could cause blindness. In the 17th century in London, about 10% of all deaths were caused by this one disease[6].

Folk medicine recorded in Europe in the 16th and 17th centuries shows that some sort of inoculation was frequently practiced. Thomas Bartholin, who was physician to Christian V of Denmark and Norway, wrote of the practice in 1675. It was reported from rural

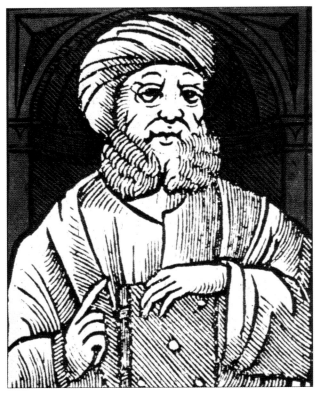

Figure 1 Rhazes (Abu Bakr Muhammad ibn Zakariya) (865–932), Persian philosopher and alchemist who described measles and smallpox as different diseases. He also was a proponent of the theory that immunity is acquired. Rhazes is often cited as the premier physician of Islam

France and Wales. The universal folk expression seems to have been 'buying the smallpox', and a widely held superstition was that the inoculation would not be successful without a symbolic transaction, of giving a small coin, fruit, nut or sweetmeat for each 'purchase'.

Historically, the intracutaneous inoculation of pus from lesions of smallpox victims into healthy, non-immune subjects to render them immune to smallpox was known as *variolation*. In China, lesional crusts were ground into a powder and inserted into the recipient's nostrils. These procedures protected some individuals, but often led to life-threatening smallpox infection in others.

The first scholarly observation of this custom may be one made by a Greek physician, Emmanuele Timoni, living in Constantinople, who had taken a medical degree at Oxford. He circulated several copies of a manuscript describing inoculation of smallpox matter and sent a copy to the Royal Society of London in 1713, which was published in the *Philosophical Transactions* in 1714. Two years later, another report, the

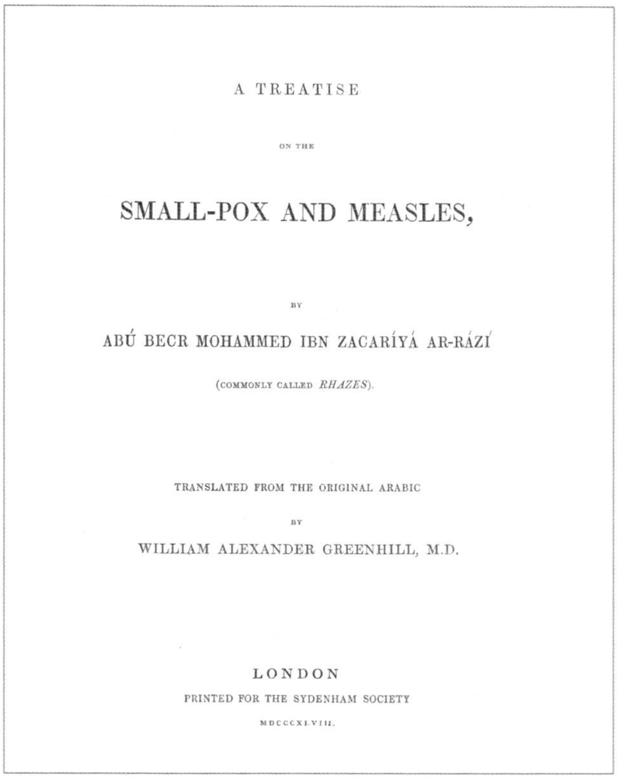

A TREATISE

ON THE

SMALL-POX AND MEASLES,

BY

ABÚ BECR MOHAMMED IBN ZACARÍYÁ AR-RÁZÍ

(COMMONLY CALLED *RHAZES*).

TRANSLATED FROM THE ORIGINAL ARABIC

BY

WILLIAM ALEXANDER GREENHILL, M.D.

LONDON
PRINTED FOR THE SYDENHAM SOCIETY
MDCCCXLVIII.

Figure 2 Rhazes' famous treatise on the smallpox and measles. Title page from work translated by William Alexander Greenhill

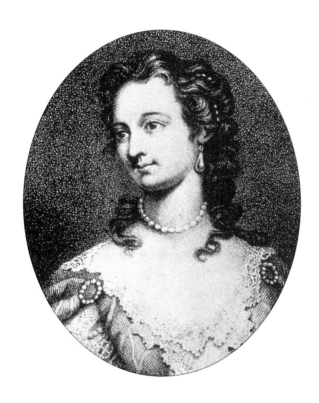

Figure 3 Lady Mary Wortley Montagu (1689–1762), often credited as the first to introduce inoculation as a means of preventing smallpox in England in 1722. After observing the practice in Turkey where her husband was posted as Ambassador to the Turkish court, she had both her young son and her daughter inoculated and interested the Prince and Princess of Wales in the practice. Accounts of inoculation against smallpox are found in her *Letters*, 1777. From Robert Halsband, author of a biography *The Life of Lady Mary Wortley Montagu*. Oxford, Clarendon: 1956

first separately published treatise on inoculation, was sent by Jacob Pylarini, who was the Venetian Consul in Smyrna. It also appeared in the *Philosophical Transactions*. Perhaps because her actions were publicized by Voltaire, or because of her own literary talents, Lady Mary Wortley Montagu is often cited as the first to report the custom in England (Figure 3). She had suffered a disfiguring case of smallpox as a young woman in England, before accompanying her husband to Constantinople, where he was posted as Ambassador to the Turkish court from 1716 to 1718. She had her young son inoculated and reported enthusiastically on the success of the treatment in a letter to a friend in England in April, 1717. On her return to England, she also had her 4-year-old daughter inoculated by Mr Charles Maitland in April, 1721. She was a friend of the Prince and Princess of Wales, according to some reports, and they lent their prestige to popularizing the treatment in England. It is very possible that Sir Hans Sloane, who was editor of the *Philosophical Transactions*, president of the Royal Society and physician to George II, had more influence in interesting the Princess of Wales in investi-

gating the worth of inoculation, than did Lady Mary. Sir Hans supervised the original experiments which were conducted in England with the inoculation, using six criminals from Newgate Prison, who were inoculated by Mr Maitland in 1721[6]. Educated people began to use the term inoculation, from the Latin *inoculare*, to graft, or variolation (Latin *varus*, a pimple), the scholarly name for smallpox[4].

In the American colonies, Cotton Mather, who regularly received communications from the Royal Society, read the reports of Timoni and Pylarini in the *Philosophical Transactions*. He also heard of the practice of inoculation from a slave who told of similar folk customs in southern Tripoli, in Africa. In 1721, when smallpox broke out in Boston, he enlisted the aid of Zabdiel Boylston, a physician, who first inoculated his own 6-year-old son and two slaves. Being successful, he went on to inoculate about 240 Bostonians. In spite of the opposition of other doctors, inoculation continued to be used, particularly when epidemics occurred[6].

There was a storm of controversy about inoculation in England. Disease in general was often viewed as punishment meted out by God, who might see fit to chastise and mold his servants by various tribulations, and to take matters into human hands was seen as sinful. Since the disease produced was true smallpox, it could cause a more virulent attack of the disease than expected. The patient could certainly pass the smallpox on to others in the natural way if not isolated, giving rise to another epidemic. The practice took hold slowly, first among the nobility and wealthy class. The first inoculation hospital was opened in London in 1746, at the time of a serious epidemic. A pronouncement was made by the College of Physicians in 1755, commending the practice[6]. James Kirkpatrick, a Scottish physician who had practiced in the Carolinas, was a successful and vocal promoter of inoculation who represented himself as reviving the practice in England in the 1740s[6]. Robert Sutton and six of his seven sons took advantage of a good opportunity and became wealthy and famous for their 'method' of inoculation from about 1757[7]. Their technique called for a period of preparation by rest and special light diet, and segregation during the course of the disease in one of their nursing facilities, an expensive process. They set up practices in different parts of southern England. Inoculation went through the same slow process of growth and promotion in France.

Several members of the nobility of Europe were attacked by smallpox. Maria Theresa of Austria survived a case in 1759. Queen Mary of England died in 1694 and the Duke of Gloucester died in 1700. Voltaire, who was in exile in England during the time when inoculation was first introduced, 1726–29, and who himself had had smallpox, was a correspondent of Catherine the Great of Russia. He encouraged her to try the new treatment to protect herself. British physicians had been popular in the Russian court since the 16th century. Dr Thomas Dimsdale of Hertford wrote a popular and successful book, *The present method of inoculating for the smallpox*, which must have helped bring him to the attention of the Russian ambassador Mussin-Pushkin, who arranged for him to go to Russia to attend Catherine. Dr Dimsdale performed the inoculation successfully, and later also inoculated the Grand Duke,

Catherine's young son and several others. He was given the title of Baron, a gift of £10 000 and an annuity of £1500 for life. The episode led to a period of westernization and modernization in Russian medicine in addition to popularizing inoculation there[8].

The contemporary literature on inoculation was extensive. The arguments for and against it raged in pamphlets, sermons by the clergy and communications to the learned societies of England and France. Sir Hans Sloane and Voltaire wrote accounts in the 1730s. Charles La Condamine published a *Memoire sur l'inoculation de la petite verole*, an excellent summary of the introduction of inoculation in France in 1754. William Woodville, of the Smallpox and Inoculation Hospital of London, wrote a detailed history of the introduction of inoculation into Britain, *A History of the Inoculation of the Smallpox in Great Britain*, London, 1796. After a thorough discussion of the antiquity of the folk customs, he gave a complete account of the various reports on early trials, the process of experimentation and investigation in Great Britain, including detailed lists of the patients and their various doctors and reviewed a number of books and pamphlets on the subject. His Volume I ends with a promise to discuss the Suttons and their business venture in a second volume. He is said to have prepared a draft of the second part, but unfortunately abandoned it when Jenner published his *Inquiry* in 1798.

Edward Jenner (1749–1823) is often credited as the founder of immunology for his contribution of the first reliable method of conferring lasting immunity to a major contagious disease (Figure 4). As a young man, he studied under John Hunter, and continued to collaborate with him in various natural history studies for many years. He spent most of his career as a country doctor in Berkeley, in southern England (Figures 5 and 6). It was fairly common knowledge in the country then that an eruptive skin disease of cattle (Figure 7), cowpox, and a similar disease in horses called grease, conferred immunity to smallpox on those who milked and cared for the animals and caught the infection from them. A few other people had also experimented with inducing an experimental infection of cowpox in humans to produce this immunity. However, it is to Jenner, with his careful observation and record of 23 cases and his initiative in describing his work in a small privately printed work, that we must give credit for initiating the technique of vaccination. He vaccinated an 8-year-old boy James Phipps with matter taken from the arm of the milkmaid Sarah

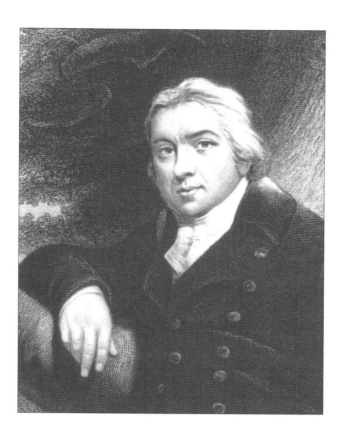

Figure 4 Edward Jenner (1749–1822), often credited as the founder of immunology for his contribution of the first reliable method of conferring lasting immunity to a major contagious disease. He studied medicine under John Hunter, and for most of his career was a country doctor in Berkeley in southern England. Although it was common knowledge among the country folk that an eruptive skin disease of cattle, cowpox, and a similar disease in horses called 'grease', conferred immunity to smallpox on those who cared for the animals and contracted the infection from them, Jenner carefully observed and recorded 23 cases. The results of his experiments were published, establishing his claim of credit for initiating the technique of vaccination. He vaccinated an 8-year-old boy, James Phipps, with matter taken from the arm of the milkmaid, Sarah Nelmes, who was suffering from cowpox. After the infection subsided, he inoculated the child with smallpox and found that the inoculation had no effect. His results led to widespread adoption of vaccination in England and elsewhere in the world, leading ultimately to the eradication of smallpox

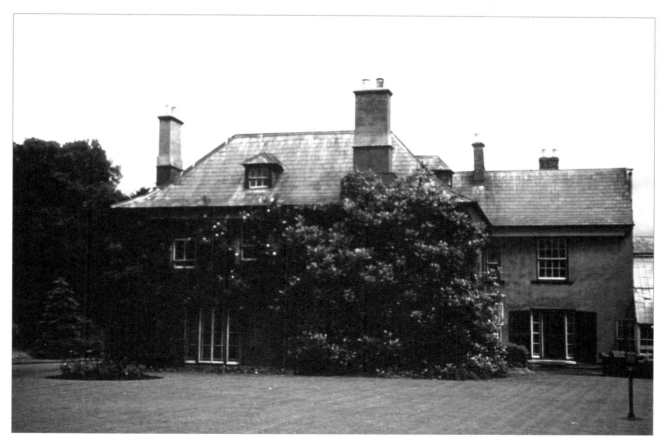

Figure 5 Edward Jenner's home at Berkeley, Gloucestershire

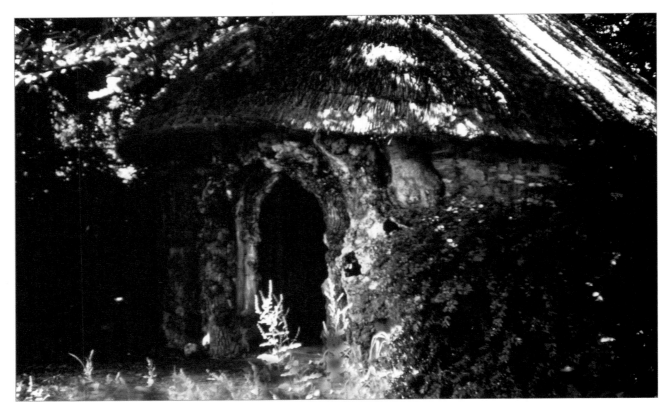

Figure 6   The vaccination hut on the Jenner estate

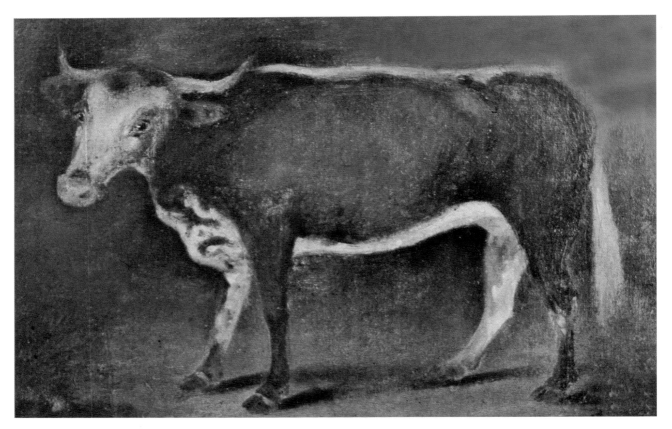

Figure 7   'Blossom', a cow infected with cowpox which was transmitted to milkmaids

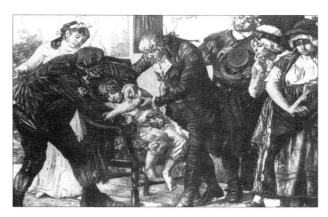

Figure 8 Dr Edward Jenner inoculating pus from the hand of Sarah Nelmes into the arm of James Phipps

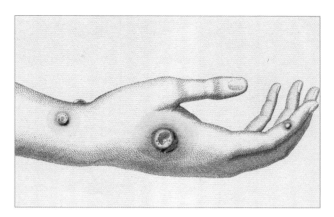

Figure 9 The hand of Sarah Nelmes. a milkmaid infected with cowpox

Nelmes (Figures 8–10), who was suffering from cowpox. After the infection subsided, he inoculated the child with smallpox and found, as he expected, that the inoculation had no effect. He observed the several related viruses causing similar eruptive diseases in animals and termed them collectively 'viruses', which in time led to the use of this word in its modern sense. He observed and described an anaphylactic reaction in one of his patients, and made a correct observation in another case that a concurrent infection with herpes interfered with vaccination. His excellent colored illustrations of the typical lesion were accurate and showed that cowpox was a separate disease. The new procedure was known as vaccination (Latin *vacca*: cow)[9–11] (Figure 11).

Jenner's discovery was soon adopted by many physicians (Figures 12–16). A Royal Commission was set up to investigate his claim, and ruled in his favor. The British Parliament voted for him to receive two large grants in gratitude. He spent a great portion of his life thereafter in defending and publicizing his new method. He modified his views in the face of experience, for example coming to the view that revaccination might become necessary and that absolutely total protection could not be produced. It was soon learned that the vaccine could be dried and transported from place to place in quills, or using threads soaked in the matter (Figure 17). For distant transmittal by ocean voyage, a group of immigrant children were sent and the disease passed serially among them. By 1801, the vaccine had been sent overland as far as Basra and thence by ship to India, where many thousands were vaccinated. In Massachusetts, Benjamin Waterhouse introduced vaccination to the USA with vaccine sent by

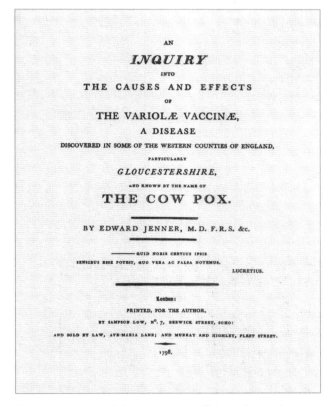

Figure 10 Jenner's famous report of his studies on immunization against smallpox

Jenner in 1800. President Jefferson vaccinated his family and neighbors with vaccine from Waterhouse, and wrote, encouraging the adoption of the practice elsewhere in the country[12]. By 1840, the practice of inoculating with smallpox was officially banned in England. Edward Jenner's introduction of vaccination with cowpox to protect against smallpox rendered variolation obsolete.

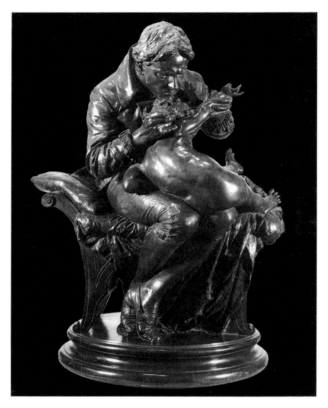

Figure 11 Bronze statue of Jenner vaccinating his own son against smallpox with cowpox lymph

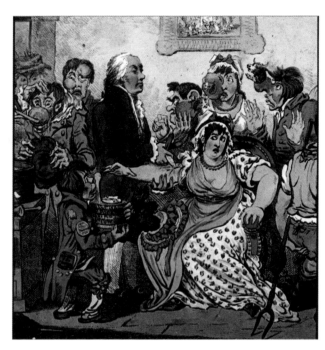

Figure 12 L. Gillray cowpox cartoon, 'The Cowpox or the wonderful effects of the new inoculation'

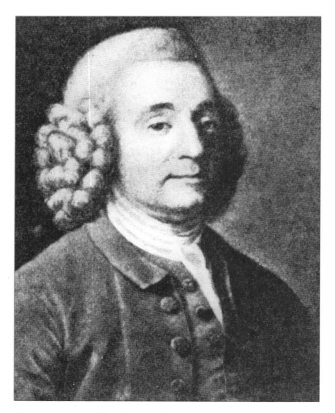

Figure 13 Dr Dimsdale, a pioneer in smallpox vaccination

KINE POCK INOCULATION.

Rules to be attended to during the Vaccination.

1. THE diet to be the same as before vaccination.
2. Scratching or rubbing the arm, or shoving up the sleeve should be avoided as much as possible.
3. In case an itching sensation of the vaccinated part should give the patient uneasiness, a little vinegar applied to the part will give immediate relief.
4 No matter to be transferred from the person inoculated to another person. Taking it from another often becomes a snare to individuals, and the source of spurious matter. But even those, who by chance have had the genuine disease in that way, have no certainty of it—and who would wish to have it upon uncertainties?
5. Women, who do house work, should avoid washing and baking on the 7th and 8th days, the usual time for the symptoms.
6. No danger of washing the hands and face in cold water during the disease.
7. Women may without hesitation receive the Kine Pock in all circumstances without exception, at home or travelling by land or water.
8. No danger of vaccinating children at the period of teething.
9. Labouring men and mechanics need not abstain from their customary employment, provided their indisposition does not require it.
10. Children should never be lifted by the arms,* especially when under the inoculation. The arm should not be bound up, nor confined in tight sleeves.

OBSERVATIONS.

1. It occasions no other disease. On the contrary, it has often been known to improve health; and to remedy those diseases, under which the patient before laboured.
2. It leaves behind no blemish, but a *blessing*;—one of the greatest ever bestowed on man;—*a perfect security against the future infection of the small-pox.*
N. B. Save the scab for examination. B. WATERHOUSE.

* No prudent person, who is aware of the tenderness of the bone of a young child, would ever lift one by its arms, or lead a child a mile by one arm.

Cambridge, July 3, 1809.

Figure 14 Kine pock inoculation: published observations

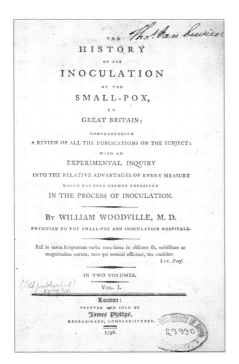

Figure 15 Dr William Woodville's famous history of inoculation against smallpox

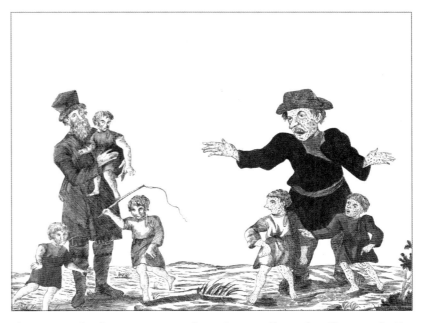

Figure 16 Smallpox cartoon, artist unknown. From the Clement C. Fry Collection, Yale Medical Library, contributed by Jason S. Zielonka, published in *J Hist Med* 1972;27:447. Legend translated: Smallpox disfigured father says, 'How shameful that your pretty little children should call my children stupid and should run away, refusing to play with them as friends...' Meanwhile, the children lament: 'Father dear, it appears to be your fault that they're avoiding us. To tell the truth, it looks as though you should have inoculated us against smallpox'

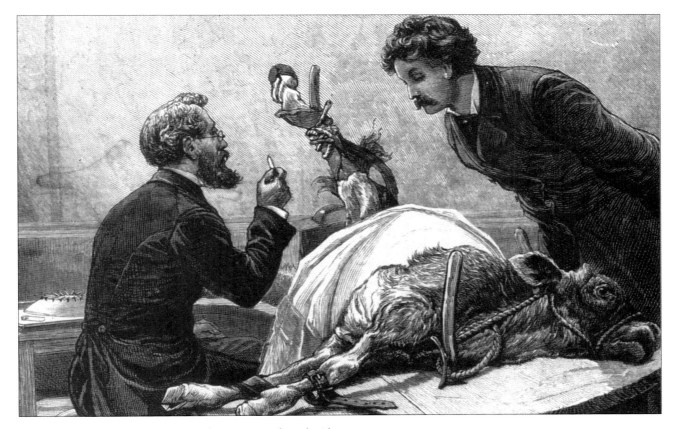

Figure 17 The collection of lymph from a cow infected with cowpox

Vaccination is immunization against infectious disease through the administration of vaccines for the production of active (protective) immunity in man or other animals.

Cowpox is a bovine virus disease that induces vesicular lesions on the teats. It is of great historical significance in immunology because Edward Jenner observed that milkmaids who had cowpox lesions on their hands failed to develop smallpox. He used this principle in vaccinating humans with the cowpox preparation to produce harmless vesicular lesions at the site of inoculation (vaccination). This stimulated protective immunity against smallpox (variola) because of shared antigens between the vaccinia virus and the variola virus.

Vaccinia refers to a virus termed *Poxvirus officinale* derived from cowpox and used to induce active immunity against smallpox through vaccination. It differs from both cowpox and smallpox viruses in minor antigens.

Smallpox vaccine was an immunizing preparation prepared from the lymph of cowpox vesicles obtained from healthy vaccinated bovine animals. This vaccine is no longer used, as smallpox has been eradicated throughout the world.

Smallpox vaccination involves the induction of active immunity against smallpox (variola) by immunization with a related agent, vaccinia virus, obtained from vaccinia vesicles on calf skin. Shared, and therefore cross-reactive, epitopes in the vaccinia virus provide protective immunity against smallpox. This ancient disease has now been eliminated worldwide, with the only laboratory stocks maintained in Atlanta (USA) and Moscow (Russia). These stocks are supposed to have been destroyed by both agencies once the virus was sequenced. Smallpox vaccination was first developed by the English physician Edward Jenner, whose method diminished the mortality from 20% to less than 1%. Following application of vaccinia virus by a multiple pressure method, vesicles occur at the site of application within 6–9 days. Maximum reactivity is observed by day 12. Initial vaccinations were given to 1- to 2-year-old infants with revaccination after 3 years. Children with cell-mediated immunodeficiency syndromes sometimes developed complications such as generalized vaccinia spreading from the site of inoculation. Postvaccination encephalomyelitis also occurred occasionally in adults and in babies less than 1 year old. The procedure was contraindicated in subjects experiencing immunosuppression due to any cause.

Progressive vaccinia describes an adverse reaction to smallpox vaccination in children with primary cell-mediated immunodeficiency, such as severe combined immunodeficiency. The vaccination lesion would begin to spread from the site of inoculation and cover extensive areas of the body surface, leading to death.

Postvaccinal encephalomyelitis is a demyelinating encephalomyelitis that occurs approximately 2 weeks following vaccination of infants less than 1 year of age, as well as adults, with vaccinia virus to protect against smallpox. This rare complication of the smallpox vaccination frequently led to death.

Chronic progressive vaccinia (vaccinia gangrenosa) (historical) is an unusual sequela of smallpox vaccination in which the lesions produced by vaccinia on the skin became gangrenous and spread from the vaccination site to other areas of the skin. This occurred in children with cell-mediated immunodeficiency.

Generalized vaccinia is a condition observed in some children being vaccinated against smallpox with vaccinia virus. There were numerous vaccinia skin lesions that occurred in these children who had a primary immunodeficiency in antibody synthesis. Although usually self-limited, children who also had atopic dermatitis in addition to the generalized vaccinia often died.

Vaccination had its opponents into the 20th century[13,14]. It is one of the outstanding achievements of modern medicine that, through the efforts of the World Health Organization, smallpox was finally

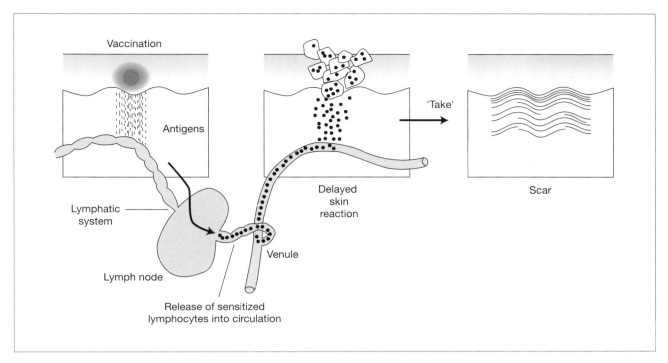

Figure 18 Vaccination against smallpox

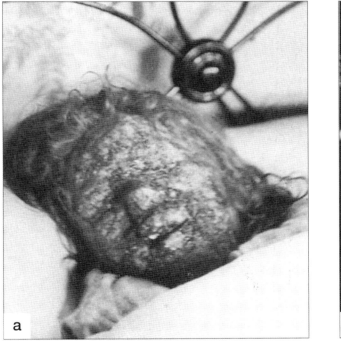
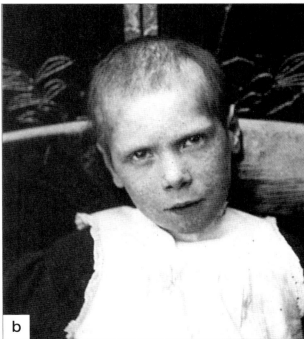

Figure 19 Small eruptions on the face of a smallpox patient (a) and the same child following recovery (b)

eradicated and continues to exist only in cultures in a few reference laboratories (Figures 18–23).

Even though naturally occurring smallpox was eradicated in 1977, recent terrorist attacks around the world, including the United States, have raised the specter that deadly biological weapons might be crafted from stocks of the virus that remain in known or clandestine laboratories.

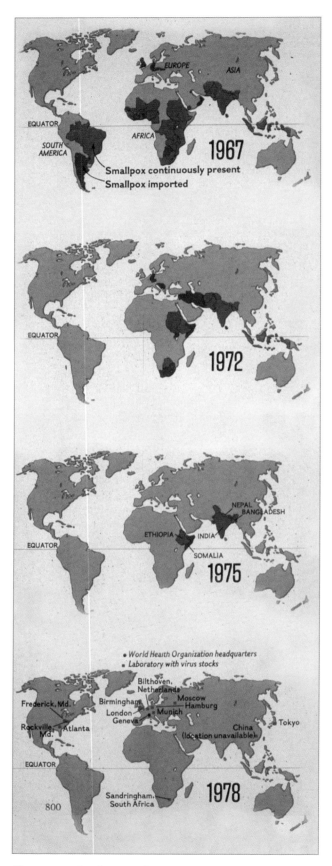

Figure 20 Smallpox eradication map

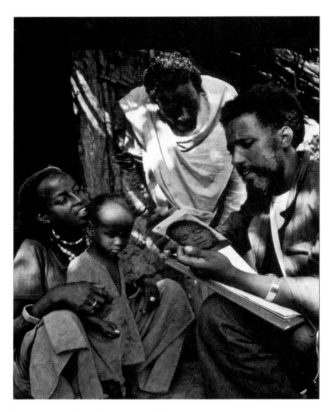

Figure 21 Smallpox surveillance

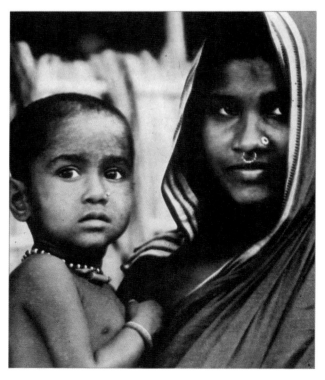

Figure 22 Rahima Banu of Bangladesh, the world's last case of naturally occurring variola major. Photo courtesy of World Health Organization. Rahima's rash began on October 16, 1975

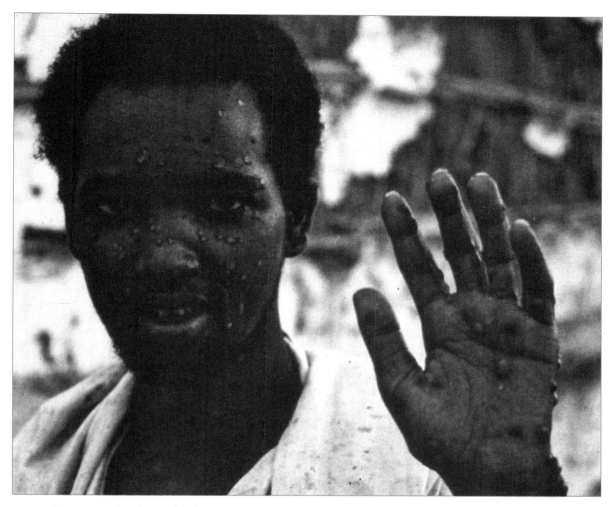

Figure 23   Ali Maow Maalin, the world's last case of naturally occurring smallpox. Photo courtesy of Dr Jason Weisfeld. Maalin's rash began on October 26, 1977 in Merka Town, Somalia

REFERENCES

1.   Murray JAH, ed. *A New English Dictionary on Historical Principles*. Oxford: Clarendon Press, 1888–1928

2.   Silverstein AM, Bialasiewicz AA. A history of theories of acquired immunity. *Cell Immunol* 1980;51:151–67

3.   *The Encyclopaedia Britannica: a Dictionary of Arts, Sciences, Literature and General Information*, 11th edn. Cambridge: Cambridge University Press, 1910

4.   Langer WL. Immunization against smallpox before Jenner. *Sci Am* 1976;234:112–17

5.   Silverstein AM. Cellular versus humoral immunity; determinants and consequences of an epic 19th century battle. *Cell Immunol* 1979;48:208–21

6.   Miller G. *The Adoption of Inoculation for Smallpox in England and France*. Philadelphia: University of Pennsylvania Press, 1957

7.   van Zwanenbert D. The Suttons and the business of inoculation. *Med Hist* 1978;22:71–82

8.   Clendenning PH. Dr. Thomas Dimsdale and smallpox inoculation in Russia. *J Hist Med* 1973:28:1109–25

9.   Baxby D. Edward Jenner, William Woodville, and the origins of vaccina virus. *J Hist Med* 1979;34:134–62

10. Lefanu WR. Edward Jenner. *Proc R Soc Med* 1973;66:664–8

11. McCrae J. Jenner, family doctor, naturalist and first immunologist. *Clin Paediatr* 1972;11:49–56

12. Cohn LH. Contributions of Thomas Jefferson to American medicine. *Am J Surg* 1979;138:286–92

13. Carrell JL. *The Speckled Monster: Historical Tale of Battling Smallpox*. New York: Dutton, 2003

14. Hopkins DR. *The Greatest Killer, Smallpox in History*. Chicago: The University of Chicago Press, 1983

CHAPTER 2

Germ theories and the advent of classical immunology

Although not very well understood, diseases were perceived as being contagious from very early times. The Bible contains many references to epidemics and the spread of disease, and the quarantine regulations which were enforced in an attempt to control them. In Europe, with the rise of trade, public health measures were instituted which were aimed at halting the spread of infection. Because the mechanisms of disease transmission were unknown, many of the regulations were useless and caused unnecessary hardship, which made them very unpopular.

An early understanding of the concept of specific infections was shown by Girolamo Fracastoro, who in 1546 wrote *De contagione, contagionis morbis et eorum curatione*. He speaks in this work of imperceptible particles which cause disease, some by contact, some through secondary objects such as clothing and some at a distance. He understood that the 'seeds' or 'germs' of infection generate and propagate other germs precisely like themselves, and recognized that there was a similarity, not well understood, between putrefaction and contagion. Best known for his poem *Syphilis*, he also recognized typhus, rabies, diphtheria and tuberculosis[1].

Leeuwenhoek was the first to see and describe microscopic organisms, although he did not speculate on their origin or their relationship to disease. J. B. von Helmont in 1662 recognized that recovery from disease produced what he described as 'balsamic' blood, which had some mysterious power of resisting infection[2]. Spallanzani studied the properties of microscopic living things and the effect of heat in killing them. His demonstrations effectively demolished the theories of spontaneous generation, although there continued to be speculation about the subject up to Pasteur's day.

Jacob Henle (1809–85) in 1840 wrote a small essay on miasmic, contagious and miasmic–contagious diseases. He understood that something was introduced into the body which produced disease and which was eliminated from the body upon recovery. He thought it would be necessary to separate the contagious material and culture it, thus showing that it had an independent existence[1].

The French physiologist Francois Magendie (1783–1855) showed that decomposing blood was lethal when injected intravenously, and innocuous when taken by mouth. He proved by experiment that gas from decomposing material did not produce disease in laboratory animals. He observed the phenomenon of anaphylaxis in rabbits in 1839, although he had no means of interpreting what had happened[3,4].

Agnostino Bassi (1773–1856) was the first to prove that microscopic living organisms, fungi, were the cause of a disease of silkworms. Villemin in 1865 demonstrated that tuberculosis was a specific disease entity, transmissible from man to rabbits by inoculation. Davaine observed the rod-shaped organism of anthrax, and transmitted the disease using blood containing the bacteria. In 1870, Klebs observed bacteria in wounds. He postulated that there was a single organism which caused all sorts of pathological conditions. Ferdinand Cohn (1828–98) attempted a classification of bacteria into four main tribes, laying a foundation for bacteriology. It was one of Cohn's students, Robert Koch (1843–1910) (Figures 1–3), who brilliantly proved that a specific organism caused a specific disease in an animal. He instituted many of the procedures which are common in bacteriology today. His postulates, arising out of the criteria implicit in Henle's essay on contagion, became part of the central dogma of bacteriology.

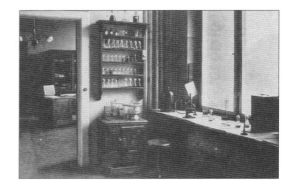

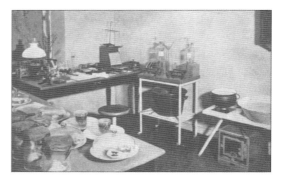

Figure 3 Robert Koch's laboratory, Institute for Infectious Diseases, Berlin

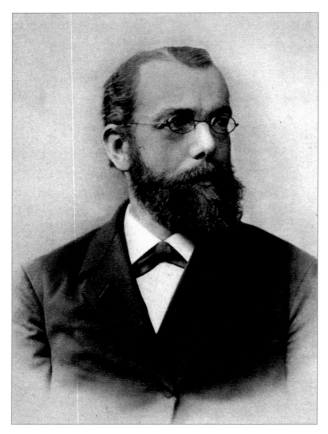

Figure 1 Robert Koch

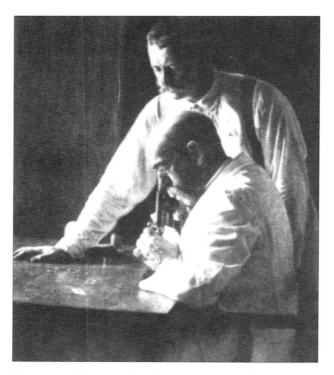

Figure 2 Robert Koch's laboratory, Institute for Infectious Diseases, Berlin

The most valuable outgrowth of his extensive research in tuberculosis for immunology was the concept of delayed hypersensitivity, an allergy of infection upon which the principles of skin testing were founded. As valuable as his many discoveries in relation to disease was the training of a large group of students and co-workers, who went on to make some of the major discoveries in early immunology. By common consent the greatest pure bacteriologist, he was awarded the Nobel Prize in 1905 for his research in tuberculosis[3].

Robert Koch (1843–1910), German bacteriologist awarded the Nobel Prize in 1905 for his work on tuberculosis. Koch made many contributions to the field of bacteriology. Along with his postulates for proof of etiology, Koch instituted strict isolation in culture methods in bacteriology. He studied the life cycle of anthrax and discovered both the cholera vibrio and the tubercle bacillus. The Koch phenomenon and Koch–Weeks bacillus both bear his name.

In the meantime, in France, Louis Pasteur (1822–95), (Figures 4–7), who was trained as a chemist, had solved problems of economic importance to France in taking up the study of selected silkworm diseases and fermentation

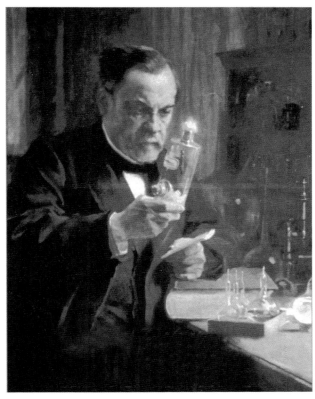

Figure 4 Louis Pasteur at work in his laboratory (The Edelfeldt painting)

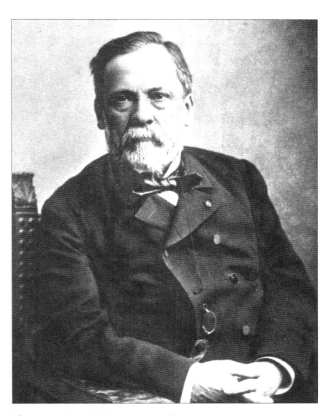

Figure 5 Louis Pasteur, portrait

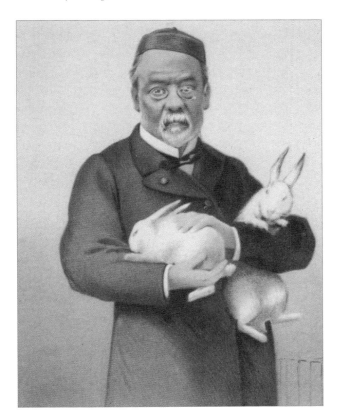

Figure 6 Louis Pasteur, a caricature

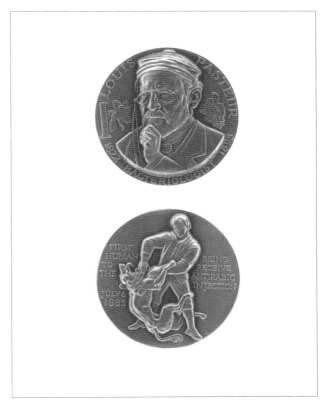

Figure 7 Louis Pasteur medallion commemorating his vaccine for rabies

in relation to beer and wine. He turned his attention to the study of anthrax and confirmed the findings of Koch, then investigated chicken cholera, whose bacteriological cause was already known. When by chance he allowed some of his cultures to grow old, he found that the chickens treated with this culture did not die, and were subsequently able to withstand injections of virulent cultures. He had discovered that attenuated bacterial cultures could produce immunity. He also observed that the anthrax bacillus would grow but not produce spores at 42°C, and that this resulted in a non-virulent form of anthrax which would produce immunity in animals.

In May of 1881, he carried out a large-scale public demonstration of anthrax immunization of sheep, a goat and several cattle, with an equal number of control animals, proving the correctness of his deductions. He paid tribute to Jenner by naming the new technique 'vaccination'. He went on to produce a vaccine for rabies by drying the spinal cords of rabbits, and using the material to prepare a series of 14 injections of increasing virulence. To attenuate the rabies virus, spinal cords of rabbits, which had died from 'fixed virus' injection, were suspended in dry, sterile air. The spinal cords became almost non-virulent in approximately 14 days. Dogs injected with emulsions of progressively less attenuated spinal cord were protected against inoculation with the most virulent form of the virus. The injection of dogs with infected spinal cord dried for 14 days, followed the next day by 13-day-old material, and so on until fresh cord was used, protected against contraction of rabies, even when the most virulent virus was injected into the brain. Thus, immunity against rabies was established in 15 days. Pasteur's first human subject was a child, Joseph Meister, whose life was saved by the treatment. Meister later spent many years as the door porter of the Institut Pasteur in Paris, which was built with funds contributed from all over the world in order that the control of this terrifying disease might be facilitated.

Louis Pasteur (1822–1895), French, 'Father of Immunology'. One of the most productive scientists of modern times, Pasteur's contributions included the crystallization of L- and O-tartaric acid, disproving the theory of spontaneous generation, studies of diseases in wine, beer and silkworms, and the use of attenuated bacteria and viruses for vaccination. He used attenuated vaccines to protect against anthrax, fowl cholera and rabies. He successfully immunized sheep and

cattle against anthrax, terming the technique vaccination in honor of Jenner. He produced a vaccine for rabies by drying the spinal cord of rabbits and using the material to prepare a series of 14 injections of increasing virulence. A child's (Joseph Meister's) life was saved by this treatment. *Les Maladies des Uers a Soie*, 1865; *Etudes sur le Vin*, 1866; *Etudes sur la Biere*, 1876; *Oeuvres*, 1922–39.

A step forward in the production of vaccines was made by Daniel E. Salmon (1850–1914) and Theobald Smith (1859–1934) (Figure 8), in the Veterinary Division of the US Department of Agriculture in 1886, when they found that pigeons inoculated with heat-killed cultures of hog cholera bacilli developed immunity[5]. They reasoned from this discovery that immunity could be induced by exposure of the body to chemical substances or toxins produced by bacteria causing the disease. George Nuttal (1862–1937) (Figure 9), in studying the blood of various animals, found that it and other body fluids were able to cause bacteria to disintegrate[6]. Hans Buchner (1850–1902) carried the study further and discovered that the bactericidal properties were to be found in cell-free serum, and that this property was destroyed by heat. He named the substance *alexine* (Greek: to ward off or protect)[7]. Experiments at the Institut Pasteur by Emile Roux (1853–1933) (Figures 10 and 11) and Alexandre Yersin (1863–1943) showed that the bacterium-free filtrate of the diphtheria bacillus culture contained an exotoxin which produced the disease[8]. While these insights into the humoral mechanisms of immunity were being developed, an original and dynamic personality appeared in the scientific community in Paris.

Elie (Illya) Metchnikoff (also spelled Mechnikov) (1845–1916) (Figures 12–16), was born at Avanovska, Ukraine on May 15, 1845. He showed an interest in natural sciences from childhood, and completed his 4-year university studies in 2 years. The son of an officer in the Imperial Guard, he attended the University of Kharkov, graduating in 1864. He studied with several researchers in Germany and Italy and began publishing original observations at a young age. He returned to Russia in 1867 as professor of zoology and comparative anatomy at the University of Odessa. He was plagued with eye trouble and bouts of depression, and lost his young wife to tuberculosis

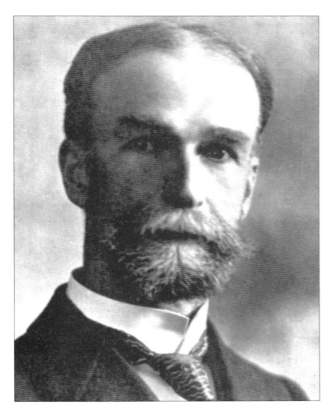

Figure 8 Theobald Smith

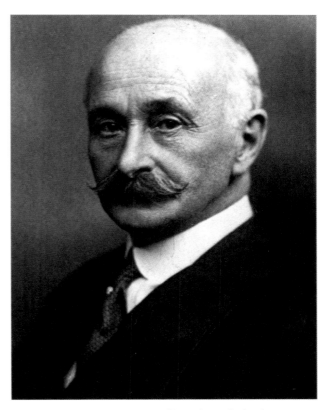

Figure 9 George H. F. Nuttalll, author of *Blood Immunity and Blood Relationships*

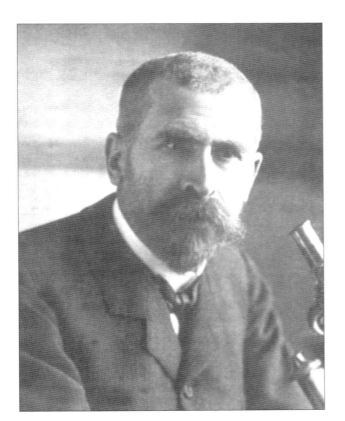

Figure 10 Emile Roux, close associate of Louis Pasteur

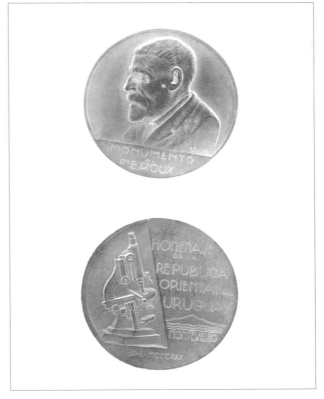

Figure 11 Emile Roux medallion

despite his devoted efforts to save her life. His second marriage, to a much younger neighbor, was happy, and the world is indebted to her for a biography of her famous husband. He was not temperamentally suited to a teaching career and left to do private study in Messina, where he first studied phagocytes, examining the transparent larvae of starfish. He observed that cells surrounded and engulfed foreign particles that had been introduced into the larvae. He further discovered that special ameba-like cells surrounded bacteria introduced into starfish larvae and fungal spores introduced into water fleas (*Daphnia*) and engulfed them. He observed the digestive powers of the mesodermal cells in starfish larvae and connected the process with the cause of immunity against infectious disease. He returned to Odessa, and while there, made further studies of the water flea, *Daphnia*, infected by a parasite, from which he built a theory of cellular immunity involving phagocytosis. He was appointed director of the Bacteriological Institute in Odessa, but being unhappy in this position, again traveled to the West, first visiting the Hygiene Institute of Robert Koch, who showed no interest. When he visited Pasteur in Paris, he was invited to remain, and spent the rest of his life at the Institut Pasteur. He found that many of the white blood cells or leukocytes are phagocytic, defending the body against acute infection by engulfing invading microorganisms. After discovering the role of phagocytes in host defense, he devoted much of his subsequent career to elaborating and championing his cellular theory of immunity. He attracted a number of students to his laboratory, including Jules Bordet (Figures 17 and 18), and published many papers, a series of *Lectures on the comparative pathology of inflammation* and a thorough and balanced review of the whole field of comparative and human immunity, *L'immunité dans les maladies infectieuses*. He was a colorful and influential personality in the early attempts to understand the mechanisms of immunity[9].

He shared the Nobel Prize in Medicine or Physiology for 1908 with Paul Ehrlich for his work in immunology, and made many more contributions to immunity and bacteriology. Metchnikoff became interested in longevity and aging in his later years, and advocated the consumption of yogurt. He believed that lactic acid-producing bacteria in the gut prolonged life span.

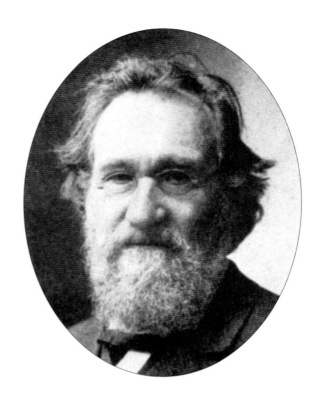

Figure 12   Elie Metchnikoff

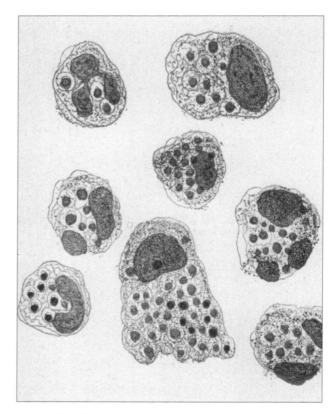

Figure 13   Drawings of leukocytes by Metchnikoff in his famous book, *Immunity Against Infective Diseases*

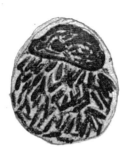
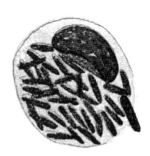
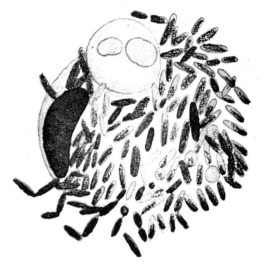

Fig. 43. — Macrophage de cobaye, rempli de bacilles de la peste humaine.

Fig. 44. — Macrophage de cobaye avec des bacilles pesteux qui commencent à sortir du protoplasma.

Fig. 45. — Macrophage de cobaye éclaté, à la suite du développement de bacilles pesteux dans son intérieur.

Figure 14   Drawings of leukocytes by Metchnikoff in his famous book, *Immunity Against Infective Diseases*

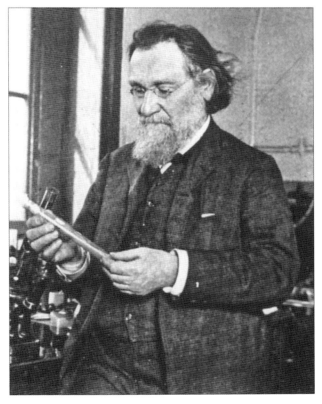

Figure 15   Elie Metchnikoff

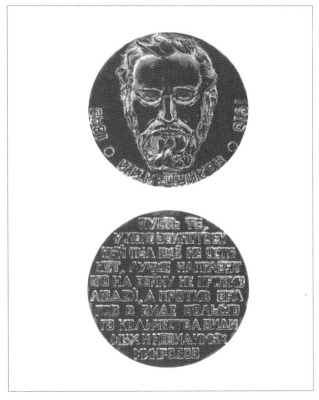

Figure 16   Elie Metchnikoff medallion commemorating his research

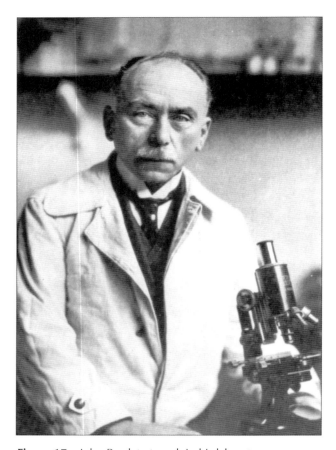

Figure 17   Jules Bordet at work in his laboratory

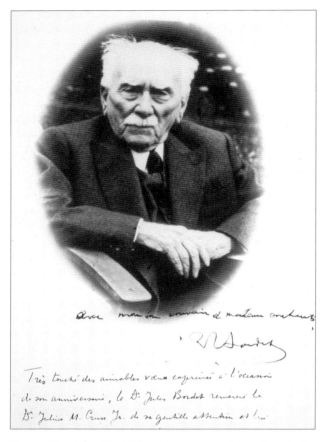

Figure 18   Jules Bordet in old age, portrait inscribed to Dr Julius M. Cruse

A new human bacterial pathogen was discovered every year from 1879 to 1888 and beyond. It was the golden age of bacteriology. In the laboratory of Robert Koch (Figure 19), a whole circle of younger men were trained and set to work on important research. Diphtheria toxin, demonstrated by Roux and Yersin, was the first molecule identified as an antigen. Diphtheria was a serious disease at that time, and several people attempted to create artificial immunity to the disease. Carl Fraenkel (1861–1915) induced immunity with heat-killed broth cultures, and published his finding in December, 1890. One day later, Emil von Behring (1854–1917) (Figures 20–23) and Shibasaburo Kitasato (1852–1931) (Figure 24) published their account of raising immune serum in rabbits and mice against tetanus toxin, which not only protected them from lethal doses but could be transferred by means of the immune serum to the bodies of other animals. In a footnote, the word 'anti-toxic' was used and was immediately adopted. A week later, von Behring published a further paper on immunization against diphtheria. The

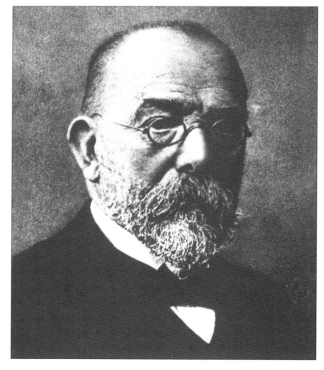

Figure 19   Robert Koch (1843–1910)

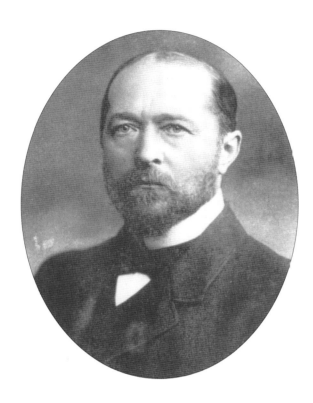

Figure 20   Emil von Behring

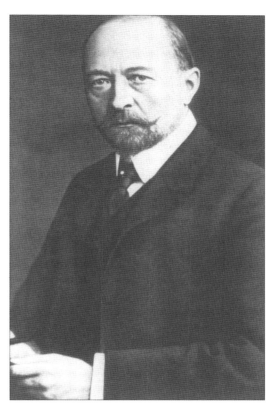

Figure 21   Emil von Behring

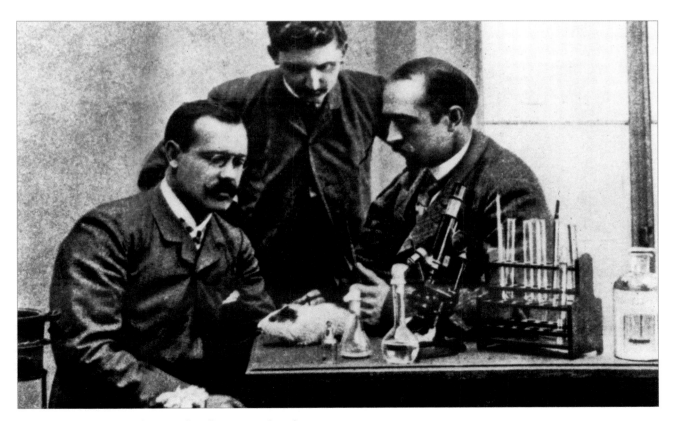

Figure 22   Emil von Behring with colleagues in the aboratory

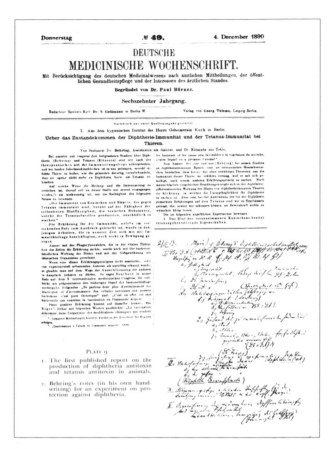

Figure 23 Published article by von Behring on diphtheria antitoxin with notes in his handwriting

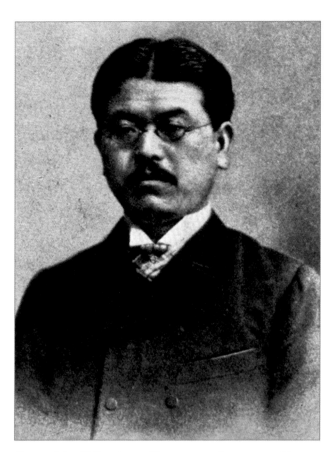

Figure 24 Shibasaburo Kitasato, co-discoverer with von Behring of diphtheria antitoxin

first child treated with diphtheria antitoxin was in von Bergmann's clinic in Berlin; the injection was given on Christmas night, 1891, by Geissler. von Behring was awarded the first Nobel Prize for Medicine or Physiology for his development of antiserum therapy in 1901[3].

Emil Adolph von Behring (1854–1917), German bacteriologist who worked at the Institute for Infectious Diseases in Berlin with Kitasato and Wernicke in 1890–92 and demonstrated that circulating antitoxins against diphtheria and tetanus toxins conferred immunity. He demonstrated that the passive administration of serum containing antitoxin could facilitate recovery. This represented the beginning of serum therapy, especially for diphtheria. He received the first Nobel Prize in Medicine in 1901 for this work. *Die Blutserumtherapie*, 1902; *Gesammelte Abhandlungen*, 1914; *Behring, Gestalt und Werk*, 1940; *Emil von Behring zum Gedächtnis*, 1942.

There followed a period of productive studies on the properties of blood serum. Richard Pfeiffer (1858–1945) (Figure 25) observed that cholera vibrios were lysed in the peritoneum of immunized guinea pigs, and showed the same process *in vitro*. This became known as the 'Pfeiffer phenomenon'[10]. Jules Bordet (1870–1961) (Figure 17), studying in Metchnikoff's laboratory, found that he could repeat the experiment and that there were two distinct substances in the serum, one heat-labile, which seemed to be similar to Buchner's alexine, and a second component which was heat-stable. The lytic action was found by Bordet to be applicable to cells other than bacteria. Thus, red blood cells were also lysed, and studies of hemolysis continued to reveal fundamental facts about the immune response. Bordet was awarded the Nobel Prize for Medicine or Physiology in 1919 for his studies on complement[11]. In 1889, A. Charrin (1856–1907) and J. Roger had observed that immune sera agglutinated a suspension of bacteria[12].

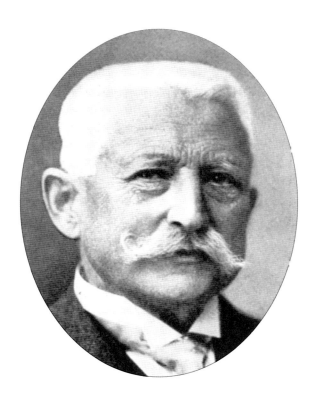

Figure 25   Richard Pfeiffer

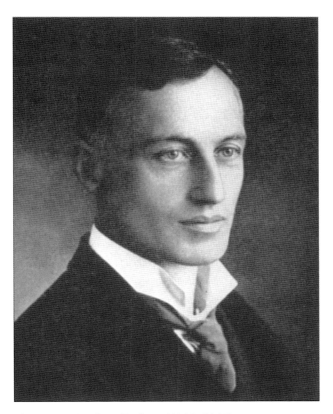

Figure 26   Herbert Durham (1866–1945)

In 1896, Herbert Durham (1866–1945) (Figure 26), an English graduate student working in Max von Grüber's (Figure 27) laboratory in Vienna, made a thorough study of the agglutination of bacteria by the blood; von Grüber (1853–1927) and Durham published several papers on the subject[13]. Within a few months, Fernand Widal (1862–1929), at the Faculté de Médecine in Paris, turned the process around and used the agglutination of known cultures of bacteria to diagnose disease using patient blood serum, later to be known as the Grüber–Widal test for typhoid fever[14]. In 1901, Bordet with a colleague, Octave Gengou, developed the complement-fixation reaction[15], the basis of many subsequent tests for infection, notably the Wassermann test for syphilis, which von Wassermann (1866–1915) and associates developed in 1906[16].

Another of the scientists who received early training in Koch's laboratory was Paul Ehrlich (1854–1915) (Figure 28), the pioneer in immunochemistry and one of the most original scientific minds of his time. His research had a profound influence on the direction taken by immunology. Although educated as a physician, Ehrlich had considerable expertise in chemistry.

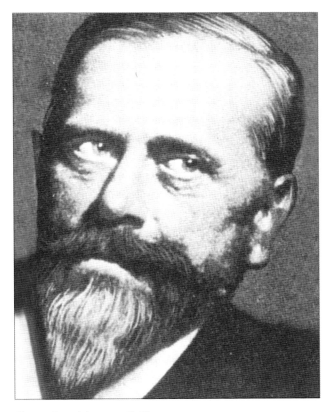

Figure 27   Max von Grüber

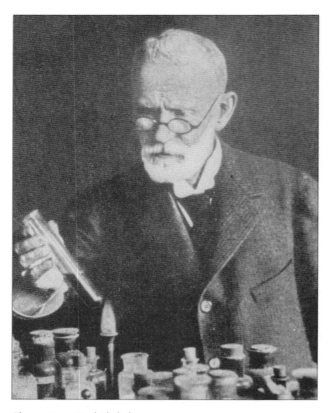

Figure 28 Paul Ehrlich

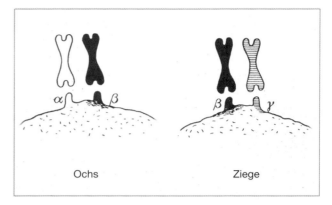

Figure 29 Ehrlich's diagram of 'toxophore' and 'haptophore' groups

He was one of the first to recognize the limitations of the available knowledge of his day in solving the complex biochemical and genetic aspects of antibody formation and solving the riddle of cancer, which is only now beginning to be elucidated. One of his early projects was a study of the vegetable toxins abrin and ricin. He raised antibodies to the two poisons in laboratory animals, and from his studies concluded that the antibody–antigen union was essentially a chemical process with constant amounts combining. He was able to assist von Behring by working out a satisfactory method of standardizing diphtheria antitoxin, a problem Behring had not been able to solve. Ehrlich began then to visualize the way antibody and antigen combine and developed his famous side-chain theory, which postulated that a toxin had two combining sites, the toxophore and the haptophore groups[17] (Figures 29 and 30). Molecules of protoplasm were equipped with side-chains with a nutritive function. When they were blocked by the haptophoric group of a toxin, excess side-chains were secreted by the cell, constituting what was known as antitoxin in the peripheral blood (Figures 31–33). His theory stimulated much debate and a vast amount of research. We perceive his uncanny intuition

upon noting diagrams such as those shown in these figures by observing the Y-shaped receptor on a cell, which is remarkably similar to the modern-day model for immunoglobulin such as IgG (Figure 34). Ehrlich's life work fell into three phases, an early histology period when he worked mostly with biological stains to differentiate cells and tissues, a middle period comprising his studies on immunity and a late period at the end of his career which he devoted mostly to chemotherapy. He discovered a specific treatment for syphilis in the arsenical compound numbered 606, Salvarsan, with Sachahiro Hata (1873–1938) (Figures 35 and 36), who had come to his laboratory in Frankfurt to teach the transmission of syphilis in laboratory animals and learn some principles of chemotherapy. His entire attention was drawn to supervising the production and use of this important drug, the 'magic bullet' which could selectively destroy bacteria without harming the body. Ehrlich also trained a whole generation of younger men who continued to do research in immunology[18] (Figures 37 and 38). He shared the 1908 Nobel Prize in Medicine with Metchnikoff for their studies on immunity. Fruits of these labors led to treatments for trypanosomiasis and syphilis.

Paul Ehrlich presented his famous *side-chain theory* in the Croonian Lecture before the Royal Society of Great Britain in 1900[19]. According to this theory, the cell was believed to possess highly complex chemical aggregates with attached groupings, or 'side-chains', the normal function of which was to anchor nutrient substances to the cell before internalization (Figures 31–33). These side-chains, or receptors, were considered to permit cellular interaction with substances in the extracellular environment. Antigens were postulated to stimulate the

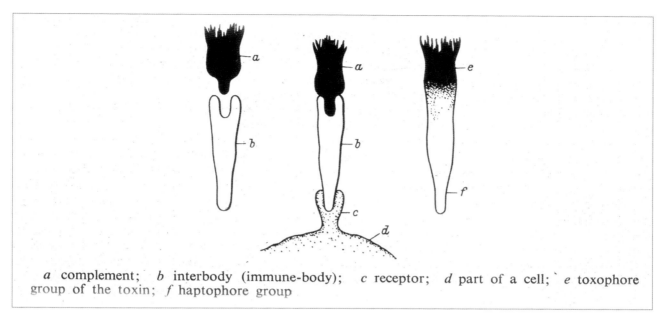

a complement; *b* interbody (immune-body); *c* receptor; *d* part of a cell; *e* toxophore group of the toxin; *f* haptophore group

Figure 30 Ehrlich's diagram of 'toxophore' and 'haptophore' groups

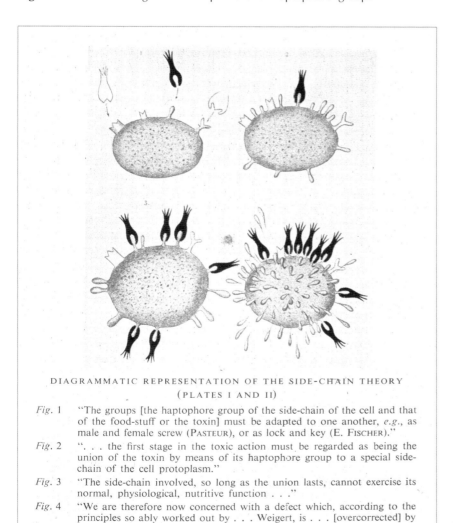

DIAGRAMMATIC REPRESENTATION OF THE SIDE-CHAIN THEORY
(PLATES I AND II)

Fig. 1 "The groups [the haptophore group of the side-chain of the cell and that of the food-stuff or the toxin] must be adapted to one another, *e.g.*, as male and female screw (PASTEUR), or as lock and key (E. FISCHER)."

Fig. 2 ". . . the first stage in the toxic action must be regarded as being the union of the toxin by means of its haptophore group to a special side-chain of the cell protoplasm."

Fig. 3 "The side-chain involved, so long as the union lasts, cannot exercise its normal, physiological, nutritive function . . ."

Fig. 4 "We are therefore now concerned with a defect which, according to the principles so ably worked out by . . . Weigert, is . . . [overcorrected] by regeneration."

Figure 31 The Ehrlich side-chain theory of antibody formation

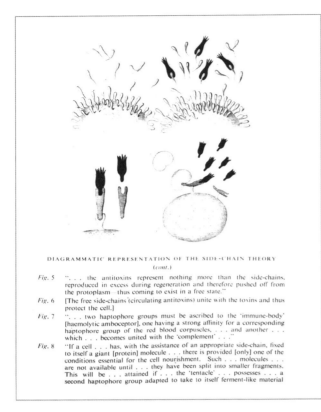

DIAGRAMMATIC REPRESENTATION OF THE SIDE-CHAIN THEORY
(cont.)

Fig. 5   ". . . the antitoxins represent nothing more than the side-chains, reproduced in excess during regeneration and therefore pushed off from the protoplasm – thus coming to exist in a free state."

Fig. 6   [The free side-chains (circulating antitoxins) unite with the toxins and thus protect the cell.]

Fig. 7   ". . . two haptophore groups must be ascribed to the 'immune-body' [haemolytic amboceptor], one having a strong affinity for a corresponding haptophore group of the red blood corpuscles, . . . and another . . . which . . . becomes united with the 'complement' . . ."

Fig. 8   "If a cell . . . has, with the assistance of an appropriate side-chain, fixed to itself a giant [protein] molecule . . . there is provided [only] one of the conditions essential for the cell nourishment.   Such . . . molecules . . . are not available until . . . they have been split into smaller fragments. This will be . . . attained if . . . the 'tentacle' . . . possesses . . . a second haptophore group adapted to take to itself ferment-like material

Figure 32   The Ehrlich side-chain theory of antibody formation

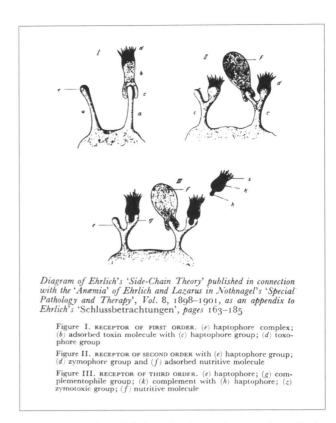

Diagram of Ehrlich's 'Side-Chain Theory' published in connection with the 'Anæmia' of Ehrlich and Lazarus in Nothnagel's 'Special Pathology and Therapy', Vol. 8, 1898–1901, as an appendix to Ehrlich's 'Schlussbetrachtungen', pages 163–185

Figure I. RECEPTOR OF FIRST ORDER. (*e*) haptophore complex; (*b*) adsorbed toxin molecule with (*c*) haptophore group; (*d*) toxophore group

Figure II. RECEPTOR OF SECOND ORDER with (*e*) haptophore group; (*d*) zymophore group and (*f*) adsorbed nutritive molecule

Figure III. RECEPTOR OF THIRD ORDER. (*e*) haptophore; (*g*) complementophile group; (*k*) complement with (*h*) haptophore; (*z*) zymotoxic group; (*f*) nutritive molecule

Figure 33   The Ehrlich side-chain theory of antibody formation

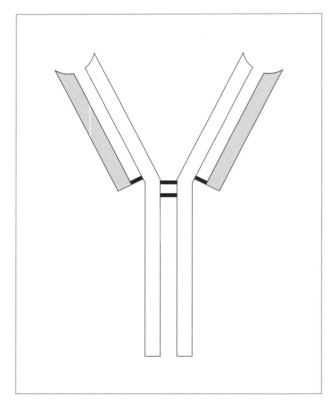

Figure 34   Y-shaped structure of immunoglobulin molecule comprising two heavy and two light polypeptide chains

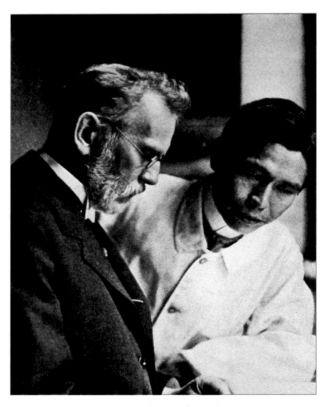

Figure 35   Professor Paul Ehrlich with Dr Hata in the laboratory

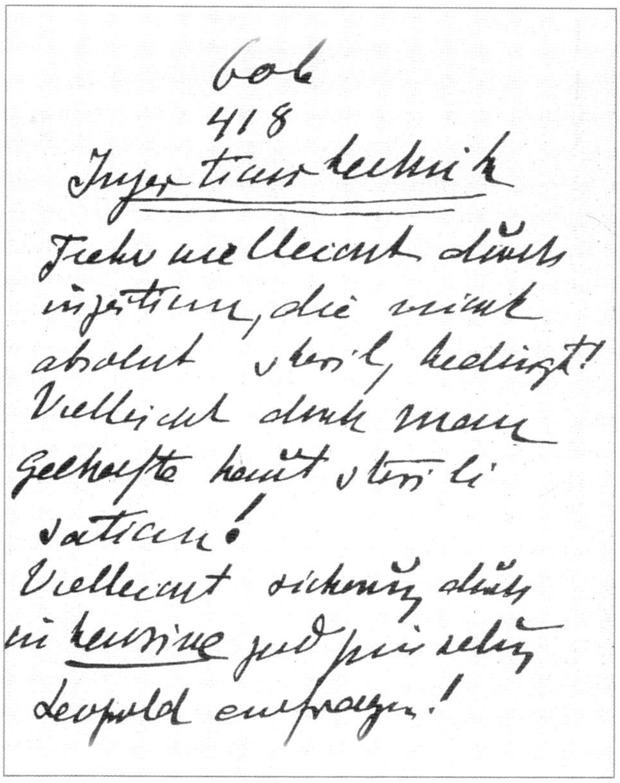

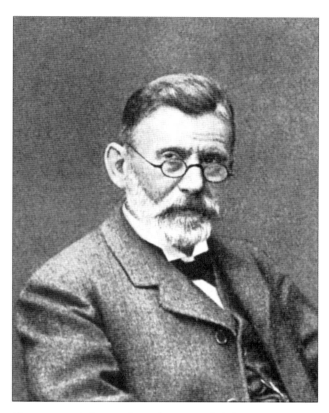

Figure 36 Ehrlich's instructions concerning '606' or Salvarsan, the first effective treatment for syphilis

Figure 37 Geheimrath Professor Dr Ehrlich

cell by attachment to these receptors. Because antigens played no part in the normal economy of the cell, the receptors were diverted from their normal function. Stimulated by this derangement of its normal mechanism, the cell produced excessive new receptors, of the same type as those thrown out of action. The superfluous receptors shed by the cell into the extracellular fluids constituted specific antibodies with the capacity to bind homologous antigens. Ehrlich endowed each of his receptors with a special chemical grouping, the *haptophore group*, which entered into chemical union with a corresponding group of the antigen, as in neutralization of a toxin by antitoxin (Figure 33). When, however, the antigen was altered in some other recognizable way, as in agglutination or precipitation, Ehrlich postulated another grouping in the receptor, the *ergophore group*, which determined the particular change in the antigen after the antibody was anchored by its haptophore group. In certain cases, it was necessary to postulate receptors that united an antigen to complement. Ehrlich proposed receptors with two haptophore groups, one of which became attached to the antigen to be acted upon, and one to the complement that was the

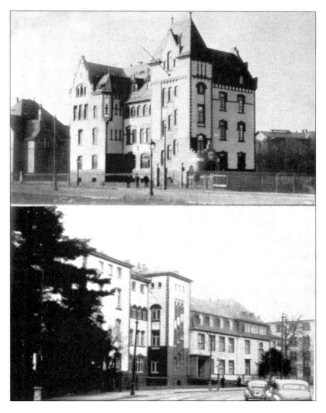

Figure 38 The Paul Ehrlich Institut, Frankfurt-am-Main

acting substance. Both of these groups were to be regarded as strictly specific in their chemical affinities. The one that combined with the cell or other antigen was called the *cytophilic group*, the one that combined with complement the *complementophilic group*; Ehrlich named this type of receptor an *amboceptor*, because both groups were supposed to be of the *haptophore* type.

Ehrlich regarded these receptors as definite chemical structures. When it was discovered that antigens such as toxins could be detoxified without losing their antitoxin-binding capacity, he assumed that a *toxophore group* had been altered, whereas the *haptophore group* remained intact. Similarly, he postulated the existence of a modified complement, in which an intact *haptophore group* was associated with an *ergophore group* that had lost its efficacy. Ehrlich varied the functional activity of the various groups to account for new phenomena. The quantitative aspects of toxin neutralization by antitoxin could not be reconciled with the *side-chain theory* in its simple form. To retain the concept of firm union between antigen and antibody in constant proportions, Ehrlich postulated a large number of different toxin components with varying degrees of affinity for antitoxin. Similarly, some of his studies on hemolysins made it necessary to assume the intervention of receptors of considerable structural complexity. The consequent coining of a host of new terms for components whose existence was extremely doubtful served to confuse the problem rather than to clarify it. In spite of these failings, Ehrlich's theory had the merit of emphasizing chemical specificity as the essential feature of the antigen–antibody reaction.

Obermayer and Pick, two Viennese chemists, in 1903 investigated the effects on specificity of coupling various chemical groupings to proteins[20]. Nitric acid, nitrous acid or iodine treatment of proteins altered their specificity to the point that they were rendered antigenic in the species of origin. Later experiments demonstrated that alteration of protein specificity by such treatment was based upon modification of aromatic amino acids, as opposed to alteration of protein specificity by the introduced groups alone.

This work fired the imagination of Karl Landsteiner (Figures 39–41), who with some associates in 1918 coupled organic radicals to proteins[21]. The ability of a particular chemical to act as a determinant of specificity was tested by coupling it to an aromatic amine such as aniline. The product of this reaction was diazotized and coupled to a protein to form a conjugated antigen or

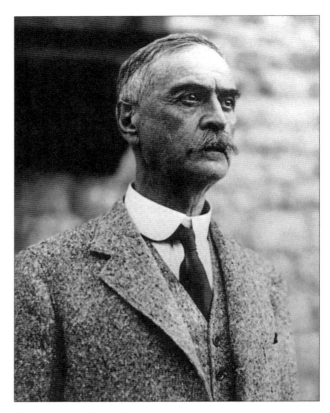

Figure 39 Karl Landsteiner

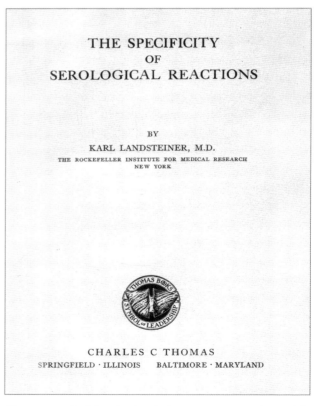

THE SPECIFICITY
OF
SEROLOGICAL REACTIONS

BY

KARL LANDSTEINER, M.D.
THE ROCKEFELLER INSTITUTE FOR MEDICAL RESEARCH
NEW YORK

CHARLES C THOMAS
SPRINGFIELD · ILLINOIS   BALTIMORE · MARYLAND

Figure 40 Karl Landsteiner's famous monograph (English translation)

30

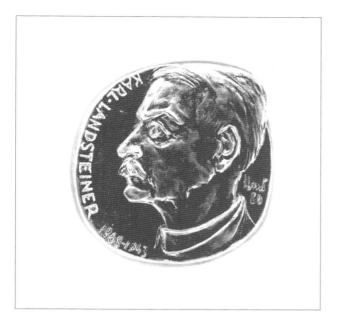

Figure 41 Landsteiner medallion commemorating the International Congress of Immunology

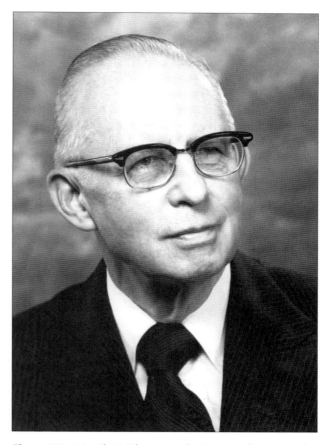

Figure 42 Merril W. Chase, Landsteiner's colleague at the Rockefeller Institute for Medical Research, New York

azoprotein. From these studies the chemical basis for serologic specificity was proved. Not only the nature of radicals coupled to proteins but also the position of the attachment site on the ring (ortho, meta or para) was shown to be of paramount importance for specificity[21].

Ehrlich had attempted to develop a selective theory of antibody formation with his *side-chain theory*, which required that every cell involved in antibody production be capable of reacting against every known antigen in nature. However, it was precisely this weakness in the hypothesis that allowed Landsteiner to discredit it by raising antibodies against haptens manufactured in the chemical laboratory, and which had never appeared before in nature[22]. It was inconceivable that there would be preformed receptors for antigens that the animal body would never see. As Landsteiner had invalidated the first cell selection theory of antibody formation, it is ironic that his work subsequently contributed to the re-emergence of a selective hypothesis. He proposed natural diversity and accidental affinity[22]. Together with Chase (Figure 42), he initiated a return to cellular immunology in 1942[23].

Merrill Chase (1905–2004), American immunologist who worked with Karl Landsteiner at the Rockefeller Institute for Medical Research, New York. He investigated hypersensitivity, including delayed-type hypersensitivity and contact dermatitis. He was the first to demonstrate the passive transfer of tuberculin and contact hypersensitivity and also made contributions in the fields of adjuvants and quantitative methods.

With the abandonment of Ehrlich's selective theory, Breinl and Haurowitz[24] (Figure 43) and Mudd[25] proposed an instructive hypothesis, which the chemists favored. Pauling[26] (Figure 44) proposed a template theory of antibody formation that required that the antigen must be present during the process of antibody synthesis. According to the *refolding template theory*, uncommitted and specific globulins could become refolded upon the antigen, serving as a template for it (Figure 45). The cell thereupon released the complementary antibodies, which thenceforth rigidly retained their shape through disulfide bonding. This theory had to be abandoned when it became clear that the specificity of antibodies in all cases is a result of the particular arrangement of their primary amino acid sequence. *De novo* synthesis template theories that recognized the necessity for antibodies to be synthesized by amino

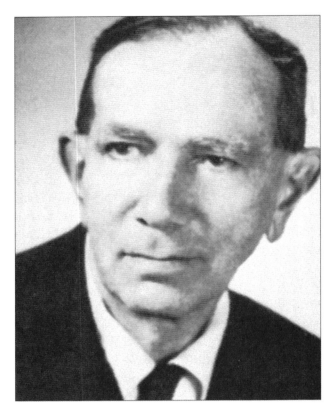

Figure 43 Felix Haurowitz, an early proponent of the instructive theory of antibody formation

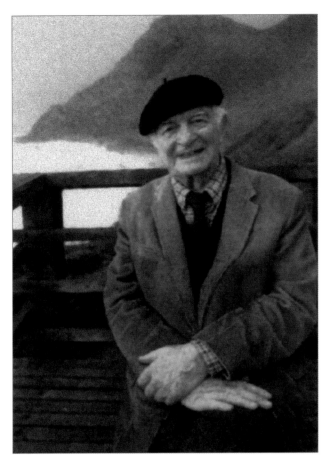

Figure 44 Linus Pauling, proponent of the template theory of antibody formation

acid, in the proper and predetermined order, still had to contend with the serious objection that proteins cannot serve as informational models for the synthesis of other proteins.

> **Felix Haurowitz (1896–1988)**, a noted protein chemist from Prague who later came to the USA. He investigated the chemistry of hemoglobins. In 1930 (with Breinl) he advanced the instruction theory of antibody formation. *Chemistry and Biology of Proteins*, 1950; *Immunochemistry and Biosynthesis of Antibodies*, 1968.

Burnet (Figures 46 and 47) and Fenner[27] at the Walter and Eliza Hall Institute were beginning to take a view of antibody production that was different from that proposed by chemists adhering to the template theory of antibody synthesis. The second edition of their classic monograph entitled *The Production of Antibodies*, published in 1949 (Figure 48), contains an

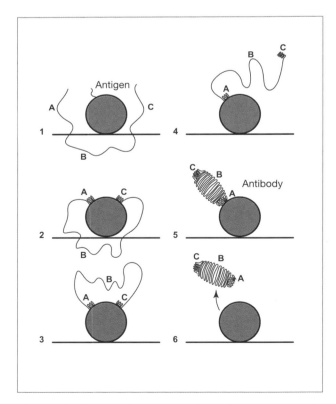

Figure 45 The template theory (schematic representation)

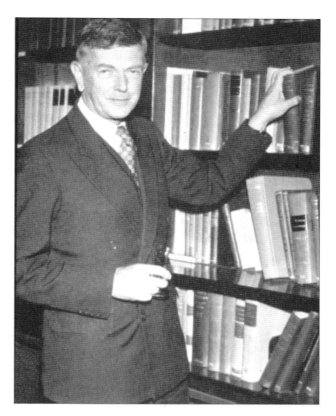

Figure 46   Sir Macfarlane Burnet

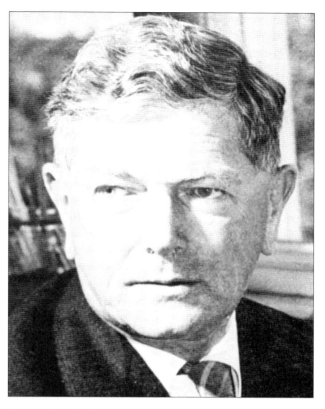

Figure 47   Sir Macfarlane Burnet

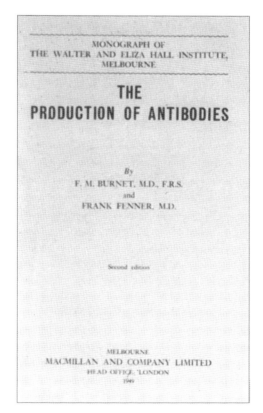

MONOGRAPH OF
THE WALTER AND ELIZA HALL INSTITUTE,
MELBOURNE

THE
PRODUCTION OF ANTIBODIES

By
F. M. BURNET, M.D., F.R.S.
and
FRANK FENNER, M.D.

Second edition

MELBOURNE
MACMILLAN AND COMPANY LIMITED
HEAD OFFICE 'LONDON
1949

Figure 48   Burnet and Fenner's famous monograph on antibody formation

exposition of their developing concepts. Burnet advocated but later abandoned a self-marker hypothesis to explain antibody production.

Frank Macfarlane Burnet (1899–1975), Australian virologist and immunologist who shared the Nobel Prize with Peter B. Medawar in 1960 for the discovery of acquired immunological tolerance. Burnet was a theoretician who made major contributions to the developing theories of self-tolerance and clonal selection in antibody formation. Burnet and Fenner's suggested explanation of immunologic tolerance was tested by Medawar *et al.*, who confirmed the hypothesis in 1953 using inbred strains of mice. *The Production of Antibodies* (with Fenner), 1949; *Natural History of Infectious Diseases*, 1953; *Clonal Selection Theory of Antibody Formation*, 1959; *Autoimmune Diseases* (with Mackay), 1962; *Cellular Immunology*, 1969; *Changing Patterns* (autobiography), 1969.

The template theory of antibody production that had been popular with the chemists and prevailed for so many years could no longer explain new biologic revelations that included immunologic tolerance, and it had never explained the anamnestic (memory) immune response. The *coup de grâce* to this hypothesis was the observation that mature antibody-synthesizing cells contained no antigen. Burnet proposed lymphoid cells genetically programmed to synthesize one type of antibody[28] (Figures 49–51).

As pointed out by Talmage[29], events in the 1950s that made the template theories of Breinl and Haurowitz[24] and of Pauling[26] untenable included four significant developments. The first was Jerne's demonstration in 1951 that antibody avidity increased rapidly in an anamnestic response[30]. The greater is the avidity of antibody produced on an antigen template, the slower should be its rate of turnover on the template.

David Wilson Talmage (1919–), American physician and investigator who in 1956 developed the cell selection theory of antibody formation. His work was a foundation for Burnet's subsequent clonal selection theory. After training in immunology with Taliaferro in Chicago where he became a Professor in 1952, Talmage subsequently became Chairman of Microbiology, 1963; Dean of Medicine, 1968; and Director of the

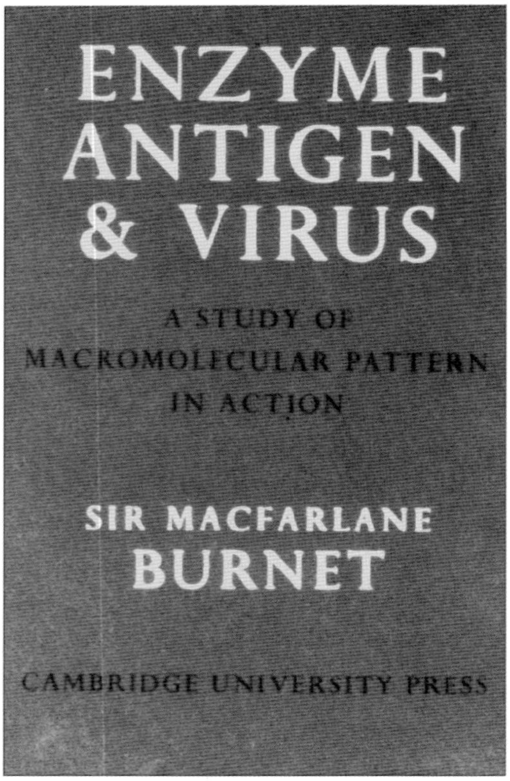

Figure 49 One of Burnet's classic monographs

Webb–Waring Institute in Denver, 1973. In addition to his investigations of antibody formation, he also studied heart transplantation tolerance. *The Chemistry of Immunity in Health and Disease* (with Cann), 1961.

Niels Kaj Jerne (1911–94), Danish immunologist who proposed a selection theory of antibody formation, the functional network of antibodies and lymphocytes and distinction of self from non-self by T lymphocytes. He shared the 1984 Nobel Prize in Medicine or Physiology with Georges Köhler and Cesar Milstein.

Niels Kaj Jerne was born in London to Danish parents. His ancestors were from western Jutland. He studied at Leiden, Holland, where he completed his baccalaureate when he was 16, but spent the next 12 years deciding on a profession. At the age of 28, he began the study of medicine in Copenhagen with the plan to become a village doctor. After taking a part-time job in a scientific laboratory, he became interested in science, especially immunology. Jerne followed in his father's footsteps by moving frequently. His doctoral dissertation was on the theoretical foundation for the study of antibody avidity. He earned his MD in 1951. Jerne worked at the State Serum Institute in Copenhagen between 1943 and 1954. Thereafter, he left for America, working at the California Institute of Technology in Pasadena where he wrote a paper that was the death-knell for the instructionist theories of antibody synthesis and a forerunner of the clonal selection theory. He next accepted a staff position with the World Health Organization in Geneva, Switzerland, where he coined new immunological terms such as 'epitope' and 'idiotype'. He also served as a Professor of Biophysics at the University of Geneva between 1960 and 1962. Thereafter, he went to the United States to serve for 4 years as Professor and Chairman of the Department of Microbiology at the University of Pittsburgh, where he developed a plaque assay for antibody forming cells. In 1966 he was appointed Director of the Paul Ehrlich Institute at the University of Frankfurt, Germany, where he began formulating a theory on the role of self-antigens in the generation of antibody diversity. Jerne became Director of the Basel Institute for Immunology in 1969, where he developed a network theory of the immune system. He was elected a Fellow of the Royal Society in 1980, and after retiring from the Basel Institute, served for a year at the Institut Pasteur in Paris. He then took up residence in France.

Further reading

Steinburg CM, Lefkovits I, eds. *The Immune System. 1. Past and Future. 2. The Present.* Basel: S. Karger Publishers, 1981 (Festschrift for Jerne's 70th birthday)

Jerne NK. The natural selection theory of antibody formation. *Proc Natl Acad Sci USA* 1955;41:849

Jerne NK. Towards a network theory of the immune system. *Arch Immunol (Paris)* 1974;125C:373-89

Silverstein AM. *A History of Immunology.* San Diego: Academic Press, 1989

Burnet and Fenner[27] showed the logarithmic increase in antibody synthesis, and Barr and Glenny[31] and William and Lucy Taliaferro[32] demonstrated the logarithmic normal distribution of peak antibody titers induced in rabbits. These findings indicated that a replicating antigenic substance induced antibody formation. Owen[33] demonstrated chimerism in dizygotic cattle twins in which blood cells of one twin were tolerated immunologically by the other. Billingham and associates[34] demonstrated actively acquired immunologic tolerance in mice by exposing a fetus to antigen before or at birth. Taliaferro and Talmage[35] and Roberts and Dixon[36] demonstrated that the capacity to synthesize antibody could be transferred passively from an immune to a previously non-immune animal with viable lymphoid cells. This weight of evidence rendered the antigen template theory obsolete, and necessitated the proposal of alternative explanations. These included Burnet and Fenner's[27] and Schwect and Owen's[37] indirect template theories.

Jerne[38] (Figure 52) proposed a natural selection theory of antibody formation in 1955 based on various antibody populations. Substituting replicating cells for

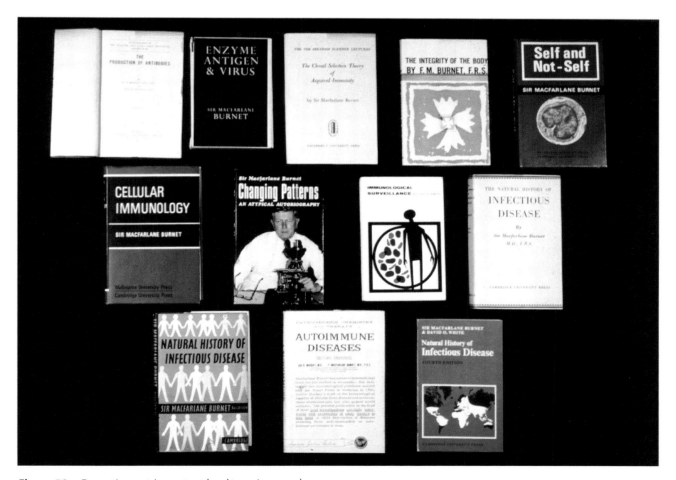

Figure 50 Burnet's most important books on immunology

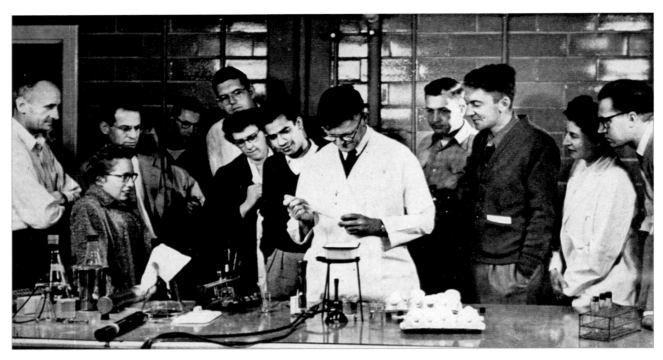

Figure 51   Sir Macfarlane Burnet with students in a laboratory at the University of Wisconsin, Madison

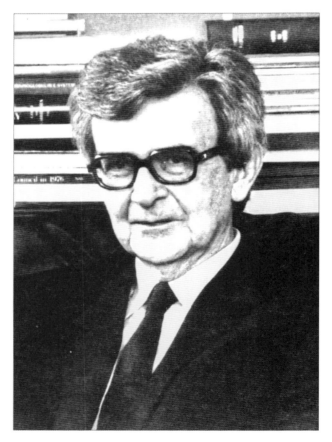

Figure 52   Niels K. Jerne, author of the 'natural selection theory of antibody formation' and of the 'network theory of immunity'

the antibody populations, Talmage[39] published a cell selection theory in 1956 (Figure 53). He communicated his ideas to Burnet in Australia who had independently formulated a similar concept. Clearly acknowledging Talmage's contribution, Burnet named his own version of the cell selection hypothesis the 'clonal selection theory of acquired immunity'[28] (Figure 54).

Burnet postulated the presence of numerous antibody-forming cells, each capable of synthesizing its own predetermined antibody. One of these cells, after having been selected by the best-fitting antigen, multiplies and forms a clone of cells that continue to synthesize the same antibody. Provided that one accepted the existence of very many different cells, each capable of synthesizing an antibody of a different specificity, all known facts of antibody formation were easily accounted for. An important element of the clonal selection theory as proposed by Burnet was the hypothesis that the many cells with different antibody specificities arise through random somatic mutations, during a period of hypermutability, early in the animal's life. Also early in life, the 'forbidden' clones of antibody-forming cells (i.e. the cells that make antibody to the animal's own antigens) are destroyed after encountering these autoantigens. This process accounts for an animal's tolerance of its own antigens.

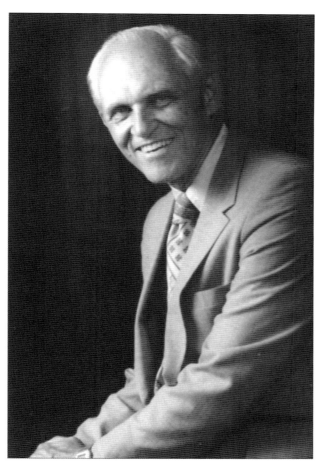

Figure 53 **Figure 53**   David W. Talmage, who proposed the cell selection theory of antibody formation in 1956

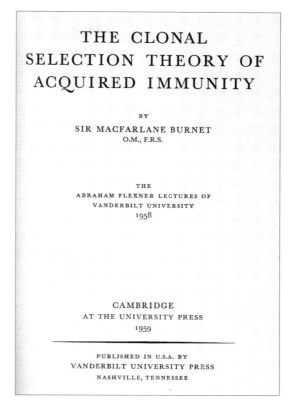

Figure 54   Burnet's classic monograph proposing his clonal selection theory of antibody formation

Antigen would have no effect on most lymphoid cells, but would selectively stimulate those cells already synthesizing the corresponding antibody at a low rate. The cell surface antibody would serve as receptor for antigen and proliferate into a clone of cells producing antibody of that specificity. Burnet introduced the 'forbidden clone' concept to explain autoimmunity. Cells capable of forming antibody against a normal self-antigen were 'forbidden' and eliminated during embryonic life. Since that time various modifications of the clonal selection hypothesis have been offered.

Burnet[40] suggested a concept of 'clonal deletion' as a means to eliminate precursor lymphocytes capable of reacting with self-antigens before birth. This concept provided for the permanent removal of self-reactive lymphocytes with the possibility that so-called 'forbidden clones' might develop by spontaneous mutation in the later life of the individual. Therefore, tolerance to some self-antigens is maintained even when the antigen is removed, whereas tolerance to other self-antigens

may be terminated. Thus, natural tolerance or unresponsiveness could result from the elimination of immunocompetent cell clones specific for self-antigens, or clones of immunocompetent cells rendered unresponsive by early exposure to self-antigenic determinants.

Nossal and Pike[41] demonstrated 'clonal anergy' by functionally inactivating B-lymphocyte precursors from the bone marrow with excessive but critical concentrations of antigens bearing appropriate numbers of carrier determinants. This phenomenon may occur *in vivo* as well as *in vitro*. B cells suppressed functionally by these carefully adjusted concentrations of antigen persist but do not proliferate or form antibody. For clonal anergy to be able to explain self-tolerance could require the maintenance of significant concentrations of antigen during an individual animal's lifetime, and should be true for T as well as B cells.

Early criticism of the cell selection theory was based on its failure to explain antibody specificity for the limitless antigens in nature[29]. Studying the specificity of antibodies against synthetic haptens, Landsteiner[22] had shown that antisera demonstrated the features of specificity, universality, cross-reactivity and diversity. Thus, it became apparent that an animal could synthesize antibodies in great numbers. Considering the astronomical number of antigens in nature and the fact that a single antiserum contained multiple antibodies for each antigen against which the animal was immunized, it appeared necessary for each antibody molecule to be tailor-made using the antigen template as a pattern. To explain this problem, a different concept of specificity was developed in which antibodies were suggested to be derived from a large set of natural globulins with some reactivities in common. The chance reactivity of each globulin with a few molecules of all antigenic determinants would endow each individual animal with a group of globulin molecules that could react with essentially every antigenic determinant possible. Fifty thousand separate globulins were suggested to be able to explain the observation of specificity and cross-reactivity.

The demonstration of immunoglobulin structure and its genetic basis also contributed to solving the riddle of Landsteiner's observations. Separate antibodies are encoded by a unique combination of a few genes just as antisera consist of a unique mixture of antibodies. Several hundred genes could encode several million antibodies rather than 50 000 genes encoding 50 000 antibodies[42].

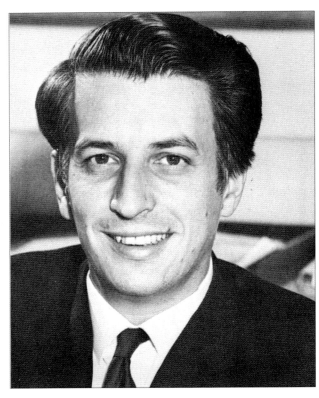

Figure 55 Sir Gustav Nossal, Director of the Walter and Eliza Hall Institute, Melbourne, who made seminal contributions to prove clonal selection

Gustav Joseph Victor Nossal (1931–), Australian immunologist whose seminal works have concentrated on antibodies and their formation. He served as director of the Walter and Eliza Hall Institute of Medical Research in Melbourne. *Antibodies and Immunity*, 1969; *Antigens, Lymphoid Cells and the Immune Response* (with Ada), 1971.

Evidence in support of the cell selection theory accumulated rapidly. Nossal (Figures 55 and 56) and Lederberg[43] found that individual antibody-synthesizing cells could produce antibody of only one specificity. In addition, surface immunoglobulins were demonstrated on circulating lymphocytes in newborn and fetal pigs[44]. Spleen cells responding to a single antigen could be eliminated without altering the response to a second antigen[45]. Of special significance was the demonstration by Raff and colleagues[46] that all surface immunoglobulin on antigen-binding lymphocytes formed caps when incubated with a single antigen. This showed that all of the immunoglobulin on the surface of a single lymphocyte was of one specificity.

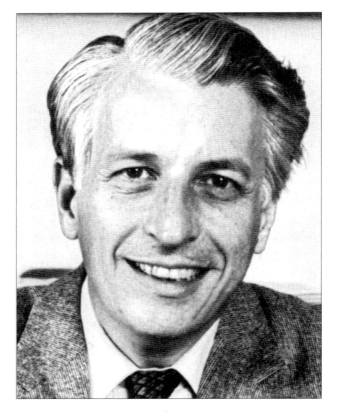

Figure 56 Sir Gustav Nossal

Joshua Lederberg (1925–), American biochemist who made a significant contribution to immunology with his work on the clonal selection theory of antibody formation. He received a Nobel Prize in 1958 (with Beadle and Tatum) for genetic recombination and organization of genetic material in bacteria.

Even though criticism of the cell selection theory continued, the subsequent accumulation of scientific evidence in its favor facilitated its acceptance. A principal source of support was Köhler and Milstein's[47] demonstration in 1975 of hybridoma technology for the formation of monoclonal antibodies. Even though monoclonal antibodies had been well known for years in myeloma patients, the widespread use of hybridoma technology by multiple investigators synthesizing monoclonal antibodies to all sorts of antigens led to their popular use in research. Clearly, monoclonal antibodies provided convincing evidence of the validity of the cell selection hypothesis. In addition to the rapid advances in cellular immunology in the 1970s was the progress in molecular immunology. Immunoglobulin structure and the genes encoding these molecules were defined. Diversity was shown to be due to the random rearrangement of numerous separate variable genes in different cells. Thus, the clonal selection theory has proved compatible with the accumulated scientific evidence.

The **Ehrlich side-chain theory (historical)** was the first selective theory of antibody synthesis developed by Paul Ehrlich in 1900. Although elaborate in detail, the essential feature of the theory was that cells of the immune system possess the genetic capability to react to all known antigens, and that each cell on the surface bears receptors with surface haptophore side-chains. On combination with antigen, the side-chains would be cast off into the circulation, and new receptors would replace the old ones. These cast-off receptors represented antibody molecules in the circulation. Although far more complex than this explanation, the importance of the theory was in the amount of research stimulated to try to disprove it. Nevertheless, it was the first effort to account for the importance of genetics in immune responsiveness at a time when Mendel's basic studies had not even yet been 'rediscovered' by de Vries.

Ehrlich's theory assumed that each antibody-forming cell had the ability to react to every antigen in nature. The demonstration by Landsteiner that antibodies could be formed against substances manufactured in the laboratory that had never existed before in nature led to abandonment of the side-chain theory. Yet its basic premise as a selective hypothesis rather than an instructive theory was ultimately proved correct.

The **indirect template theory (historical)** was a variation of the template hypothesis which postulated that instructions for antibody synthesis were copied from the antigen configuration into the DNA encoding the specific antibody. This was later shown to be untenable, and is of historical interest only.

The **self-marker hypothesis (historical)** was a concept suggested by Burnet and Fenner in 1949 in an attempt to account for the failure of the body to react against its own antigens. They proposed that cells of the body contained a marker that identified them to the host's immunologically competent cells as self. This recognition system was supposed to prevent the immune cells of the host from rejecting its own tissue cells. This hypothesis was later abandoned by the authors and replaced by the clonal selection theory of acquired immunity which Burnet proposed in 1957.

The **template theory (historical)** was an instructive theory of antibody formation which required that the antigen must be present during the process of antibody synthesis. According to the refolding template theory, uncommitted and specific globulins could become refolded on the antigen, serving as a template for it. The cell thereupon would release the complementary antibodies, which thenceforth would rigidly retain their shape through disulfide bonding. This theory had to be abandoned when it became clear that the specificity of antibodies in all cases is due to the particular arrangement of their primary amino acid sequence. The template theory could not explain immunological tolerance or the anamnestic (memory) immune response.

The **instructive theory (of antibody formation)** was a hypothesis that postulated acquisition of antibody specificity after contact with a specific antigen. According to one template theory of antibody formation, it was necessary that the antigen be present during the process of antibody synthesis. According to the refolding template theory, uncommitted and specific globulins could become refolded upon the antigen, serving as a template for it. The cell released the complementary antibodies, which rigidly retained their shape through disulfide bonding. This theory had to be abandoned when it was shown that the specificity of antibodies in all cases is due to the particular arrangement of their primary amino acid sequence. *De novo* synthesis template theories that recognized the necessity for antibodies to be synthesized by amino acids, in the proper and predetermined order, still had to contend with the serious objection that proteins cannot serve as informational models for the synthesis of proteins. Instructive theories were abandoned when immunologic tolerance was demonstrated and when antigen was shown not to be necessary for antibody synthesis to occur. The template theories had never explained the anamnestic (memory) immune response. Antibody specificity depends upon the variable region amino acid sequence, especially the complementarity-determining or hypervariable regions.

The **selective theory** is a hypothesis that describes antibody synthesis as a process in which antigen selects cells expressing receptors specific for that antigen. The antigen–cell receptor interaction leads to proliferation and differentiation of that clone of cells which synthe-

sizes significant quantities of antibodies of a single specificity. Selective theories included the side-chain theory of Paul Ehrlich proposed in 1899, the natural selection theory proposed by Niels Jerne in 1955 and the cell selection theory proposed by Talmage and by Burnet in 1957. Burnet termed his version of the theory the clonal selection theory of acquired immunity. The basic tenets of the clonal selection theory have been substantiated by the scientific evidence. The selective theories maintained that cells are genetically programmed to react to certain antigenic specificities prior to antigen exposure. They are in sharp contrast to the instructive theories which postulated that antigen was necessary to serve as a template around which polypeptide chains were folded to yield specific antibodies. This template theory was abandoned when antibody was demonstrated in the absence of antigen (Figure 57).

The **recombinatorial germ line theory** was a hypothesis proposed by Dreyer and Bennett which postulated that variable-region and constant-region immunoglobulin genes were separated and rejoined in DNA levels. This concept was an important step toward understanding the generation of diversity in the production of antibody molecules, a puzzle finally solved by Tonegawa (Figures 58–61) with significant contributions by Leroy Hood (Figure 62).

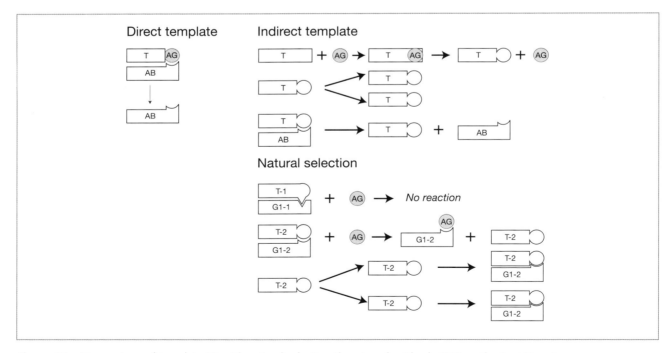

Figure 57 Comparison of template (T) with natural selection theories of antibody (AB) synthesis. AG, antigen

Susumu Tonegawa (1939–) received the 1987 Nobel Prize in Medicine or Physiology for his research on the generation of antibody diversity. Doubting that all genes needed for antibody diversity could be present in the germ line, most scientists postulated somatic mutation involving a very limited number of germ line genes. Dreyer and Bennett fostered a two gene/one polypeptide chain theory in 1965, which proposed that the combination of multiple variable-region genes with a single constant region gene for a particular isotype might require less DNA.

Susumu Tonegawa (1939–), Japanese-born immunologist working in the United States. He received the Nobel Prize in 1987 for his research on immunoglobulin genes and antibody diversity. Tonegawa and many colleagues were responsible for the discovery of immunoglobulin gene C, V, J and D regions and their rearrangement.

In 1976, Tonegawa and Hozumi demonstrated that embryonic DNA contained separate constant (C)-region and variable (V)-region genes. Tonegawa and his associates observed that an intron separates these two genes when joined in a differentiated cell. Following the

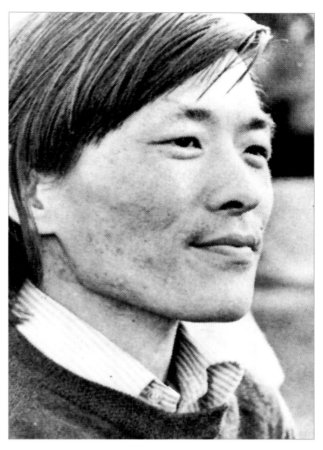

Figure 58   Susumu Tonegawa

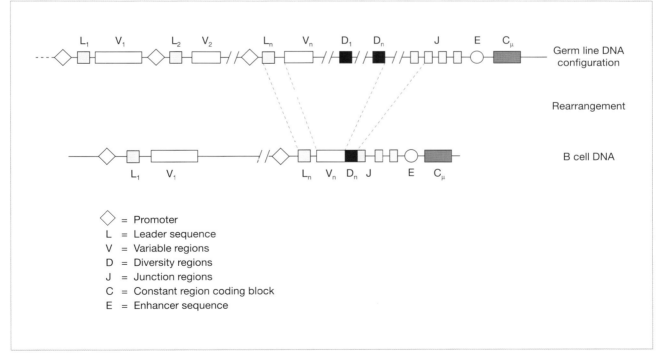

Figure 59   Immunoglobulin gene rearrangement

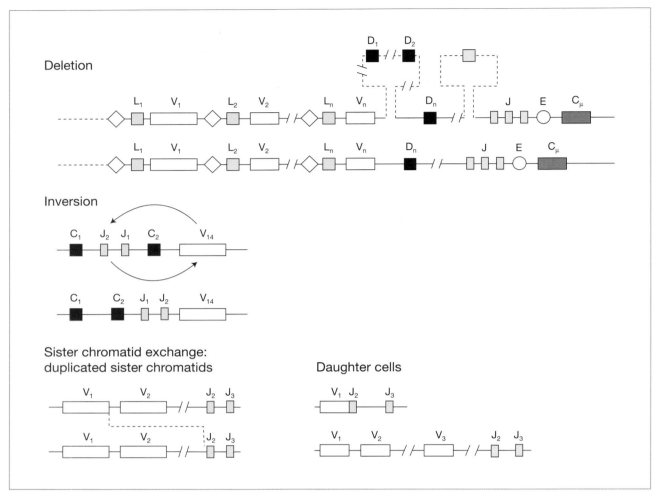

Figure 60 Immunoglobulin gene rearrangement (see Figure 59 for key)

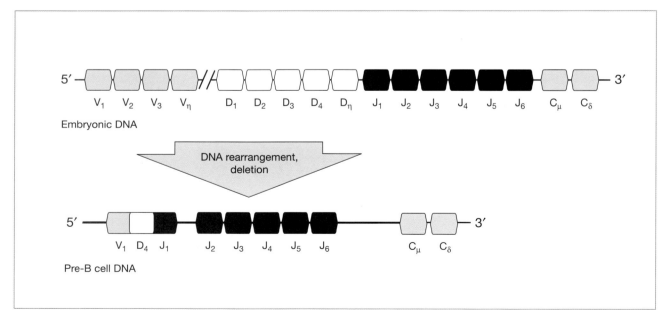

Figure 61 Gene rearrangement (see Figure 59 for key)

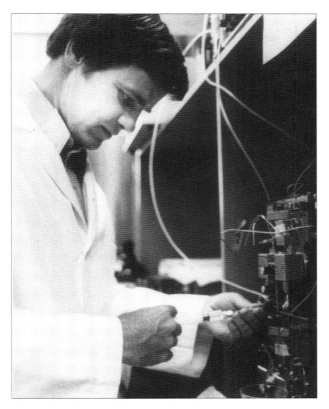

Figure 62 Leroy Hood, pioneer in immunogenetics and molecular immunology

finding by Tonegawa and by Leder that more amino acids were present in the variable region polypeptide chain than the V-region light-chain DNA could encode, a J (joining) segment was discovered to account for the missing DNA. The union of a single constant region segment with one of several J segments and one of numerous V-region segments could generate a broad variety of different light chains.

Tonegawa and Leroy Hood proved that three separate DNA segments must be combined to complete the heavy-chain variable-region sequence. They found yet another diversity (D) group of DNA segments in addition to the V and J segments. Besides the numerous V, D and J elements, splicing in the middle of a triplet codon, leading to a translational shift, contributed to even greater heavy-chain variability. Hood went on to demonstrate mutations in these gene segments. This elegant body of scientific evidence elucidated finally one of immunology's most mystifying conundrums.

Immunoglobulin genes encoding heavy and light polypeptide chains of antibody molecules are found on different chromosomes (i.e. chromosome 14 for heavy chain, chromosome 2 for κ light chain and chromosome 22 for λ light chain). The DNA of the majority of cells does not contain one gene that encodes a complete immunoglobulin heavy or light polypeptide chain. Separate gene segments that are widely distributed in somatic cells and germ cells come together to form these genes. In B cells, gene rearrangement leads to the creation of an antibody gene that encodes a specific protein. Somatic gene rearrangement also occurs with the genes that encode T cell antigen receptors. Gene rearrangement of this type permits the great versatility of the immune system in recognizing a vast array of epitopes. Three forms of gene segments join to form an immunoglobulin light-chain gene. The three types include light-chain variable region (V_L), joining (J_L) and constant region (C_L) gene segments. V_H, J_H, and C_H as well as D (diversity) gene segments assemble to encode the heavy chain. Heavy and light chain genes have a closely similar organizational structure. There are 100–300 $V\kappa$ genes, five $J\kappa$ genes and one C gene on the κ locus of chromosome 2. There are 100 V_H genes, 30 D genes, six J_H genes and 11 C_H genes on the heavy chain locus of chromosome 14. Several $V\lambda$, six $J\lambda$, and six $C\lambda$ genes are present on the λ locus of chromosome 22 in humans. V_H and V_L genes are classified as V gene families, depending on the sequence homology of their nucleotides or amino acids.

Gene diversity is the determination of the extent of an immune response to a particular antigen or immunogen as determined by mixing and matching of exons from variable, joining, diversity and constant region gene segments. S. Tonegawa (Figure 58) received the Nobel Prize for revealing the mechanism of the generation of diversity in antibody formation.

Allelic exclusion occurs when only one of two genes for which the animal is heterozygous is expressed, whereas the remaining gene is not. Immunoglobulin genes manifest this phenomenon. Allelic exclusion accounts for the ability of a B cell to express only one immunoglobulin or the capacity of a T cell to express a T cell receptor of a single specificity. Investigations of allotypes in rabbits established that individual immunoglobulin molecules have identical heavy chains and light chains. Immunoglobulin-synthesizing cells produce only a single class of heavy chain and one type of light chain at a time. Thus, by allelic exclusion, a cell that is synthesizing antibody expresses just one of two alleles encoding an immunoglobulin chain at a particular locus.

Junctional diversity occurs when gene segments join imprecisely; the amino acid sequence may vary and affect variable region expression, which can alter codons at gene segment junctions. These include the V–J junction of the genes encoding immunoglobulin κ and λ light chains and the V–D, D–J and D–D junctions of genes encoding immunoglobulin heavy chains or the genes encoding T cell receptor and β and δ chains.

Recombination activating genes (RAG-1 and RAG-2) are genes that activate immunoglobulin (Ig) gene recombination. Pre-B cells and immature T cells contain them. It remains to be determined whether RAG-1 and RAG-2 gene products are requisite for rearrangements of both Ig and T cell receptor (TCR) genes. In the absence of these genes, no Ig or TCR proteins are produced, which blocks the production of mature T and B cells.

Gene rearrangement refers to genetic shuffling that results in elimination of introns and the joining of exons to produce mRNA (Figures 59–61). Gene rearrangement within a lymphocyte signifies its dedication to the formation of a single cell type, which may be immunoglobulin synthesis by B lymphocytes or production of a β chain receptor by T lymphocytes. Neoplastic transformation of lymphocytes may be followed by the expansion of a single clone of cells, which is detectable by Southern blotting. RNA splicing is the method whereby RNA sequences that are non-translatable (known as introns) are excised from the primary transcript of a split gene. The translatable sequences (known as exons) are united to produce a functional gene product.

Clonal selection refers to antigen-mediated activation and proliferation of members of a clone of B lymphocytes bearing receptors for the antigen or for major histocompatibility complexes (MHCs) and peptides derived from the antigen in the case of T lymphocytes.

The **clonal selection theory** is a selective theory of antibody formation proposed by F. M. Burnet who postulated the presence of numerous antibody-forming cells, each capable of synthesizing its own predetermined antibody (Figure 63). One of the cells, after having been selected by the best-fitting antigen, multiplies and forms a clone of cells which continue to synthesize the same antibody. Considering the existence of many different cells, each capable of synthesizing an antibody of a different specificity, all known facts of antibody formation are easily accounted for. An important element of the clonal selection theory was the hypothesis that many cells with different antibody specificities arise through random somatic mutations during a period of hypermutability early in the animal's life. Also early in life, the 'forbidden' clones of antibody-forming cells (i.e. the cells that make antibody to the animal's own antigen) are still destroyed after encountering these autoantigens. This process accounted for an animal's tolerance of its own antigens. Antigen would have no effect on most lymphoid cells, but it would selectively stimulate those cells already synthesizing the corresponding antibody at a low rate. The cell surface antibody would serve as receptor for antigen and proliferate into a clone of cells, producing antibody of that specificity. Burnet introduced the 'forbidden clone' concept to explain autoimmunity. Cells capable of forming antibody against a normal self-antigen were 'forbidden' and eliminated during embryonic life. During fetal development, clones that react with self-antigens are destroyed or suppressed. The subsequent activation of suppressed clones reactive with self-antigens in later life may induce autoimmune disease. D. W. Talmage proposed a cell selection theory of antibody formation, which was the basis for Burnet's clonal selection theory.

Other workers were also interested in concepts of how antigen and antibody combine. Svante Arrhenius (1859–1927), of Stockholm, visited Ehrlich. He and one of Ehrlich's colleagues, the Danish bacteriologist Thorvald Madsen (Figure 64), formed an opinion from their studies that the reaction was a reversible equilibrium between the substances as when a weak acid and weak base are combined according to the ordinary law of mass action. Evidence to support this had come from Jan Danysz (1860–1928), who found that the toxicity of

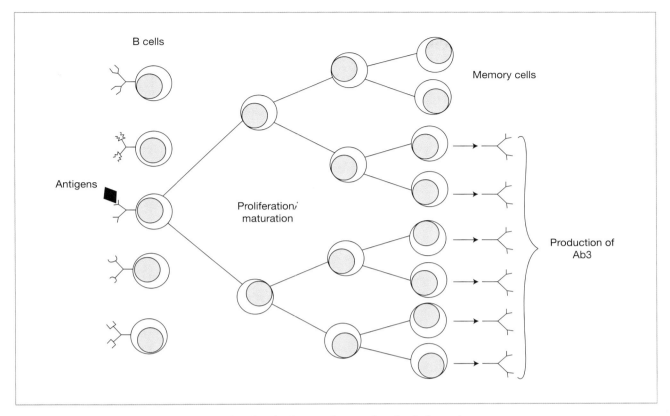

Figure 63 Schematic representation of the clonal selection theory of antibody formation

antigen was neutralized by a stated quantity of antibody when they were mixed but that the mixture remained toxic if half the antigen was added later, the 'Danysz phenomenon'. Bordet had a still different view of the way the antigen–antibody union took place, considering that the two substances acted like colloids, having varying proportions akin to adsorptive phenomena[11]. A solution to the problem had to await more sophisticated understanding of the structure and nature of macromolecules and the forces responsible for their behavior.

The humoral–cellular immunity controversy had occupied much attention through the last decade of the 19th century. In 1903, the English pathologist, Sir Almroth Wright (1861–1947) (Figures 65 and 66), and his co-worker Stewart Douglas (1871–1936), showed the existence of thermolabile substances in both normal and immune serum, which they termed 'opsonins' (Greek opsono: I provide food for), that attach themselves to bacteria and facilitate their phagocytosis. This finding is often cited as reconciling the two schools of thought[11]. However, the mainstream of research for many years continued to be the study of antibodies as the renaissance in cellular immunology emerged only in the 1960s[48].

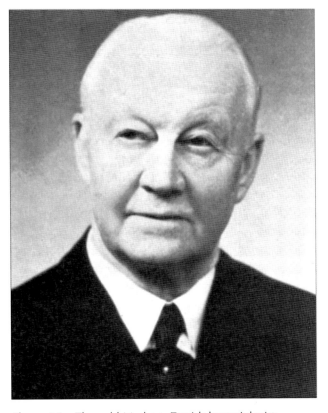

Figure 64 Thorvald Madsen, Danish bacteriologist

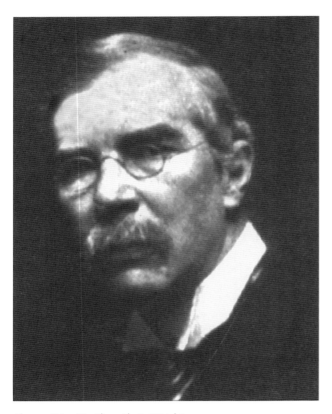

Figure 65 Sir Almroth E. Wright

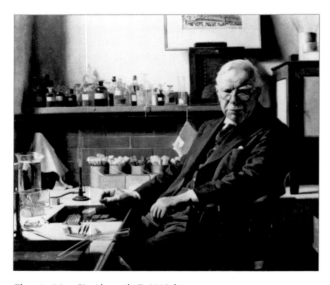

Figure 66 Sir Almroth E. Wright

Almroth Edward Wright (1861–1947), British pathologist and immunologist who graduated as a Doctor of Medicine from Trinity College Dublin in 1889. He became Professor of Pathology at the Army Medical School in Netley in 1892. He later became associated with the Institute of Pathology at St Mary's Hospital

Medical School, London, in 1902. Together with Douglas, he formulated a theory of opsonins and perfected an antitoxoid inoculation system. He studied immunology in Frankfurt-am-Main under Paul Ehrlich and made important contributions to the immunology of infectious diseases and immunization. He played a significant role in the founding of the American Association of Immunologists. *Pathology and Treatment of War Wounds*, 1942; *Researches in Clinical Physiology*, 1943; *Studies in Immunology*, (2 vol.), 1944.

REFERENCES

1. Brock TD, ed. *Milestones in Microbiology*. Englewood Cliffs, NJ: Prentice-Hall, 1961

2. Silverstein AM, Bialasiewicz AA. A history of theories of acquired immunity. *Cell Immunol* 1980;51:151–67

3. Bulloch W. *The History of Bacteriology*. London: Oxford University Press, 1938

4. Morton LT. *A Medical Bibliography: an Annotated Check-list of Texts Illustrating the History of Medicine*, 3rd edn. Philadelphia: JB Lippincott, 1970

5. Salmon DE, Smith T. The bacterium of swine-plague. *Proc Biol Soc Washington* 1886;3:29, also *Am Mon Micro J* 1886;7:204–5

6. Nuttall GHF. Experimente über de bacterienfeindlichen Einflusse des thierischen Korpers. *Z Hyg InfektKr* 1888;4:353–94

7. Buchner H. Ueber die bakterientodtende Wirkung des zellenfreien Blutserums. *Zentralbl Bakteriol* 1889;5:817–23

8. Roux E, Yersin A. Contribution a l'étude de la dipterie. *Ann Inst Pasteur* 1888;2:629–61; also 1889;3:273–88; 1890;4:385–426

9. Brieger G. Introduction. In Metchnikoff E, ed. *Immunity to infective diseases* (transl. by Binnie FG). The Sources of Science, no. 61. New York: Johnson Reprint, 1968

10. Pfeiffer RFJ, Isayev BI. Über die specifische Bedeutung der Choleraimmunitat (Bakterilyse). *Z Hyg InfektKr* 1894;17:355–400; also 1894;18:1–16

11. Humphrey JH, White RG. *Immunology for Students of Medicine*, 3rd edn. Philadelphia: Davis, 1970

12. Charrin A, Rogers J. Note sur le développement des microbes pathogens dans le serum des animaux vaccines. *CR Soc Biol* 1889;41:667–99

13. von Grüber M, Durham HE. Eine neue Methode zur raschen Erkennung des Choleravibrio und des Typhusbacillus. *Münch Med Wschr* 1896;43:285–6

14. Widal GFI, Sicard A. Recherches de la reaction agglutinante dans le sang et le serum desséches des typhiques et dans le serosité des vesicatoires. *Bull Mem Soc Med Hop Paris* 1896;13:681–2

15. Bordet J, Gengou O. Sur l'existence de substance sensibilisatrices dans la plupart des serums antimicrobiens. *Ann Inst Pasteur* 1901;15:289–302

16. Wassermann A, Neisser A, Bruck C. Eine Serodiagnostische Reaktion bei Syphilis. *Deutsche Med Wschr* 1906;32:745–6

17. Ehrlich P. *Das Sauerstoff-Bedurfniss des Organismus. Eine farbenanalytische Studie*. Berlin: A Hirschwald, 1885

18. Marquardt M. *Paul Ehrlich*. New York: Henry Schuman, 1951

19. Ehrlich P. On immunity with special reference to cell life. *Proc R Soc Lond* 1900;66:424

20. Obermayer F, Pick EP. Über Veranderungen des Brechungsvermogens von Glykosiden und Eiweisskorpern durch Fermente, Sauren und Bakterien. *Beitr Z Chem Phys Path Brnschwg* 1903;VII:331

21. Landsteiner K. Über die Abhängigkeit der serologischen Spezifität von der chemischen Struktur. (Darstellung von Antigenen mit bekannter chemischer Konstitution der specifischen Grüppen) XII Mitteilung über Antigene. *Biochem Z* 1918;86:343

22. Landsteiner K. *Die Spezifität der Serologischen Reaktionen*. Berlin: Springer-Verlag, 1933

23. Landsteiner K, Chase MW. Experiments on the transfer of cutaneous sensitivity to simple compounds. *Proc Soc Exp Biol Med* 1942;49:488

24. Breinl F, Haurowitz F. Chemische Untersuchung des Prazipitätes aus Hamoglobin und Anti-Hamoglobin Serum und über die Natur der Antikorper. *Z F Physiol Chem* 1930;192:45

25. Mudd S. Hypothetical mechanism of antibody formation. *J Immunol* 1932;23:423

26. Pauling L. A theory of the structure and process of formation of antibodies. *J Am Chem Soc* 1940;62:2643

27. Burnet FM, Fenner F. *The Production of Antibodies*, 2nd edn. Melbourne: The MacMillan Co, 1949

28. Burnet F. A modification of Jerne's theory of antibody production using the concept of clonal selection. *Aust J Sci* 1957;20:67–8

29. Talmage DW. Is this theory necessary? In Mazumdar PMH, ed. *Immunology 1930–1980*. Toronto: Wall & Thompson, 1989:67

30. Jerne NK. A study of avidity. *Acta Pathol Microbiol Scand* 1951;87(Suppl):1

31. Barr M, Glenny AT. Some practical applications of immunological principles. *J Hyg* 1945;44:135

32. Taliaferro W, Taliaferro L. The role of spleen in hemolysin production in rabbits receiving multiple antigen injections. *J Infect Dis* 1951;89:143

33. Owen R. Immunogenetic consequences of vascular anastomoses between bovine twins. *Science* 1945;102:400

34. Billingham R, Brent L, Medawar P. Actively acquired tolerance of foreign cells. *Nature (London)* 1953;172:603

35. Taliaferro W, Talmage D. Absence of amino acid incorporation into antibody during the induction period. *J Infect Dis* 1955;97:88

36. Roberts JC, Dixon FJ. The transfer of lymph node cells in the study of the immune response to foreign proteins. *J Exp Med* 1955;102:379

37. Schweet R, Owen RD. Concepts of protein synthesis in relation to antibody formation. *J Cell Comp Physiol* 1957;50(Suppl 1):199

38. Jerne NK. The natural selection theory of antibody formation. *Proc Natl Acad Sci* USA 1957;41:849

39. Talmage DW. The acceptance and rejection of immunological concepts. In Paul WE, Garrison CG, Metzger H, eds. *Annual Review of Immunology*. Palo Alto, CA: Annual Reviews, Inc., 1986;4:1

40. Burnet FM. Autoimmune disease. II. Pathology of the immune response. *Br Med J* 1959;ii:720

41. Nossal GJV, Pike BL. Single cell studies on the antibody-forming potential of fractionated, hapten-specific B lymphocytes. *Immunology* 1976;30:189

42. Hood LE, Weissman LL, Wood WB, Wilson JH. *Immunology*, 2nd edn. Menlo Park, CA: Benjamin Cummings, 1984:81

43. Nossal GJV, Lederberg J. Antibody production by single cells. *Nature (London)* 1958;181:1419

44. Binns RM, Feinstein AA, Gurner BW, Coombs RRA. Immunoglobulin determinants on lymphocytes of adult, neonatal and foetal pigs. *Nature (London)* 1972;229:114

45. Dutton RS, Mishell RJ. Cell populations and cell proliferation in vitro response of normal spleen to heterologous erythrocytes: analysis by the hot pulse method. *J Exp Med* 1967;126:443

46. Raff MC, Feldmann M, dePetris S. Monospecificity of bone marrow-derived lymphocytes. *J Exp Med* 1973;137:1024–30

47. Köhler G, Milstein C. Continuous cultures of fused cells secreting antibody of predefined specificity. *Nature (London)* 1975;256:495

48. Silverstein AM. Cellular versus humoral immunity; determinants and consequences of an epic 19th century battle. *Cell Immunol* 1979;48:208–21

CHAPTER 3

Immunochemistry (molecular immunology)

The fundamental position that immunology occupies among the natural sciences is no better demonstrated than by the fact that distinguished chemists outside the field of biomedical science have been fascinated by the basic biological significance of such topics as antibody formation and antigen–antibody interaction. Indeed, it was the Nobel Laureate in Chemistry Svante Arrhenius who coined the term 'immunochemistry' in 1905 when he was invited to the University of California at Berkeley to present a series of lectures on the chemistry of immune reactions[1] (Figures 1 and 2).

Svante Arrhenius (1859–1927), photographed in Figure 1 with Paul Ehrlich, 1903. He coined the term 'immunochemistry' and hypothesized that antigen–antibody complexes are reversible. He was awarded the Nobel Prize for Chemistry, 1903. *Immunochemistry*. New York: MacMillan Publishers, 1907.

Obermayer and Pick, two Viennese chemists, in 1903 investigated the effects on specificity of coupling various chemical groupings to proteins[2]. Nitric acid, nitrous acid or iodine treatment of proteins altered their specificity to the point that they were rendered antigenic (i.e. immunogenic) in species to which they were not originally alien. Later experiments demonstrated that alteration of protein specificity by such treatment was based upon modification of aromatic amino acids as opposed to alteration of protein specificity by the introduced groups alone.

There can be little doubt that this work fired the imagination of Karl Landsteiner (Figures 3 and 4), who, with some associates in 1918, coupled organic radicals to proteins[3]. Landsteiner devised a method whereby an immune response could be directed against small molecules of known structure. He referred to these substances as 'haptens', which by themselves were too small to initiate an immune response, but were capable of reacting with the products of an immune response. He chemically coupled these haptens to large biological macromolecules, such as ovalbumin, which he termed 'carriers', producing conjugated antigens capable of stimulating an immune response. The non-valent hapten in pure form, together with serum antibodies,

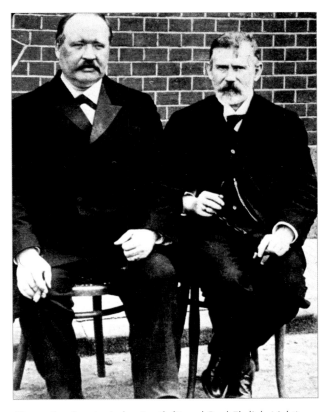

Figure 1   Svante Arrhenius (left) and Paul Ehrlich (right)

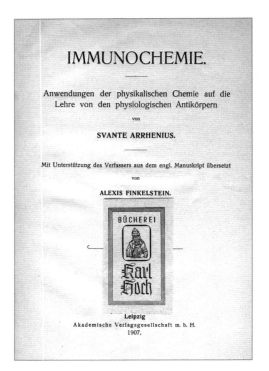

IMMUNOCHEMIE.

Anwendungen der physikalischen Chemie auf die
Lehre von den physiologischen Antikörpern

von

SVANTE ARRHENIUS.

Mit Unterstützung des Verfassers aus dem engl. Manuskript übersetzt

von

ALEXIS FINKELSTEIN.

BÜCHEREI

Karl Hoch

Leipzig
Akademische Verlagsgesellschaft m. b. H.
1907.

Figure 2 S. Arrhenius' lectures on immunochemistry delivered at the University of California, Berkeley, in 1905

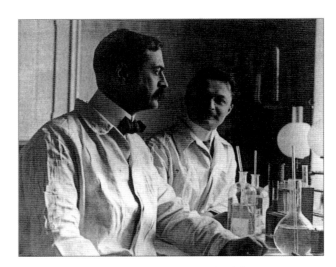

Figure 3 Karl Landsteiner at work in his laboratory

could then be used to study antibody– hapten interactions without the complications of multideterminant macromolecular antigens. The ability of a particular chemical to act as a determinant of specificity was tested by coupling it to an aromatic amine such as aniline. The product of this reaction was diazotized and coupled to a protein to form a conjugated antigen or azoprotein. From these studies, which dominated Landsteiner's research activities until his death in 1943, the chemical basis for serological specificity was proved. Not only the nature of the radical coupled to a protein, but also the position of the attachment site on the ring (*ortho*, *meta* or *para*), was shown to be of critical importance with respect to specificity. Landsteiner found cross-reactivity with immune antibodies to related haptens (Figure 5). This represented the 'golden age of immunochemistry', when the views of chemists prevailed over those of biologists.

Ehrlich had attempted to develop a selective theory of antibody formation with his side-chain theory, which required that every cell involved in antibody production be capable of reacting against every known antigen in nature. However, it was precisely this weakness in the hypothesis that allowed Landsteiner to deal it a death blow by raising antibodies against haptens (partial

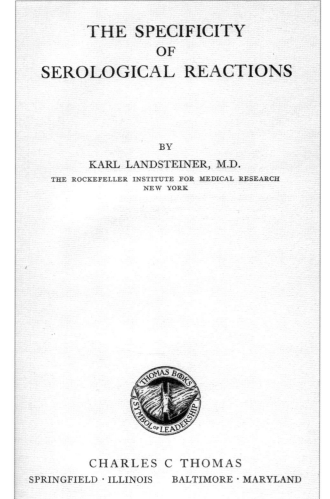

Figure 4 The English translation of Landsteiner's famous monograph

Immune sera for meta-amino-benzene sulfonic acid after absorption with	Azoproteins made from chicken serum and			
	Ortho-amino-benzene sulfonic acid	Meta-amino-benzene sulfonic acid	Meta-amino-benzene arsenic acid	Meta-amino-benzoic acid
o-Aminobenzene sulfonic acid	o	++±	±	+
	o	+++±	±	+
m-Aminobenzene arsenic acid	+±	+++	o	+
	++	++++	o	+±
m-Aminobenzoic acid	+±	+++	±	o
	++	++++	±	±
Unabsorbed immune serum	++	+++±	+	+±
	+++	++++	++	++±

Reading: first line, after standing 1 hour at room temperature; second line, after standing overnight in the icebox

Figure 5 Cross-reactivity with immune antibodies to related haptens. Since the test antigens contained the same proteins, unrelated to the horse serum used for immunization, the protein component could not be responsible for the differential reactions

antigens) which he had manufactured in the chemical laboratory and which had never appeared before in nature. He pointed out that it was inconceivable that nature would provide receptors for antigens which the animal body would never see. It is important to remember the limitations not only of chemical knowledge of the period, but also that Hugo de Vries had rediscovered Mendel's basic work in genetics only 23 years earlier[4]. Arrhenius was not the only famous chemist to become interested in immunological phenomena. Wells authored an important book on chemical aspects of immunity in the 1920s (Figures 6–8). The British chemical pathologist, J. R. Marrack, published a critical review of the chemistry of antigens and antibodies in 1934 (revised 1938), and proposed a lattice theory of antigen–antibody interaction (Figures 9–12). The description of forces involved in antigen–antibody interaction and the demonstration of the necessity of sterophysical complementarity of reaction sites were made in 1940 by Linus Pauling, another Nobel Laureate in Chemistry[5]. As had Felix Haurowitz and Breinl in 1930[6] and Mudd in 1932[7], Pauling proposed a template theory of antibody formation which required that the antigen must be present during the process of antibody formation. This view prevailed among many immunologists until the demonstration that it was inadequate to explain such newly discovered phenomena as immunological tolerance which represented the basis of successful tissue transplantation. Working with Pressman (Figure 13) and Campbell, he provided strong evidence for the bivalence of antibodies and the significance of molecular shapes in binding of antibody to antigen. The development of precise methods of quantitation of antibody and the discovery and characterization of nonprecipitating antibodies (incomplete or functionally univalent antibodies) was made between 1930 and 1935 by Heidelberger and Kendall[8]. To O. T. Avery's (Figure 14) nitrogen-free 'specific soluble substance' derived from pneumococcal polysaccharide, Heidelberger (Figures 15–17) added homologous antibody in a precipitin reaction to yield a precipitate. This permitted him to measure antibody, since the precipitate contained antibody nitrogen exclusively.

Heidelberger, Kendall and Kabat resolved the question of whether antibodies were globulins and whether precipitins and agglutinins were the same or separate entities. In fact, specific precipitation, agglutination and complement fixation were demonstrated to be different

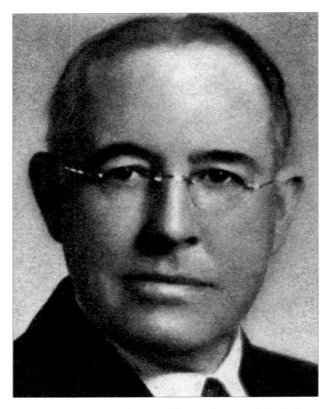

Figure 6 Harry Gideon Wells, Professor of Pathology, University of Chicago

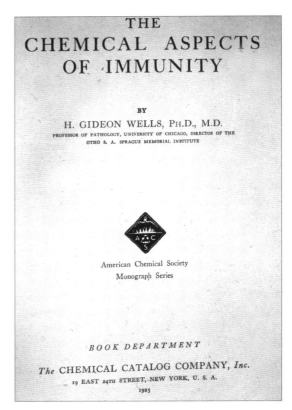

Figure 7 H. G. Wells' early monograph on the chemistry of immunity in the 1920s

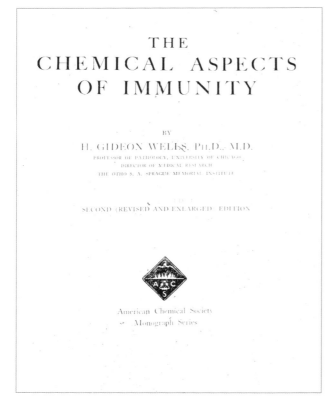

Figure 8 Revision of Wells' monograph

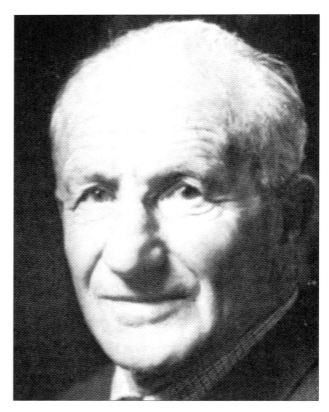

Figure 9 John Richardson Marrack

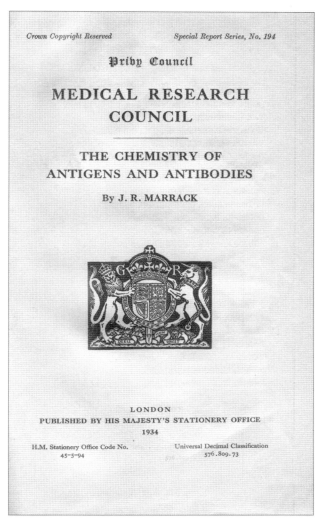

Figure 10   Dr Marrack's important report to the Br tish government on the chemistry of antigens and antibodies in 1934

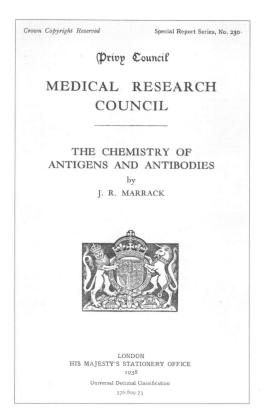

Figure 11   Revision of Dr Marrack's book in 1938

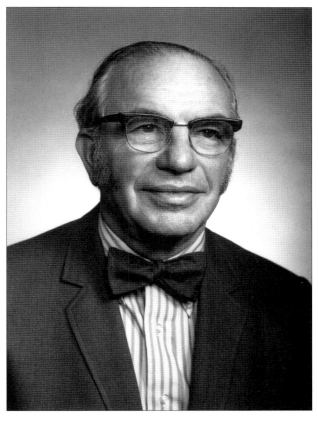

Figure 13   David Pressman, colleague of Linus Pauling

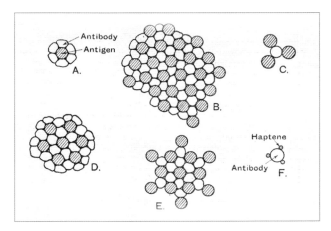

Figure 12   Marrack's proposal of a lattice network theory of antigen–antibody interaction

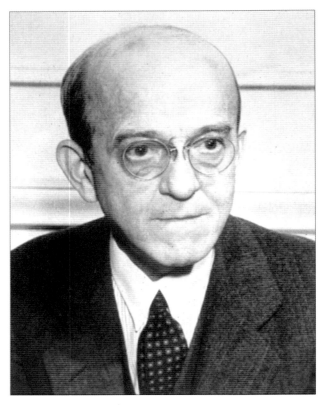

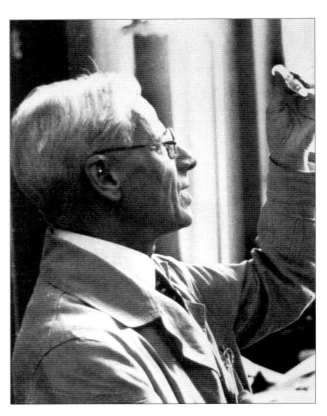

Figure 14 Oswald T. Avery, Rockefeller Institute for Medical Research, New York

Figure 15 Michael Heidelberger

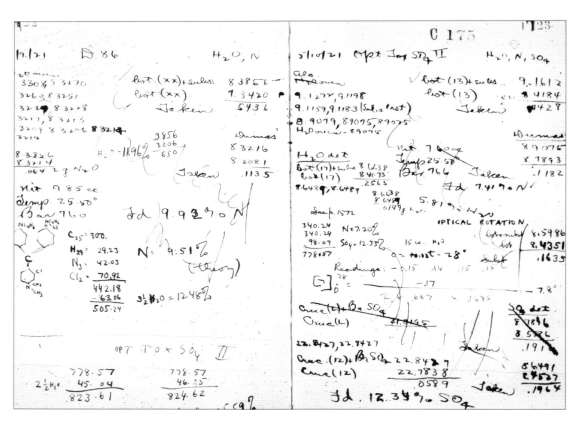

Figure 16 Pages in Michael Heidelberger's laboratory notebook

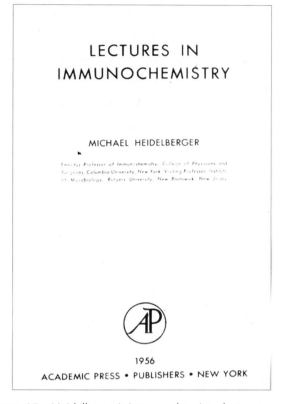

Figure 17 Heidelberger's immunochemistry lectures

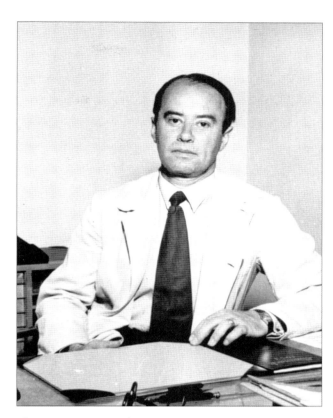

Figure 18 Arne Tiselius

manifestations of a single antibody. Heidelberger and associates were able to isolate and analyze antibodies. In 1934, they developed a 70% pure antibody preparation which proved to be a globulin with the aid of a newly developed ultracentrifuge in Sweden. The Heidelberger team proved that complement was a real nitrogen-containing substance, or substances, with weight. This discovery, together with Pillemer and Ecker's independent purification of the first component, enabled other investigators to purify and analyze the complement system. In his long and distinguished career, Professor Heidelberger served as the dean of American immunochemists who trained Elvin Kabat, Manfred Mayer and a host of other investigators.

The electrophoretic method of separating serum proteins and the assignment of antibody activity to the globulin fraction was proposed by Tiselius (Figure 18). In the same year Kabat (Figures 19–21) and Tiselius demonstrated by electrophoresis and ultracentrifugation that 19S antibody is found early and 7S antibody late in the immune response[9]. In 1959, Rodney Porter working in England demonstrated that antibody molecules could be split into fragments by the enzyme

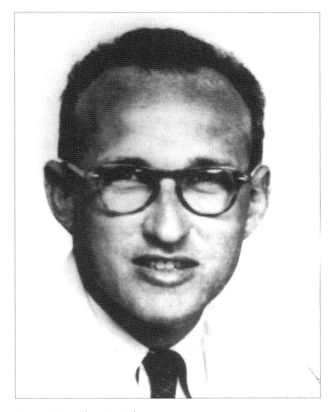

Figure 19 Elvin A. Kabat as a young man

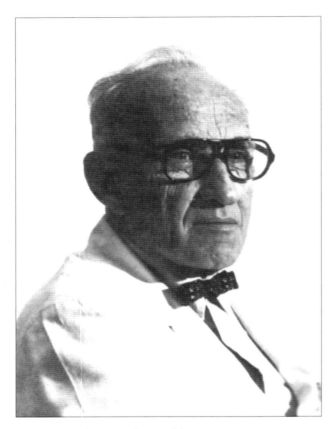

Figure 20 Elvin A. Kabat in old age

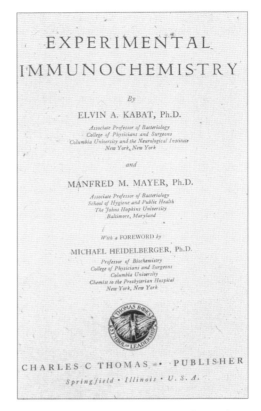

EXPERIMENTAL
IMMUNOCHEMISTRY

By

ELVIN A. KABAT, Ph.D.

*Associate Professor of Bacteriology
College of Physicians and Surgeons
Columbia University and the Neurological Institute
New York, New York*

and

MANFRED M. MAYER, Ph.D.

*Associate Professor of Bacteriology
School of Hygiene and Public Health
The Johns Hopkins University
Baltimore, Maryland*

With a FOREWORD *by*

MICHAEL HEIDELBERGER, Ph.D.

*Professor of Biochemistry
College of Physicians and Surgeons
Columbia University
Chemist to the Presbyterian Hospital
New York, New York*

CHARLES C THOMAS · PUBLISHER

Springfield · Illinois · U. S. A.

Figure 21 Kabat's famous monograph (with Manfred Mayer) on experimental immunochemistry

papain (Figures 22 and 23). He found that those fragments which remained in the supernatant of his reaction mixture retained the capacity to interact with antigen, whereas that part of the molecule which crystallized had no antigen-binding property. He subsequently designated these as Fab and Fc fragments, i.e. fragment antigen-binding and fragment crystallizable, respectively[10]. In 1969, Gerald Edelman (Figures 24 and 25) reported the results of his primary sequence analysis of a human myeloma protein (namely immunoglobulin G, IgG)[11]. The isolation of sufficient homogeneous antibody from the serum of a patient with multiple myeloma over a significant period of time had overcome the previous difficulty of attempting to analyze heterogeneous antibodies. For their work in demonstrating the fundamental structure of immunoglobulin molecules, Porter and Edelman received the Nobel Prize in Medicine in 1972. However, many other investigators including Henry Kunkel (Figure 26), Hugh Fudenberg and Frank Putnam had laid the groundwork for this discovery. Valentine demonstrated immunoglobulin structure by electron microscopy (Figure 27). Alfred Nisonoff's

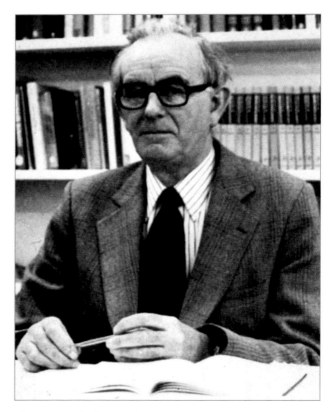

Figure 22 Rodney R. Porter

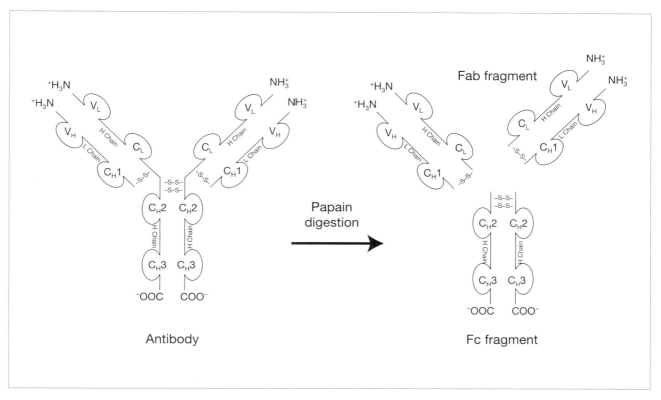

Figure 23   Papain digestion of immunoglobulin G (IgG) into two Fab and one Fc fragments

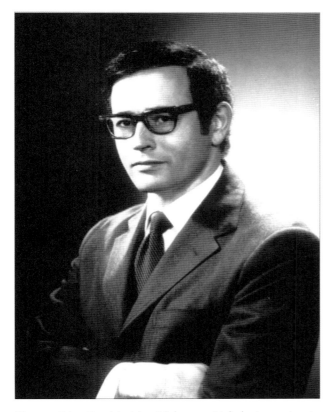

Figure 24 Gerald M. Edelman, Nobel Laureate in Medicine or Physiology

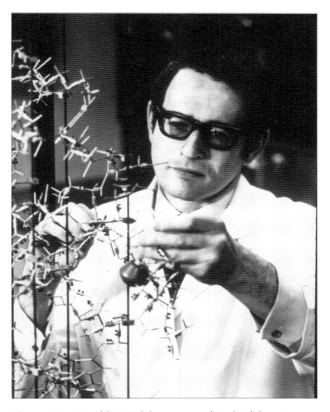

Figure 25   Gerald M. Edelman at work in his laboratory

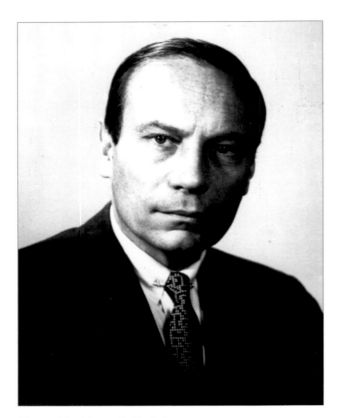

Figure 26   Henry G. Kunkel

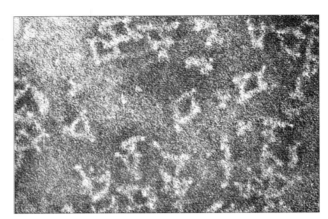

Figure 27   Valentine and Green's demonstration of antibody structural morphology by electron microscopy. From reference 12

fundamental studies on immunoglobulin structure resulted in part from his preparation of F(ab')$_2$ fragments of IgG as a consequence of pepsin digestion (Figure 28). Kunkel was Edelman's mentor at the Rockefeller Institute for Medical Research. Much activity was then initiated to sequence the heavy and light chains comprising immunoglobulin molecules[13]. It was shown that man possesses three major and two minor classes of immunoglobulin, each determined by the specificity of the heavy chain. These were designated as IgG, IgM, IgA, IgD and IgE. After this period of activity in the 1960s, interest in immunochemistry began to wane and cellular immunology came to the forefront of research. Even the journal entitled *Immunochemistry* was renamed *Molecular Immunology*.

Jan Gosta Waldenström (1906–96), Swedish physician who described macroglobulinemia, which now bears his name. He received the Gairdner Award in 1966.

Michael Heidelberger (1888–1991), a founder of immunochemistry, was born on 29 April 1888 in New

York City. Following completion of his PhD in organic chemistry at Columbia, and postdoctoral training with Richard Willstätter in Zurich, he returned to a position at the Rockefeller Institute for Medical Research in New York City. He and Jacobs discovered tryparsamide which proved very effective in the treatment of African sleeping sickness. In Van Slyke's laboratory at the Rockefeller, he perfected a technique for the preparation of crystalline oxyhemoglobin. This brought him into contact with Karl Landsteiner, with whom he published two classic articles comparing immunologic and solubility techniques for distinguishing hemoglobins of different species. Professor O. T. Avery requested his assistance with the biochemical analysis of 'specific soluble substance' of pneumococci. He purified Avery's broth concentrate until the components were free of nitrogen, showing that it was indeed 'specific soluble substance'. He precipitated the preparation with antiserum and recovered the same polysaccharide. This led to extensive future investigations by Heidelberger, Goebel, Avery and others on the specificity of naturally occurring antigens. Precipitin analyses permitted estimation of the quantities of numerous antigens in native materials without the need for tedious isolation and purification. Heidelberger accepted an appointment as Associate Professor of Medicine at Columbia Physicians and Surgeons where he and Kendall developed a quantitative theory defining the precipitin reaction of polysaccharides. Together with Kabat and Kendall, he demonstrated that antibodies were globulins and that specific precipitation, agglutination and complement fixation were different manifestations of a single antibody.

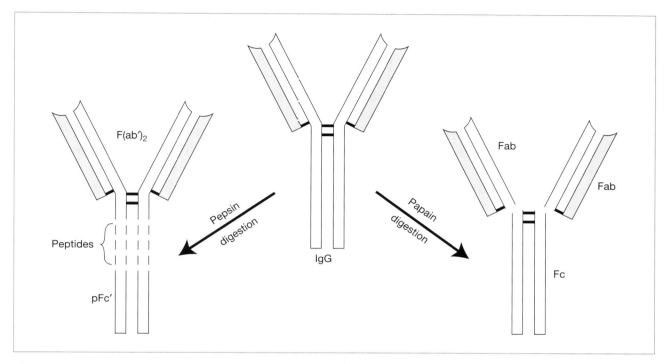

Figure 28   Pepsin digestion of IgG, by Alfred Nisonoff, into F(ab')₂ fragments

They also performed classic experiments proving complement to be a real nitrogen-containing substance, or substances, with weight. Purified antibodies developed in rabbits against types I, II and III pneumococci proved very effective in the treatment of pneumonia caused by pneumococci of the corresponding type, significantly reducing mortality.

During the post-World War II decade, accolades at home and abroad were showered upon him. He twice served as president of the American Association of Immunologists in the 1940s. Among his many honors are the Lasker, Behring and Hurwitz Awards, the Pasteur Medal of the Swedish Medical Society, the Order of Leopold II, membership in the Légion d'honneur and the Académie de Médecine of France, and the National Medal of Science, as well as a spate of honorary degrees from the world's leading universities.

After 27 years at P and S, at 67 years of age, he accepted Dr Selman Waksman's invitation to join the Institute of Microbiology at Rutgers where, for nearly a decade, he inspired the Immunochemistry Group to pursue novel and innovative research. Upon leaving Rutgers, at the age of 76, Professor Heidelberger continued his research in the Department of Pathology at New York University. He began a series of challenging

investigations on cross-reactivity of microorganisms and of plant polysaccharides, publishing many papers on immunologic relationships among their structures. Professor Heidelberger's life work was aimed at the development of rigorous quantitative techniques for purification of antibody molecules and investigations on the specificity of naturally occurring antigens.

Elvin Abraham Kabat (1914–2000) (Figures 19 and 20), American immunochemist. With Tiselius he was the first to separate immunoglobulins electrophoretically. He also demonstrated that globulins can be distinguished as 7S or 19S. Other contributions include research on antibodies to carbohydrates, the antibody-combining site and the discovery of immunoglobulin chain variable regions. He received the National Medal of Science. *Experimental Immunochemistry* (with Mayer), 1948; *Blood Group Substances: Their Chemistry and Immunochemistry, Structural Concepts in Immunology and Immunochemistry*, 1956, 1968.

Arne W. W. Tiselius (1902–71) (Figure 18), Swedish chemist who was educated at the University of Uppsala where he also worked in research. In 1934 he was at the Institute for Advanced Study in Princeton, he worked for the Swedish National Research Council in 1946 and he became President of the Nobel Foundation in 1960. Awarded the Nobel Prize in Chemistry in 1948, he perfected the electrophoresis technique and classified antibodies as K globulins together with Elvin A. Kabat. He also developed synthetic blood plasmas.

John Richardson Marrack (1899–1976) (Figure 9), British physician who served as Professor of Chemical Pathology at Cambridge and at the London Hospital. He hypothesized that antibodies are bivalent, labeled antibodies with colored dyes and proposed a lattice theory of antigen–antibody complex formation in fundamental physicochemical studies.

Herman Nathaniel Eisen (1918–), American physician whose research contributions range from equilibrium dialysis (with Karush) to the mechanism of contact dermatitis.

Gerald Maurice Edelman (1929–) (Figures 24 and 25), American investigator who was professor at the Rockefeller University and shared the Nobel Prize in 1972 with Porter for their work on antibody structure. Edelman was the first to demonstrate that immunoglobulins are composed of light and heavy polypeptide chains. He also did pioneering work with Bence Jones protein, cell adhesion molecules, immunoglobulin amino acid sequence and neurobiology.

Rodney Robert Porter (1917–85) (Figure 22), British biochemist who received the Nobel Prize in 1972, with Gerald Edelman, for their studies of antibodies and their chemical structure. Porter cleaved antibody molecules with the enzyme papain to yield Fab and Fc fragments. He suggested that antibodies have a four-chain structure. Fab fragments were shown to have the antigen-binding sites whereas the Fc fragment conferred the antibody's biological properties. He also investigated the sequence of complement genes in the major histocompatibility complex (MHC). *Defense and Recognition*, 1973.

Antigens and immunogens

An infectious agent, whether a bacterium, fungus, virus or parasite, contains a plethora of substances capable of inducing an immune response. These are called immunogens or antigens. Specifically, an immunogen is a substance capable of stimulating B cell, T cell or both limbs of the immune response. An antigen is a substance that reacts with the products of an immune response stimulated by a specific immunogen, including both antibodies and/or T lymphocyte receptors. The 'traditional' definition of antigen more correctly refers to an immunogen. A complete antigen is one that both induces an immune response and reacts with the products of it, whereas an incomplete antigen or hapten is unable to induce an immune response alone but is able to react with the products of it, e.g. antibodies. Haptens could be rendered immunogenic by covalently linking them to a carrier molecule.

Following the administration of an antigen (immunogen) to a host animal, antibody synthesis and/or cell-mediated immunity or immunologic tolerance may result. To be immunogenic, a substance usually needs to be foreign, although some autoantigens represent an exception. They should usually have a molecular weight of at least 10 000 and be either proteins or polysaccharides. Nevertheless, immunogenicity depends upon the genetic capacity of the host to respond rather than merely upon the antigenic properties of an injected immunogen.

The specific parts of antigen molecules that elicit immune reactivity are known as antigenic determinants or epitopes. Even the earliest investigators in immunology recognized that low-molecular-weight substances such as simple chemicals could react with the products of an immune response but were not themselves immunogenic. These were termed haptens. Thus, a hapten is a relatively small molecule which, by itself, is unable to elicit an immune response when injected into an animal, but is capable of reacting *in vitro* with an antibody specific for it. However, a hapten may be covalently linked to a carrier macromolecule such as a foreign protein that renders it immunogenic so that it can form new antigenic determinants. Haptens often have highly reactive chemical groupings that permit them to autocouple with a substance such as a tissue protein. This type of reaction occurs in individuals who develop contact hypersensitivity to poison ivy or poison oak.

An **antigen** is a substance that reacts with the products of an immune response stimulated by a specific immunogen, including both antibodies and/or T lymphocyte receptors, and currently considered to be one of many kinds of substances with which an antibody molecule or T cell receptor may bind. These include sugars, lipids, intermediary metabolites, autocoids, hormones, complex carbohydrates, phospholipids, nucleic acids and proteins. By contrast, the 'traditional' definition of antigen is a substance that may stimulate B and/or T cell limbs of the immune response and react with the products of that response, including immunoglobulin antibodies and/or specific receptors on T cells (see immunogen definition). The 'traditional' definition of antigen more correctly refers to an immunogen. A complete antigen is one that both induces an immune response and reacts with the products of it, whereas an incomplete antigen or hapten is unable to induce an immune response alone, but is able to react with the products of it, e.g. antibodies. Haptens could be rendered immunogenic by covalently linking them to a carrier molecule. Following the administration of an antigen (immunogen) to a host animal, antibody synthesis and/or cell-mediated immunity or immunologic tolerance may result. To be immunogenic, a substance usually needs to be foreign, although some autoantigens represent an exception. They should usually have a molecular weight of at least 1000 and be either proteins or polysaccharides. Nevertheless, immunogenicity depends also upon the genetic capacity of the host to respond to, rather than merely upon the antigenic properties of, an injected immunogen.

A **superantigen** is an antigen such as a bacterial toxin that is capable of stimulating many CD4$^+$ T cells, leading to the release of relatively large quantities of cytokines. Selected bacterial toxins may stimulate all T lymphocytes in the body that contain a certain family of variable region V β T cell receptor genes. Superantigens may induce proliferation of 10% of CD4$^+$ T cells by combining with the T cell V β and to the MHC human leukocyte antigen (HLA)-DR α-1 domain. Superantigens are thymus-dependent (TD) antigens that do not require phagocytic processing.

Instead of fitting into the T cell receptor (TCR) internal groove where a typical processed peptide antigen fits, superantigens bind to the external region of the αβ TCR and simultaneously link to DP, DQ or DR molecules on antigen-presenting cells. Superantigens react with multiple TCR molecules whose peripheral structure is similar. Thus, they stimulate multiple T cells that augment a protective T and B cell antibody response. This enhanced responsiveness to antigens such as toxins produced by staphylococci and streptococci is an important protective mechanism in the infected individual. Several staphylococcal enterotoxins are superantigens and may activate many T cells resulting in the release of large quantities of cytokines that provoke pathophysiologic manifestations resembling endotoxin shock.

An **antigenic determinant** (Figure 29) interacts with the specific antigen-binding site in the variable region of an antibody molecule known as a paratope. The excellent fit between epitope and paratope is based on their three-dimensional interaction and non-covalent union. An antigenic determinant or epitope may also react with a T cell receptor for which it is specific. A single antigen molecule may have several different epitopes. Whereas an epitope interacts with the antigen-binding region of an antibody molecule or with the T cell receptor, a separate region of the antigen that combines with class II MHC molecules is known as an agretope.

Antigenic determinants may be either conformational or linear. A conformational determinant is produced by spatial juxtaposition during folding of amino acid residues from different segments of the linear amino acid sequence. Conformational determinants are usually associated with natural rather than denatured proteins. A linear determinant is one produced by adjacent amino acid residues in the covalently sequenced proteins. They are usually available for interaction with antibody only following denaturation of a protein, and are not customarily in the native configuration. Antigenic determinants or epitopes are sometimes called immunodominant groups. In contrast to the natural antigens that constitute part of a microbe, one derived exclusively by laboratory synthesis and not obtained from living cells is termed a **synthetic antigen**.

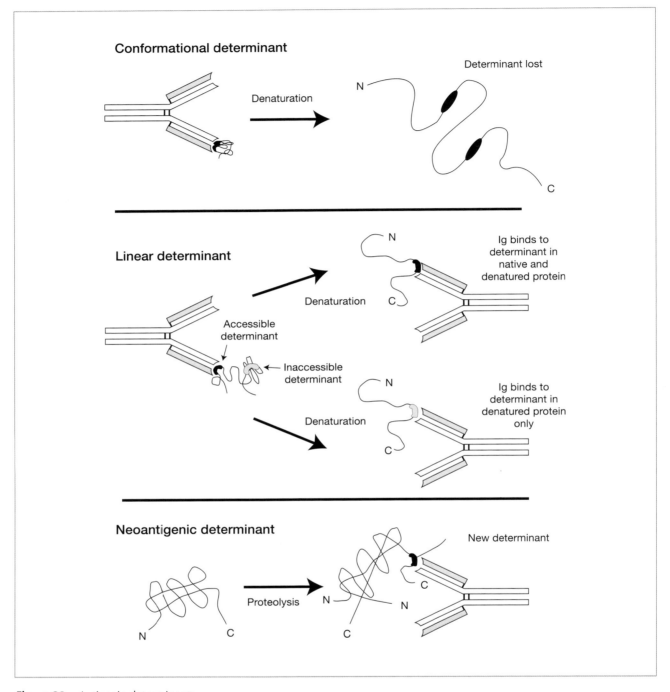

Figure 29   Antigenic determinants

A **synthetic antigen** is derived exclusively by laboratory synthesis and is not obtained from living cells (Figure 30). Synthetic polypeptide antigens have a backbone consisting of amino acids that usually include lysine. Side-chains of different amino acids are attached directly to the backbone and then elongated with a homopolymer or, conversely, attached via the homopolymer. They have contributed much to our knowledge of epitope structure and function. They have well-defined specificities determined by the particular arrangement, number and nature of the amino acid components of the molecule, and they may be made more complex by further coupling to haptens or derivatized with various compounds. The size of the molecule is less critical with synthetic antigens than with natural antigens. Thus, molecules as small

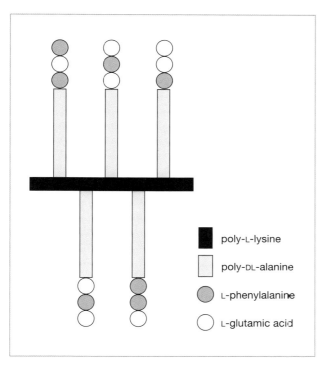

Figure 30 Synthetic polypeptide antigen with multichain copolymer (phe, G)-A-L

poly-L-lysine

poly-DL-alanine

L-phenylalanine

L-glutamic acid

as those of *p*-azobenzenearsonate coupled to three L-lysine residues (molecular weight 750) or even of *p*-azobenzenearsonate-*N*-acetyl-L-tyrosine (molecular weight 451) may be immunogenic. Specific antibodies are markedly stereospecific, and there is no cross-reaction between them, e.g. poly-D-alanyl and poly-L-alanyl determinants. Studies employing synthetic antigens demonstrated the significance of aromatic, charged amino acid residues in proving the ability of synthetic polypeptides to induce an immune response.

An antigen molecule has two or more epitopes (or antigenic determinants) per molecule. Epitopes consists of approximately six amino acids or six monosaccharides. Epitopes that stimulate a greater antibody response than others are referred to as immunodominant epitopes.

The principal chemical features of antigens include their large size, complexity and ability to be degraded by enzymes within phagocytes. Most antigens are of 10 000 or greater molecular weight. Exceptions include such substances as insulin, with a molecular weight of 5700. Antigenicity is usually more easily demonstrated with molecules of greater molecular weight. However, size alone does not make the molecule antigenic. It must have a certain amount of inter-

nal structural complexity. Linear polymers of polylysine comprising a repeating simple structure are not antigenic. The majority of protein antigens contain 20 different amino acids in an assorted arrangement. Oligosaccharides composed of both monosaccharides and complex sugars are antigenic. The antigen must also be degradable by phagocytes to be antigenic. Antigen processing includes enzymatic digestion to prepare soluble macromolecular antigen. Substances such as D-amino acid polypeptides that cannot be degraded in phagocytes are not antigenic even though they might otherwise possess the characteristics of antigens. Foreignness is another characteristic that is critical for antigenicity. We do not respond to our own self-antigens because we are immunologically tolerant of them. During development, the body becomes tolerant of self-antigens, as well as foreign antigens that may have been artificially introduced into the host prior to development of the immune system. The latter situation describes the induction of actively acquired immunologic tolerance, which was discovered by Medawar, Billingham and Brent in the 1950s in studies on skin grafting. They inoculated fetal or newborn mice with cells of a different mouse strain prior to development of immunologic competence in the recipients. Once the recipient mice reached maturity, they were able to accept skin grafts from the donor strain without rejecting them. Since that time, many studies have been conducted defining the nature of T cell and B cell tolerance. In general, T cells are rendered tolerant with lower doses of antigen and for longer periods of time than are B cells. B cell tolerance is for a relatively brief duration and requires much greater quantities of antigen than does T cell tolerance. Tolerance is a type of antigen-induced specific immunosuppression, and antigen must remain in contact with immunocompetent cells for the tolerant state to be maintained. Tolerance induction is favored by the route of administration and the physical nature of the injected antigen. For example, the intravenous route of injection of solubilized antigen favors tolerance induction. By contrast, the injection of antigen in particulate form into the skin favors the development of immunity. An antigen that induces tolerance is often referred to as a tolerogen. To mount an immune response to an antigen, a host must have appropriate immune response (Ir) genes. This has been proved in animal studies in which inbred strain-2 guinea pigs were shown to be responders, whereas strain-13 were not. Lymphocyte proteins in man encoded by Ir genes include the class II MHC molecules designated DP, DQ and DR that are found on human B cells and macrophages. This enables recognition among B cells, T cells and macrophages. Antigens may be classified as either T cell-dependent (TD) or T cell-independent (TI). TD antigens are much more complex than TI antigens; they are usually proteins, they stimulate a full complement of immunoglobulins with all five classes represented, they elicit an anamnestic or memory response and are present in most pathogenic microorganisms. This ensures that an effective immune response can be generated in a host infected with these pathogens. By contrast, the simpler TI antigens are often polysaccharides or lipopolysaccharides, elicit an IgM response only and fail to stimulate an anamnestic response, compared with T cell-dependent antigens.

Toxins are poisons that are usually immunogenic and stimulate production of antibodies termed antitoxins, with the ability to neutralize the harmful effects of the particular toxins eliciting their synthesis. The general groups of toxins include:

(1) Bacterial toxins: those produced by microorganisms such as those causing tetanus, diphtheria, botulism and gas gangrene, as well as toxins of staphylococci;

(2) Phytotoxins: plant toxins such as ricin of the castor bean, crotein and abrin derived from the Indian licorice seed, Gerukia;

(3) Zootoxins: snake, spider, scorpion, bee and wasp venom.

A **cross-reacting antigen** is an antigen that interacts with an antibody synthesized following immunogenic challenge with a different antigen. Epitopes shared between these two antigens or epitopes with a similar stereochemical configuration may account for this type of cross-reactivity. The presence of the same or of a related epitope between bacterial cells, red blood cells or other types of cells may cause cross-reactivity with an antibody produced against either of them.

Carbohydrate antigens The best known carbohydrate antigen is the 'specific soluble substance' of the capsule of *Streptococcus pneumoniae*, which is immunogenic in humans. Heidelberger developed the first effective vaccines against purified pneumococcal polysaccharide in the early 1940s, which were effective in the treatment of pneumonia caused by these microorganisms, yet interest in the vaccine waned as antibiotics were developed for treatment. With increased resistance of bacteria to antibiotics, however, there is a renewed interest in immunization with polysaccharide-based vaccines. Polysaccharides alone are relatively poor immunogens, especially in infants and in immunocompromised hosts. Pneumococci have 84 distinct serotypes, which further complicates the matter. Polysaccharides are classified as T cell-independent immunogens. They fail to induce immunologic memory which is needed for booster responses in an immunization protocol. Only a few B cell clones are activated, leading to restricted yet polyclonal heterogeneity. The majority of polysaccharides can induce tolerance or unresponsiveness and fail to induce delayed-type hypersensitivity. Polysaccharide immunogenicity increases with molecular weight. Those polysaccharides that are less than 50 kDa are non-immunogenic. Thus immunization with purified polysaccharides has not been as effective as desired. The covalent linkage of a polysaccharide or of its epitopes to a protein carrier, to form a conjugate vaccine, has facilitated enhancement of immunogenicity in both humans and other animals, and induces immunologic memory. Antibodies formed against the conjugate vaccine are protective, and bind the capsular polysaccharide from which they were derived. An example of this type of immunogen is Hib polysaccharide linked to tetanus toxoid, which has been successful in infant immunization.

An **immunogen** is a substance that is able to induce a humoral antibody and/or cell-mediated immune response rather than immunological tolerance. The term 'immunogen' is sometimes used interchangeably with 'antigen', yet the term signifies the ability to stimulate an immune response as well as react with the products of it, e.g. antibody. By contrast, 'antigen' is reserved by some to mean a substance that reacts with antibody. The principal immunogens are proteins and polysaccharides, whereas lipids may serve as haptens.

Immunogenicity is the ability of an antigen serving as an immunogen to induce an immune response in a particular species of recipient. Immunogenicity depends on a number of physical and chemical characteristics of the immunogen (antigen), as well as on the genetic capacity of the host response.

Antigenicity is the property of a substance that renders it immunogenic or capable of stimulating an immune response. Antigenicity was more commonly used in the past to refer to what is now known as immunogenicity, although the two are still used interchangeably by various investigators. An antigen is considered by many to be a substance that reacts with the products of immunogenic stimulation. It is a substance that combines specifically with antibodies formed or receptors of T cells stimulated during an immune response.

An **epitope** is an antigenic determinant. It is the simplest form or smallest structural area on a complex antigen molecule that can combine with an antibody or T lymphocyte receptor. It must be at least 1 kDa to elicit an antibody response. A smaller molecule such as a hapten may induce an immune response if combined with a carrier protein molecule. Multiple epitopes may be found on large non-polymeric molecules. Based on X-ray crystallography, epitopes consist of prominently exposed 'hill and ridge' regions that manifest surface rigidity. Antigenicity is diminished in more flexible sites.

An **epitype** is a family or group of related epitopes.

A **hidden determinant** is an epitope on a cell or molecule that is unavailable for interaction with either lymphocyte receptors or the antigen-binding region of antibody molecules because of stereochemical factors. These hidden or cryptic determinants neither react with lymphocyte or antibody receptors nor induce an immune response unless an alteration in the molecule's steric configuration causes the epitope to be exposed.

An **immunodominant epitope** is the antigenic determinant on an antigen molecule that binds or fits best with the antibody or T cell receptor specific for it.

2,4-Dinitrophenyl (DNP) (Figures 31 and 32) groups may serve as haptens after they are chemically linked to $-NH_2$ groups of proteins that interact with chlorodinitrobenzene, 2,4-dinitrobenzene sulphonic acid or dinitrofluorobenzene. These protein carrier–DNP hapten antigens are useful as experimental immunogens. Antibodies specific for the DNP hapten, which are generated through immunization with the carrier–hapten complex, interact with low-molecular-weight substances that contain the DNP groups.

Dinitrochlorobenzene (DNCB) (Figure 33) is a substance employed to test an individual's capacity to develop a cell-mediated immune reaction. A solution of DNCB is applied to the skin of an individual not previously sensitized against this chemical, where it acts as a hapten, interacting with proteins of the skin. Re-exposure of this same individual to a second application of DNCB 2 weeks after the first challenge results in a T cell-mediated delayed-type hypersensitivity (contact dermatitis) reaction. Persons with impaired delayed-type hypersensitivity or cell-mediated immunity might reveal an impaired response. The 2,4-dinitro-1-chlorobenzene interacts with free '-amino terminal groups in polypeptide chains, as well as with side-chains of lysine, tyrosine, histidine, cysteine, or other amino acid residues'.

A **hapten** is a relatively small molecule that by itself is unable to elicit an immune response when injected into an animal but is capable of reacting *in vitro* with an antibody specific for it. Only if complexed to a carrier molecule prior to administration can a hapten induce an immune response. Haptens usually bear only one epitope. Pneumococcal polysaccharide is an example

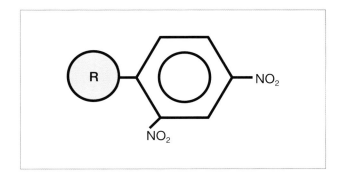

Figure 31　2,4-Dinitrophenyl (DNP)

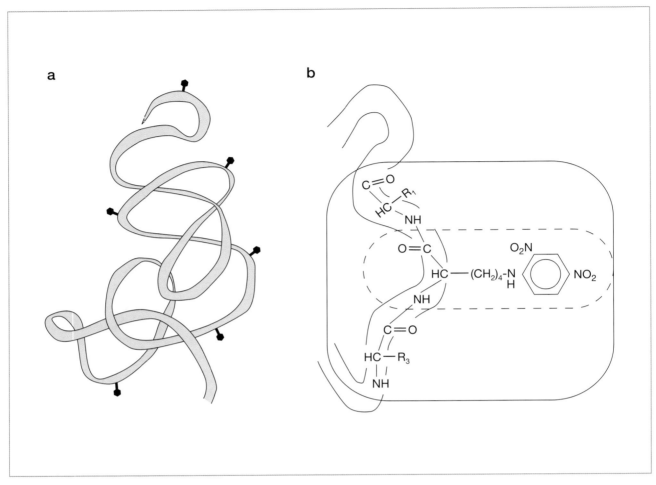

Figure 32 (a) Conjugated protein with substituents. (b) Broken line refers to the haptenic group and the solid line refers to the antigenic determinant

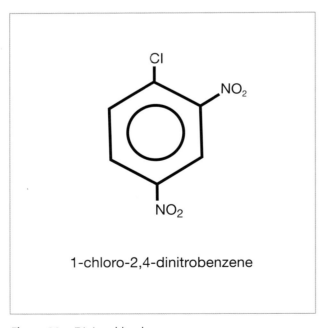

1-chloro-2,4-dinitrobenzene

Figure 33 Dinitrochlorobenzene

of a larger molecule that may act as a hapten in rabbits, but as a complete antigen in humans.

A **carrier** is an immunogenic macromolecular protein such as ovalbumin, to which an incomplete antigen termed a hapten may be conjugated either *in vitro* or *in vivo*. Whereas the hapten is not immunogenic by itself, conjugation to the carrier molecule renders it immunogenic. When self-proteins are appropriately modified by the hapten, they may serve as a carrier, *in vivo*, a mechanism operative in allergy to drugs.

Hapten–carrier conjugate refers to the combination of a small molecule covalently linked to a large immunogenic carrier molecule.

Conjugate usually refers to the covalent bonding of a protein carrier with a hapten, or it may refer to the

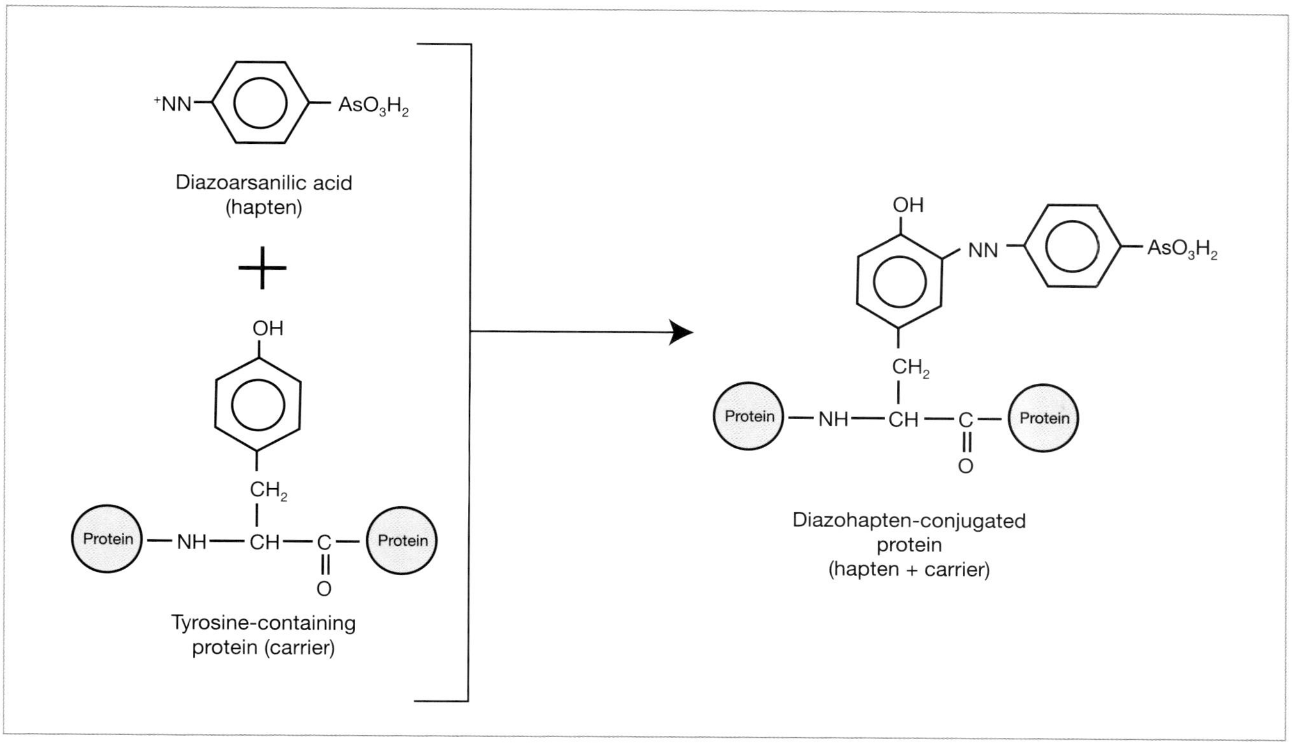

Figure 34 Hapten conjugates

labeling of a molecule such as an immunoglobulin with fluorescein isothiocyanate, ferritin or an enzyme used in the enzyme-linked immunosorbent assay.

Carrier specificity refers to an immune response, either humoral antibody- or cell-mediated immunity, that is specific for the carrier portion of a hapten–carrier complex that has been used as an immunogen. The carrier-specific part of the immune response does not react with the hapten either by itself or conjugated to a different carrier.

Schlepper is a name used by Landsteiner to refer to large macromolecules that serve as carriers for simple chemical molecules serving as haptens. The immunization of rabbits or other animals with a hapten–carrier complex leads to the formation of antibodies specific for the hapten as well as the carrier. T cells were later shown to be carrier-specific and B cells hapten-specific. Carriers are conjugated to haptens through covalent linkages, such as the diazo linkage.

Carrier effect To achieve a secondary immune response to a hapten, both the hapten and the carrier used in the initial immunization must be employed.

Hapten conjugate response The response to **hapten conjugates** (Figure 34) requires two populations of lymphocytes, T and B cells. The cells producing the antibodies are derived from B cells. T cells act as helpers in this process. B cell preparations, depleted of T cells, cannot respond to hapten conjugates. The T cells are responsive to the carrier portion of the conjugate, although in some cases they also recognize the hapten. The influence of the carrier on the ensuing response is called carrier effect. The experimental design for demonstrating the carrier effect involves adoptive transfer of hapten-sensitive B cells and of T cells primed with one or another carrier. The primed cells are those which have already had a past opportunity to encounter the antigen.

Dinitrofluorobenzene (2,4-dinitro-1-fluorobenzene) (DNFB) is a chemical employed to prepare hapten–carrier conjugates. It inserts the 2,4-dinitrophenyl group into molecules containing free $-NH_2$ groups. When placed on the skin, it leads to contact hypersensitivity.

The **hapten inhibition test** is an assay for serological characterization or elucidation of the molecular

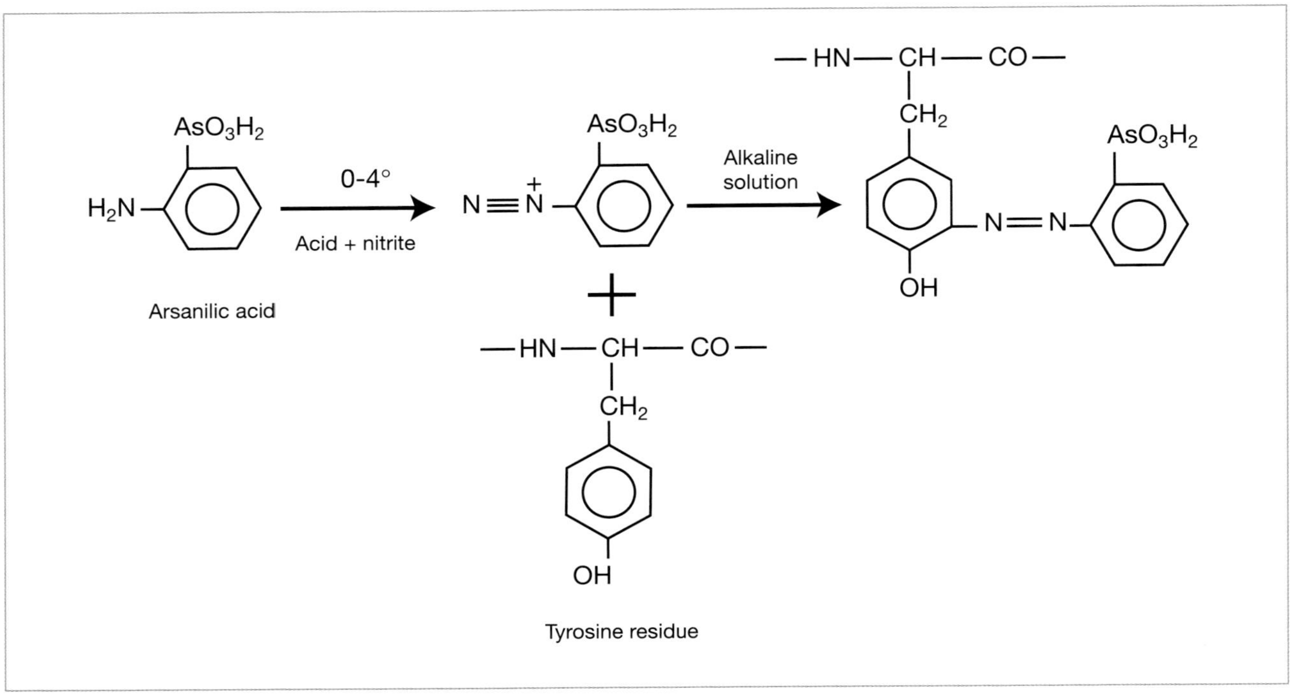

Figure 35 Diazotization

structure of an epitope by blocking the antigen-binding site of an antibody specific for the epitope with a defined hapten.

Diazotization (Figure 35) is a method to introduce the diazo group ($-N^+\equiv N^-$) into a molecule. Landsteiner used this technique extensively in coupling low-molecular-weight chemicals acting as haptens to protein macromolecules serving as carriers. Aromatic amine derivatives can be coupled to side-chains of selected amino acid residues to prepare protein–hapten conjugates, which, when used to immunize experimental animals such as rabbits, stimulate the synthesis of antibodies. Some of these antibodies are specific for the hapten, which, by itself, is unable to stimulate an immune response. First an aromatic amine reacts with nitrous acid generated through the combination of sodium nitrite with HCl. The diazonium salt is then combined with the protein at a pH that is slightly alkaline. The reaction products include monosubstituted tyrosine and histidine and also lysine residues that are disubstituted.

A **diazo salt** is a diazonium salt prepared by diazotization from an arylamine, to yield a product with a

diazo group. Diazotization has been widely used in the preparation of hapten–carrier conjugates for use in experimental immunology.

An **azoprotein** is produced by joining a substance to a protein through a diazo linkage $-N=N-$. Karl Landsteiner (in the early 1900s) made extensive use of diazotization to prepare hapten–protein conjugates to define immunochemical specificity (see also diazo reaction).

Original antigenic sin The immune response against a virus to which an individual was previously exposed, such as a parental strain, may be greater than it is against the immunizing agent, such as type A influenza virus variant. This concept is known as the doctrine of original antigenic sin.

A **thymus-dependent (TD) antigen** is an immunogen that requires T lymphocyte cooperation for B cells to synthesize specific antibodies. Presentation of thymus-dependent antigen to T cells must be in the context of MHC class II molecules. Thymus-dependent antigens include proteins, polypeptides, hapten–carrier complexes, erythrocytes and many other antigens that have diverse epitopes.

A **thymus-independent (TI) antigen** is an immuno-gen that can stimulate B cells to synthesize antibodies without participation by T cells. These antigens are less complex than thymus-dependent antigens. They are often polysaccharides that contain repeating epitopes or lipopolysaccharides (LPS) derived from Gram-negative microorganisms. Thymus-independent antigens induce IgM synthesis by B lymphocytes without coop-eration by T cells. They also do not stimulate immuno-logical memory. Murine TI antigens are classified as either TI-1 or TI-2 antigens. LPS, which activate murine B cells without participation by T or other cells, are typical TI-1 antigens. Low concentrations of LPS stimulate synthesis of specific antigen, whereas high concentrations activate essentially all B cells to grow and differentiate. TI-2 antigens include polysaccharides, glycolipids and nucleic acids. When T lymphocytes and macrophages are depleted, no antibody response devel-ops against them.

A **private antigen** is:

(1) An antigen confined to one major histocom-patibility complex (MHC) molecule;

(2) An antigenic specificity restricted to a few individuals;

(3) A tumor antigen restricted to a specific chemically induced tumor;

(4) A low-frequency epitope present on red blood cells of fewer than 0.1% of the population, e.g. I, Pt^a, By, Bp^a, etc;

(5) HLA antigen encoded by one allele such as HLA-B27.

A **public antigen (supratypic antigen)** is an epitope which several distinct or private antigens have in common. A public antigen is one such as a blood group antigen that is present in greater than 99.9% of a population. It is detected by the indirect antiglobulin (Coombs' test). Examples include Ve, Ge, Jr, Gy^a and OK^a. Antigens that occur frequently but are not public antigens include MNs, Lewis, Duffy, P, etc. In blood banking, there is a problem finding a suitable unit of blood for a tranfusion to recipients who have devel-oped antibodies against public antigens.

A **heterophile antigen** is an antigen (epitope) present in divergent animal species, plants and bacte-ria that manifest broad cross-reactivity with antibodies of the heterophile group. Heterophile antigens induce the formation of heterophile antibodies when intro-duced into a species where they are absent. Heterophile antigens are often carbohydrates.

Forssman antigen is a heterophile or heterogenetic glycolipid antigen that stimulates the synthesis of anti-sheep hemolysin in rabbits. Its broad phylogenetic distribution spans both animal and plant kingdoms. The antigen is present in guinea pig and horse organs, but not in their red blood cells. In sheep, it is found exclusively in erythrocytes. Forssman antigen occurs in both red blood cells and organs in chickens. It is also present in goats, ostriches, mice, dogs, cats, spinach and *Bacillus anthracis*, and on the gastrointesti-nal mucosa of a limited number of people. It is absent in rabbits, rats, cows, pigs, cuckoos, beans and *Salmonella typhi*. Forssman substance is ceramide tetrasaccharide. The Forssman antigen contains *N*-acylsphingo-sine (ceramide), galactose and *N*-acetyl-galactosamine. As originally defined, it is present in guinea pig kidney, is heat stable and is alcohol soluble. Forssman antigen-containing tissue is effective in absorbing the homologous antibody from serum. Antibodies to the Forssman antigen occur in the sera of patients recovering from infectious mononucleosis.

Immunoglobulin synthesis, properties, structure and function

Following enunciation of the clonal selection theory of antibody formation by Burnet in 1957, experimen-tal evidence confirms the validity of this selective theory as opposed to the instructive theory of antibody formation that prevailed during the first half of the 20th century. As immunogeneticists attempted to explain the great diversity of antibodies encoded by finite quantities of DNA, Tonegawa offered a plausible explanation for the generation of antibody diversity in his studies of immunoglobulin gene C, V, J and D regions (constant, variable, joining and diversity) and their rearrangement. It is necessary for those segments that encode genes and determine immunoglobulin H and L chains to undergo rearrangement prior to gene transcription and translation. Newly synthesized immunoglobulin molecules have different properties based upon their immunoglobulin class or isotype. Nevertheless, antigen-binding specificities reside in the Fab regions of antibody molecules, which govern their interactions with antigens *in vitro* and *in vivo*. By contrast, complement binding and activation capabilities, binding to cell surface and transport through cells reside in the Fc region of the molecule. The fate of immunoglobulin molecules also differs according to the immunoglobulin class, each with its own characteristic half-life. Only IgG is protected from catabolism by binding to a specific receptor. Some antibodies are protective, others cross the placenta from mother to fetus, whereas others participate in hypersensitivity reactions that lead to adverse effects in target tissues. Antibodies are a diverse and unique category of proteins whose antigen-binding diversity is expressed in the 10^{20} antibody molecules synthesized from the 10^{20} B lymphocytes found in the human body.

Antibodies are glycoprotein substances produced by B lymphoid cells in response to stimulation with an immunogen. They possess the ability to react *in vitro* and *in vivo* specifically and selectively with the antigenic determinants or epitopes eliciting their production or with an antigenic determinant closely related to the homologous antigen. Antibody molecules are immunoglobulins found in the blood and body fluids. Thus, all antibodies are immunoglobulins formed in response to immunogens. Antibodies may be produced by hybridoma technology in which antibody secreting cells are fused by polyethylene glycol (PEG) treatment with a mutant myeloma cell line. Monoclonal antibodies are widely used in research and diagnostic medicine and have potential in therapy. Antibodies in the blood serum of any given animal species may be grouped according to their physico-chemical properties and antigenic characteristics. Immunoglobulins are not restricted to the plasma, but may be found in other body fluids or tissues, such as urine, spinal fluid, lymph nodes, spleen, etc. Immunoglobulins do not include the components of the complement system. Immunoglobulins (antibodies) constitute approximately 1–2% of the total serum proteins in health. γ-Globulins comprise 11.2–20.1% of the total serum content in man. Antibodies are in the γ globulin fraction of serum. Electrophoretically they are the slowest migrating fraction.

Heterophile antibody is an antibody found in an animal of one species that can react with erythrocytes of a different and phylogenetically unrelated species. These are often IgM agglutinins. Heterophile antibodies are detected in infectious mononucleosis patients who demonstrate antibodies reactive with sheep erythrocytes. To differentiate this condition from serum sickness, which is also associated with a high titer of heterophile antibodies, the serum sample is absorbed with beef erythrocytes which contain Forssmann antigen. This treatment removes the heterophile antibody reactivity from the serum of infectious mononucleosis patients.

The **immunoglobulin superfamily** comprises several molecules that participate in the immune response and show similarities in structure, causing them to be named the immunoglobulin supergene family. Included are CD2, CD3, CD4, CD7, CD8, CD28, T cell receptor (TCR), MHC class I and MHC class II molecules, leukocyte function-associated antigen 3 (LFA-3), the IgG receptor and a dozen other proteins. These molecules share in common with each other an immunoglobulin-like domain, with a length of approximately 100 amino acid residues and a central disulfide bond that anchors and stabilizes antiparallel β strands into a folded structure resembling immunoglobulin. Immunoglobulin superfamily members may share homology with constant or variable immunoglobulin domain regions. Various molecules of the cell surface with polypeptide chains whose folded structures are involved in cell–cell interactions belong in this category. Single gene and multigene members are included.

Globulins are serum proteins comprising α-, β-, and γ-globulins, and are classified on the basis of their electrophoretic mobility. All three globulin fractions demonstrate anodic mobility that is less than that of albumin. α-Globulins have the greatest negative charge, whereas γ-globulins have the least negative charge. Originally, globulins were characterized based on their insolubility in water, the euglobulins, or sparing solubility in water, the pseudoglobulins. Globulins are precipitated in half-saturated ammonium sulfate solution.

γ-Globulin is an obsolete designation for immunoglobulin. These serum proteins show the lowest mobility toward the anode during electrophoresis when the pH is neutral. The γ-globulin fraction contains immunoglobulins. It is the most cationic of the serum globulins.

Antibody-binding site is the antigen-binding site of an antibody molecule, known as a paratope, that is composed of heavy chain and light chain variable regions. The paratope represents the site of attachment of an epitope to the antibody molecule. The complementarity-determining hypervariable regions play a significant role in dictating the combining site structure together with the participation of framework region residues. The T cell receptor also has an antigen-binding site in the variable regions of its α and β (or γ and δ) chains.

Euglobulin is a type of globulin that is insoluble in water, but dissolves in salt solutions. In the past, it was used to designate that part of the serum proteins that could be precipitated by 33% saturated ammonium sulfate at 4°C or by 14.2% sodium sulfate at room temperature. Euglobulin is precipitated from the serum proteins at low ionic strength.

Antibody specificity is a property of antibodies determined by their relative binding affinities, the intrinsic capacity of each antibody combining site, expressed as equilibrium dissociation (K_d) or association (K_a) for their interactions with different antigens.

Antiserum is a preparation of serum-containing antibodies specific for a particular antigen, i.e. immunogen. A therapeutic antiserum may contain antitoxin, antilymphocyte antibodies, etc. An antiserum contains a heterogeneous collection of antibodies that bind the antigen used for immunization. Each antibody has a specific structure, antigenic specificity and cross-reactivity contributing to the heterogeneity that renders an antiserum unique.

Antitoxin is an antibody specific for exotoxins produced by certain microorganisms such as the causative agents of diphtheria and tetanus. Prior to the antibiotic era, antitoxins were the treatment of choice for diseases produced by the soluble toxic products of microorganisms, such as those from *Corynebacterium diphtheriae* and *Clostridium tetani*.

Amboceptor (historical) Paul Ehrlich (circa 1900) considered anti-sheep red blood cell antibodies known as amboceptors to have one receptor for sheep erythrocytes and another receptor for complement. The term gained worldwide acceptance with the popularity of complement fixation tests for syphilis, such as the Wassermann reaction. The term is still used by some when discussing complement fixation.

Humoral immunity is immunity attributable to specific immunoglobulin antibody and is present in the blood plasma, lymph, other body fluids or tissues. The antibody may also adhere to cells in the form of cytophilic antibody. Antibody or immunoglobulin-mediated immunity acts in conjunction with complement proteins to produce either beneficial (protective) or pathogenic (hypersensitivity-tissue injuring) reactions. Antibodies that are the messengers of humoral immunity are derived from B cells. For purposes of discussion, it is separated from so-called cellular or T cell-mediated immunity. However, the two cannot be clearly distinguished since antibodies and T cells often participate in immune reactions together. However, the classification of humoral separate from cellular immunity is useful in understanding and explaining biological mechanisms.

Antibody detection Techniques employed to detect antibodies include immunoprecipitation, agglutination, complement-dependent assays, labeled anti-immunoglobulin reagents, blotting techniques and immunohistochemistry. Enzyme-based immunoassays, blotting methods and immunohistochemistry are routine procedures to detect antibodies and to characterize their specificity.

Antibody titer is the amount or level of circulating antibody in a patient with an infectious disease. For example, the reciprocal of the highest dilution of serum (containing antibodies) that reacts with antigen, e.g. agglutination, is the titer. Two separate titer determinations are required to reflect an individual's exposure to an infectious agent.

Antitoxin assay (historical) Antitoxins are assayed biologically by their capacity to neutralize homologous toxins as demonstrated by the production of no toxic manifestations following inoculation of the mixture into experimental animals, e.g. guinea pigs. They may be tested serologically by their ability to flocculate (precipitate) toxin *in vitro*.

Univalent antibody is an antibody molecule with one antigen-binding site. Although incapable of leading to precipitation or agglutination, univalent antibodies or Fab fragments resulting from papain digestion of an IgG molecule might block precipitation of antigen by a typical bivalent antibody.

Antitoxin unit A unit of antitoxin is that amount of antitoxin present in 1/6000 g of a certain dried unconcentrated horse serum antitoxin which has been maintained since 1905 at the National Institutes of Health in Bethesda, MD. The standard antitoxin unit contained sufficient antitoxin to neutralize 100 times minimum lethal dose (MLD) of the special toxin prepared by Ehrlich and used by him in titration of standard antitoxin. Both the American and the international unit of antitoxin are the same.

An **antigen-binding site** is the location on an antibody molecule where an antigenic determinant or epitope combines with it. The antigen-binding site is located in a cleft bordered by the N-terminal variable regions of heavy and light chain parts of the Fab region. It is also called paratope, and also refers to that part of a T cell receptor that binds antigen specifically.

An **antivenom** is antitoxin prepared specifically for the treatment of bite or sting victims of poisonous snakes or arthropods. Antibodies in this immune serum preparation neutralize the snake or arthropod venom. It is also called antivenin or antivenene.

Titer is an approximation of the antibody activity in each unit volume of a serum sample. The term is used in serological reactions and is determined by preparing serial dilutions of antibody to which a constant amount of antigen is added. The end-point is the highest dilution of antiserum in which a visible reaction with antigen, e.g. agglutination, can be detected.

The titer is expressed as the reciprocal of the serum dilution which defines the end-point. If agglutination occurs in the tube containing a 1:240 dilution, the antibody titer is said to be 240. Thus, the serum would contain approximately 240 units of antibody per milliliter of antiserum. The titer provides only an estimate of antibody activity. For absolute amounts of antibody, quantitative precipitation or other methods must be employed.

A **precipitin** is an antibody that interacts with a soluble antigen to yield an aggregate of antigen and antibody molecules in a lattice framework called a precipitate. Under appropriate conditions, the majority of antibodies can act as precipitins.

Antibody synthesis The 10^{12} B lymphocytes that constitute the human immune system synthesize 10^{20} antibody (immunoglobulin) molecules present inside and on the surface of these cells, and most of all in the serum. Other species have B cell and immunoglobulin molecule numbers relative to their body weight. B cells and immunoglobulin molecules are formed and degraded throughout the human life span.

A **paratope** is the antigen-binding site of an antibody molecule, the variable (V) domain, or T cell receptor that binds to an epitope on an antigen. It is the variable or Fv region of an antibody molecule and is the site for interaction with an epitope of an antigen molecule. It is complementary for the epitope for which it is specific.

A paratope is the portion of an antibody molecule where the hypervariable regions are located. There is less than 10% variability in the light and heavy chain amino acid positions in the variable regions. However, there is 20–60% variability in amino acid sequence in the so-called 'hot spots' located at light chain amino acid positions 29–34, 49–52 and 91–95 and at heavy chain positions 30–34, 51–63, 84–90 and 101–110. Great specificity is associated with this variability and is the basis of an idiotype. This variability permits recognition of multiple antigenic determinants.

Cross-reacting antibody reacts with epitopes on an antigen molecule different from the one that stimulated its synthesis. The effect is attributable to shared epitopes on the two antigen molecules.

Cytotoxic antibody is an antibody that combines with cell surface epitopes followed by complement fixation that leads to cell lysis or cell membrane injury without lysis.

Cytotrophic antibodies are IgE and IgG antibodies that sensitize cells by binding to Fc receptors on their surface, thereby sensitizing them for anaphylaxis. When the appropriate allergen cross-links the Fab regions of the molecules, it leads to the degranulation of mast cells and basophils bearing IgE on their surface.

Non-precipitating antibodies The addition of antigen in increments to an optimal amount of antibody precipitates only approximately 78% of the amount of antibody that would be precipitated by one-step addition to the antigen. This demonstrates the presence of both precipitating and non-precipitating antibodies. Although the non-precipitating variety cannot lead to the formation of insoluble antigen–antibody complexes, they can be assimilated into precipitates that correspond to their specificity. Rather than being univalent as was once believed, they may merely have a relatively low affinity for the homologous antigen. Monogamous bivalency, which describes the combination of high-affinity antibody with two antigenic determinants on the same antigen particle, represents an alternative explanation for the failure of these molecules to precipitate with their homologous antigen. The formation of non-precipitating antibodies, which usually represent 10–15% of the antibody population produced, is dependent upon such variables as heterogeneity of the antigen, characteristics of the antibody and animal species.

The equivalence zone is narrower with native proteins of 40–60 kDa and their homologous antibodies than with polysaccharide antigens or aggregated denatured proteins and their specific antibody. The equivalence zone with synthetic polypeptide antigens varies with the individual compound used. The solubility of antibody–antigen complexes and the nature of the antigen are related to these variations at the equivalence zone. The extent of precipitation is dependent upon characteristics of both the antigen and antibody. At the equivalence zone, not all antigen and antibody molecules are present in the complexes. For example, rabbit anti-BSA (bovine serum albumin) precipitates only 46% of BSA at equivalence.

Antiantibody In addition to their antibody function, immunoglobulin molecules serve as excellent protein immunogens when inoculated into another species, or they may become autoantigenic even in their own host. The Gm antigenic determinants in the Fc region of an IgG molecule may elicit autoantibodies, principally of the IgM class, known as rheumatoid factor in individuals with rheumatoid arthritis. Anti-idiotypic antibodies, directed against the antigen-binding N-terminal variable regions of antibody molecules, represent another type of antiantibody. Rabbit anti-human IgG (the Coombs' test reagent) is an antiantibody used extensively in clinical immunology to reveal autoantibodies on erythrocytes.

Anti-immunoglobulin antibodies are antibodies specific for immunoglobulin constant domains, which renders them useful for detection of bound antibody molecules in immunoassays. Anti-isotype antibodies are synthesized in a different species; antiallotype antibodies are made in the same species against allotypic variants; and anti-idiotype antibodies are induced against a single antibody molecule's unique determinants.

Skin-fixing antibody is an antibody such as IgE that is retained in the skin following local injection, as in passive cutaneous anaphylaxis. Antibody with this property was referred to previously as reagin before IgE was described.

Catalytic antibodies are not only exclusively specific for a particular ligand but are also catalytic. Approximately 100 reactions have been catalyzed by antibodies. Among these are pericyclic processes, elimination reactions, bond-forming reactions and redox processes. Most antibody-catalyzed reactions are highly stereospecific. For efficient catalysis, it is necessary to introduce catalytic functions within the antibody-combining site properly juxtaposed to the substrate. Catalytic antibodies resemble enzymes in processing their substrates through a Michaelis M complex, in which the chemical transformation takes place followed by a product dissociation (refer also to abzyme).

Chimeric antibodies are antibodies that have, e.g. mouse Fv fragments for the Ag-binding portion of the molecule, but Fc regions of human immunoglobulin which convey effector functions.

Lysins are factors such as antibodies and complement or microbial toxins that induce cell lysis. For an antibody to demonstrate this capacity, it must be able to fix complement.

Complementarity-determining region (CDR) refers to the hypervariable regions in an immunoglobulin molecule that form the three-dimensional cavity where an epitope binds to the antibody molecule. The heavy and light polypeptide chains each contribute three hypervariable regions to the antigen-binding region of the antibody molecule. Together, they form the site for antigen binding. Likewise, the T cell receptor α and β chains each have three regions with great diversity that are analogous to the immunoglobulin's CDRs. These hypervariable areas are sites of binding for foreign antigen and self-MHC molecular complexes.

Constant domain refers to the immunoglobulin C_H and C_L (heavy and light chain) regions. It is a globular compact structure that consists of two antiparallel twisted β sheets. There are differences in the number and irregularity of the β strands and bilayers in variable (V) and constant (C) subunits of immunoglobulins. C domains have a tertiary structure that closely resembles that of the domains, which comprise a five-strand β sheet and a four-strand β sheet packed facing one another. However, the C domain does not have a hairpin loop at the edge of one of the sheets. Thus, the C domain has seven or eight β strands rather than the nine that are found in the V domains. The term refers also to the constituent domains of constant regions of T cell receptor polypeptides.

Constant region is that part of an immunoglobulin polypeptide chain that has an invariant amino acid sequence among immunoglobulin chains belonging to the same isotype and allotype. There is a minimum of two and often three or four domains in the constant region of immunoglobulin heavy polypeptide chains. The hinge region 'tail endpiece' (a carboxy-terminal region) constitutes part of the constant region in selected classes of immunoglobulin. A few exons encode the constant region of an immunoglobulin heavy chain, and one exon encodes the constant region of an immunoglobulin light chain. The constant region is the location for the majority of isotypic and allotypic determinants. It is associated with a number of antibody functions. T cell receptor α, β, γ and δ chains have constant regions encoded by three to four exons. MHC class I and II molecules also have segments that are constant regions in that they show little sequence variation from one allele to another. The term refers also to the part of a TCR polypeptide chain that does not vary in sequence among different clones and is not involved in antigen binding.

The **hinge region** is an area of an immunoglobulin heavy chain situated between the first constant domain and the second constant domain (C_H1 and C_H2) in an immunoglobulin polypeptide chain. The high content of proline residues in this region provides considerable flexibility to this area, which enables the Fab region of an immunoglobulin molecule to combine with cell surface epitopes that it might not otherwise reach. Fab regions of an immunoglobulin molecule can rotate on the hinge region. There can be an angle up to 180° between the two Fab regions of an IgG molecule. In addition to the proline residues, there may be one or several half cysteines associated with the interchain disulfide bonds. Enzyme action by papain or pepsin occurs near the hinge region. Whereas γ, α and δ chains each contain a hinge region, μ and ε chains do not. The 5' part of the C_H2 exon encodes the human and mouse α chain hinge region. Four exons encode the $\gamma3$ chains of humans and two exons encode human δ chains.

A **hot spot** is a hypervariable region in DNA that encodes the variable region of an immunoglobulin molecule's heavy (V_H) and light (V_L) polypeptide chains. These are also designated complementarity-determining regions (CDRs). These are the areas for specific antigen binding, and they also determine the idiotype of an immunoglobulin molecule. The remaining background support structures of the heavy and light polypeptide chains are termed framework regions (FRs). The κ and λ light chain hot spots are situated near amino acid residues 30, 50 and 95. These are also called hypervariable regions.

A **humanized antibody** is an engineered antibody produced through recombinant DNA technology. A humanized antibody contains the antigen-binding specificity of an antibody developed in a mouse, whereas the remainder of the molecule is of human origin. To accomplish this, hypervariable genes that encode the antigen-binding regions of a mouse antibody are transferred to the normal human gene which encodes an immunoglobulin molecule that is mostly human, but expresses the antigen-binding specificity of the mouse antibody in the variable region of the molecule. This greatly diminishes any immune response to the antibody molecule itself as a foreign protein by the human host, while retaining the desired functional capacity of reacting with the specific antigen.

An **immunoglobulin** (Figure 36) is a mature B cell product synthesized in response to stimulation by an antigen. Antibody molecules are immunoglobulins of defined specificity produced by plasma cells. The immunoglobulin molecule consists of heavy (H) and light (L) chains fastened together by disulfide bonds. The molecules are subdivided into classes and subclasses based on the antigenic specificity of the heavy chains. Heavy chains are designated by lower-case Greek letters (μ, γ, α, δ and ε), and immunoglobulins are designated IgM, IgG, IgA, IgD and IgE, respectively. The three major classes are IgG, IgM and IgA, and the two minor classes are IgD and IgE, which together constitute less than 1% of the total immunoglobulins. The two types of light chains termed κ and λ are present in all five immunoglobulin classes, although only one type is present in an individual molecule. IgG, IgD and IgE have two H and two L polypeptide chains, whereas IgM and IgA consist of multimers of this basic chain structure. Disulfide bridges and non-covalent forces stabilize immunoglobulin structure. The basic monomeric unit is Y-shaped, with a hinge region rich in proline and susceptible to cleavage by proteolytic enzymes. Both H and L chains have a constant region at the carboxyl terminus and a variable region at the amino terminus. The two heavy chains are alike, as are the two light chains, in any individual immunoglobulin molecule. Approximately 60% of human immunoglobulin molecules have κ light chains, and 40% have

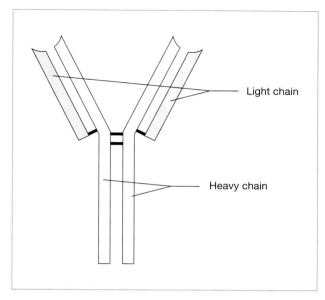

Figure 36 Immunoglobulin heavy chains that are fastened to each other or to light polypeptide chains by disulfide bonds

Light chain

Heavy chain

λ light chains. The five immunoglobulin classes are termed isotypes based on the H-chain specificity of each immunoglobulin class. Two immunoglobulin classes, IgA and IgG, have been further subdivided into subclasses based on H chain differences. The four IgG subclasses are designated as IgG1 through IgG4, and the two IgA subclasses are designated IgA1 and IgA2. Digestion of IgG molecules with papain yields two Fab fragments and one Fc fragment. Each Fab fragment has one antigen-binding site but is responsible for fixation of complement and attachment of the molecule to a cell surface. Pepsin cleaves the molecule toward the carboxy-terminal end of the central disulfide bone, yielding an F(ab')$_2$ fragment and a pFc' fragment. F(ab')$_2$ fragments have two antigen-binding sites. L chains have a single variable and constant domain, whereas H chains possess one variable and three or four constant domains. Secretory IgA is found in body secretions such as saliva, milk and intestinal and bronchial secretions. IgD and IgM are present as membrane-bound immunoglobulins on B cells, where they interact with antigen to activate B cells. IgE is associated with anaphylaxis, and IgG, which is the only immunoglobulin capable of crossing the placenta, is the major human immunoglobulin.

The **homology region** is a 105–115-amino acid residue sequence of heavy or light chains of immunoglobulins which have a primary structure that resembles that of other corresponding sequences of the same size. A homology region has a globular shape and an intrachain disulfide bond. The exons that encode homology regions are separated by introns. Light polypeptide chain homology regions are termed V_L and C_L. Heavy chain homology regions are designated V_H, C_H1, C_H2 and C_H3.

Reagin (historical) This is an obsolete term for a complement-fixing IgM antibody reacting in the Wassermann test for syphilis. It is also a name used previously for immunoglobulin E (IgE), the anaphylactic antibody in humans that fixes to tissue mast cells leading to release of histamine and vasoactive amines following interaction with a specific antigen (allergen).

Immunoglobulin function is to link an antigen to its elimination mechanism (effector system). Antibodies induce complement activation and cellular elimination mechanisms that include phagocytosis and antibody-dependent cell-mediated cytotoxicity (ADCC). This type of activation usually requires antibody molecules clustered together on a cell surface rather than as free unliganded antibody. Antibodies can combine with virus particles to render them non-infectious *in vitro* through neutralization. IgG catabolism is regulated by the IgG concentration. All immunoglobulin classes can be expressed on B cell surfaces where they act as antigen receptors, although this is mainly a function of IgM and IgD. Surface immunoglobulin has an extra C-terminal sequence compared with secreted immunoglobulin containing linker, transmembrane and cytoplasmic segments.

An **immunoglobulin heavy chain** is a 5–71-kDa polypeptide chain present in immunoglobulin molecules that serves as the basis for dividing immunoglobulins into classes. The heavy chain comprises three or four constant domains, depending upon class, and one variable domain. In addition, a hinge region is present in some chains. There is approximately 30% homology, with respect to amino acid sequence, among the five classes of immunoglobulin heavy chain in man. The heavy chain of IgM is μ, of IgG is γ, of IgA is α, of IgD is δ and of IgE is ε. A heavy chain is a principal constituent of immunoglobulin molecules. Each immunoglobulin is composed of at least one four-polypeptide chain monomer which contains two heavy and two light polypeptide chains. The two heavy chains are identical in any one molecule, as are the two light chains.

Heavy chain subclass Within an immunoglobulin heavy chain class, differences in primary structure associated with the constant region that can further distinguish these heavy chains of the same class are designated as subclasses. These differences are based on primary or antigenic structure. Heavy chain subclasses are designated as γ1, γ2, γ3, etc.

A **light chain** is a 22-kDa polypeptide chain found in all immunoglobulin molecules. Each four-chain immunoglobulin monomer contains two identical light polypeptide chains. They are joined to two like heavy chains by disulfide bonds. There are two types of light chains, designated κ and λ. An individual immunoglobulin molecule possesses two light chains that are either κ or λ, but never a mixture of the two. The types of light polypeptide chain occur in all five of the immunoglobulin classes. Each light chain has an N-terminal V region which constitutes part of the antigen-binding site of the antibody molecule. The C region or constant terminal reveals no variation except for the Km and Oz allotype markers in humans. **Km (formerly (Inv))** is the designation for the κ light chain allotype genetic markers.

An **immunoglobulin domain** (Figures 37 and 38) is an immunoglobulin heavy or light polypeptide chain structural unit that comprises approximately 110 amino acid residues. Domains are loops that are linked by disulfide bonds on constant and variable regions of heavy and light chains. Immunoglobulin functions may be linked to certain domains. There is much primary and three-dimensional structural homology among immunoglobulin domains. A particular exon may encode an immunoglobulin domain.

An **immunoglobulin fold** is an immunoglobulin domain's three-dimensional configuration. An immunoglobulin fold has a sandwich-like structure comprising two β-pleated sheets that are nearly parallel. There are four antiparallel chain segments in one sheet and three in the other. Approximately 50% of the domain's amino acid residues are in the β-pleated

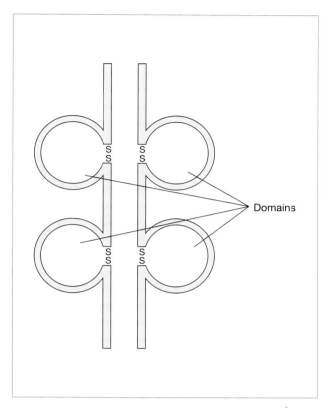

Figure 37 Domain structure of light or heavy polypeptide chains, the subunits of immunoglobulin molecules

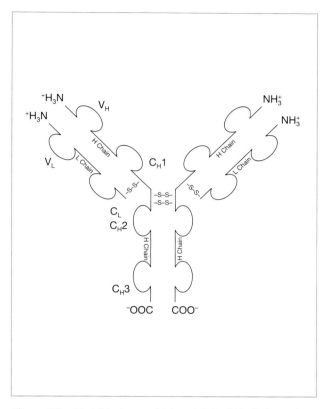

Figure 38 Variable heavy (V_H) and light (V_L) chain regions on an antibody

sheets. The other 50% of the amino acid residues are situated in polypeptide chain loops and in terminal segments. The turns are sites of invariant glycine residues. Hydrophobic amino acid side-chains are situated between the sheets.

Hypervariable regions (Figure 39) constitute a minimum of four sites of great variability which are present throughout the H and L chain V regions. They govern the antigen-binding site of an antibody molecule. Thus, grouping of these hypervariable residues into areas governs both conformation and specificity of the antigen-binding site upon folding of the protein molecule. Hypervariable residues are also responsible for variations in idiotypes between immunoglobulins produced by separate cell clones. Those parts of the variable region that are not hypervariable are termed the framework regions. Hypervariable regions are also called complementarity-determining regions (refer to hot spot). The term refers also to those portions of the T cell receptor that constitute the antigen-binding site. Each antibody heavy chain and light chain and each TCR α chain and β chain possess three hypervariable

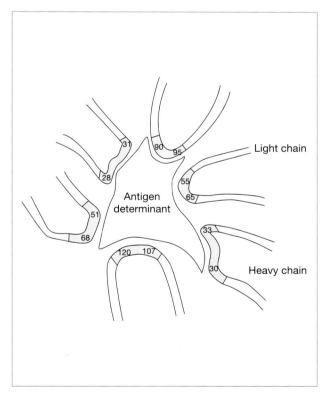

Figure 39 Depiction of the structure of the six hypervariable regions of an antibody

loops, also called CDRs. Most of the variability between different antibodies or TCRs is present within these loops.

An **immunoglobulin light chain** is a 23-kDa, 214-amino acid polypeptide chain comprising a single constant region and a single variable region that are present in all five classes of immunoglobulin molecules. The two types of light chains are designated κ and λ. They are found in association with heavy polypeptide chains and immunoglobulin molecules and are fastened to these structures through disulfide bonds.

A **J chain** is a 17.6-kDa polypeptide chain present in polymeric immunoglobulins that include both IgM and IgA. It links four-chain immunoglobulin monomers to produce the polymeric immunoglobulin structure. J chains are produced in plasma cells and are incorporated into IgM or IgA molecules prior to their secretion. Incorporation of the J chain appears to be essential for transcytosis of these immunoglobulin molecules to external secretions. The J chain constitutes 2–4% of an IgM pentamer or a secretory IgA dimer. Tryptophan is absent from both mouse and human J chains. J chains are composed of 137 amino acid residues and a single complex N-linked oligosaccharide on asparagine. Human J chain contains three

forms of the oligosaccharide which differ in sialic acid content. The J chain is fastened through disulfide bonds to penultimate cysteine residues of μ or α heavy chains. The human J chain gene is located on chromosome 4q21, whereas the mouse J chain gene is located on chromosome 5.

An **immunoglobulin class** (Figure 40) is a subdivision of immunoglobulin molecules based on antigenic and structural differences in the Fc regions of their heavy polypeptide chains. Immunoglobulin molecules belonging to a particular class have at least one constant region isotypic determinant in common. The different classes, such as IgG, IgM and IgA, designate separate isotypes. Since the light chains of immunoglobulin molecules are one of two types, the heavy chains determine immunoglobulin class. There is about 30% homology of amino acid sequence among the five immunoglobulin heavy chain constant regions in man. Heavy chains (or isotypes) also differ in carbohydrate content. Immunization of a non-human species with human immunoglobulin provides antisera that may be used for class or isotype determination. IgG is divided into four subclasses and IgA is divided into two subclasses.

An **immunoglobulin subclass** (Figure 41) is a subdivision of immunoglobulin classes according to

Ig	IgG	IgM	IgA	IgD	IgE
Serum concentration (mg/dl)	800–1700	50–190	140–420	0.3–0.4	<0.001
Total Ig (%)	85	5–10	5–15	<1	<1
Complement fixation	+	++++	−	−	−
Principal biological effect	resistance-opsonin; secondary response	resistance-precipitin; primary response	resistance prevents movement across mucous membranes	?	anaphylaxis
Principal site of action	serum	serum	secretions	?; receptor for B cells	mast cells
Molecular weight (kDa)	154	900	160 (+dimer)	185	190
Serum half-life (days)	23	5	6	2–3	2–3
Antibacterial lysis	+	+++	+	?	?
Antiviral lysis	+	+	+++	?	?
H-chain class	γ	μ	α	δ	ε
Subclass	$\gamma_1\ \gamma_2\ \gamma_3\ \gamma_4$		$\alpha_1\ \alpha_2$		

Figure 40 Table of human immunoglobulins (Ig) and their properties

Ig	IgG	IgM	IgA	IgE	IgD
H-chain class	γ	μ	α	ε	δ
Subclass	$\gamma_1\ \gamma_2\ \gamma_3\ \gamma_4$		$\alpha_1\ \alpha_2$		

Figure 41 Summary of the heavy chain designations of immunoglobulins that determine class and of their subdivisions that determine subclass

structural and antigenic differences in the constant regions of their heavy polypeptide chains. All molecules in an immunoglobulin subclass must express the isotypic antigenic determinants unique to that class, but they also express other epitopes that render that subclass different from others. IgG has four subclasses designated as IgG1, IgG2, IgG3 and IgG4. Whereas there is only 30% identity among the five immunoglobulin classes, there is three times that similarity among IgG subclasses. The IgA class is divisible into two subclasses, whereas the remaining three immunoglobulin classes have not been further subdivided into subclasses. The structural differences in subclasses are exemplified by the variations and number of inter-heavy chain disulfide bonds which the four IgG subclasses possess. The function of immunoglobulin molecules differs from one subclass to another, as exemplified by the inability of IgG4 to fix complement.

Immunoglobulin G (IgG) (Figure 42) constitutes approximately 85% of the immunoglobulins in adults. It has a molecular weight of 154 kDa based on two L chains of 22 000 Da each and two H chains of 55 000 Da each. It has the longest half-life (23 days) of the five immunoglobulin classes, crosses the placenta and is the principal antibody in the anamnestic or booster response. IgG shows high avidity or binding capacity for antigen, fixes complement, stimulates chemotaxis and acts as an opsonin to facilitate phagocytosis.

Immunoglobulin M (IgM) (Figure 43) constitutes 5–10% of the total immunoglobulins in adults and has a half-life of 5 days. It is a pentameric molecule with five four-chain monomers joined by disulfide bonds and the J chain, with a total molecular weight of

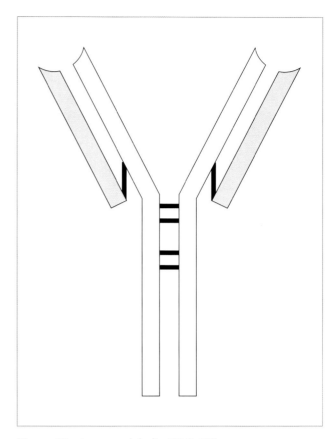

Figure 42   Immunoglobulin G2 (IgG2)

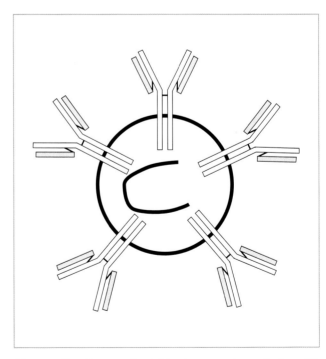

Figure 43 Pentameric IgM that consists of five 7S monomers comprising two heavy and two light polypeptide chains each, as well as one J chain per molecule

900 kDa. Theoretically, this immunoglobulin has ten antigen-binding sites. IgM is the most efficient immunoglobulin in fixing complement. A single IgM pentamer can activate the classical pathway. Monomeric IgM is found with IgD on the B lymphocyte cell surface, where it serves as the receptor for antigen. Because IgM is relatively large, it is confined to intravascular locations. IgM is particularly important for immunity against polysaccharide antigens on the exterior of pathogenic microorganisms. It also promotes phagocytosis and bacteriolysis through its complement activation activity.

Local or regional immunity was first investigated by Alexander Besredka[14], a student of Elie Metchnikoff at the Institut Pasteur, Paris, in 1919. After J. F. Heremans first reported IgA in serum in 1959, local tissue-protective secretory IgA was found to be the principal immunoglobulin of tears, saliva, colostrum, intestinal secretions, and nasal and genitourinary mucus. Thomas B. Tomasi Jr[15] and colleagues elucidated secretory IgA structure and migration in tissues, and characterized an immune system common to certain external secretions (Figure 44).

Immunoglobulin A (IgA) constitutes 5–15% of the serum immunoglobulins and has a half-life of 6 days. It has a molecular weight of 160 kDa and a basic four-chain monomeric structure. However, it can occur as monomers, dimers, trimers and multimers. It contains α heavy chains and κ or λ light chains. There are two subclasses of IgA designated as IgA1 and IgA2. In addition to serum IgA, a secretory or exocrine variety appears in body secretions and provides local immunity. For example, the Sabin oral polio vaccine stimulates secretory IgA antibodies in the gut, which provides effective immunity against poliomyelitis. IgA-deficient individuals have an increased incidence of respiratory infections associated with a lack of secretory IgA in the respiratory system. Secretory or exocrine IgA appears in colostrum; intestinal and respiratory secretions; saliva; tears; and other secretions.

Immunoglobulin class switching is the mechanism whereby an IgM-producing B cell switches isotype to begin producing IgG molecules instead. Further differentiation may lead to a B cell producing IgA.

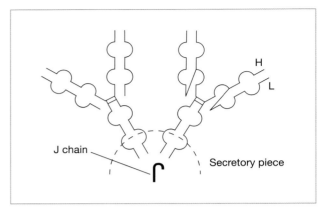

Figure 44   Secretory IgA

However, the antigen-binding specificity of the antibody molecules with a different isotype remains unchanged.

Immunoglobulin D (IgD), which has a molecular weight of 185 kDa less than 1% of serum immunoglobulins. It has the basic four-chain monomeric structure with two δ heavy chains (molecular weight 63 000 Da each) and either two κ or two λ light chains (molecular weight 22 000 each). The half-life of IgD is only 2–3 days, and the role of IgD in immunity remains elusive. Membrane IgD serves with IgM as an antigen receptor on B cell membranes.

Immunoglobulin E (IgE) constitutes less than 1% of the total immunoglobulins and has a half-life of approximately 2.5 days. This antibody has a four-chain unit structure with two ε heavy chains (molecular weight 75 000 each) and either two κ or two λ light chains per molecule (total molecular weight 190 kDa). IgE does not precipitate with antigen *in vitro* and is heat-labile. IgE is responsible for anaphylactic hypersensitivity in humans.

In **pepsin digestion** (Figure 28) a proteolytic enzyme is used to hydrolyze immunoglobulin molecules into $F(ab')_2$ fragments together with small peptides that represent what remains of the Fc fragment. Each immunoglobulin molecule yields only one $F(ab')_2$ fragment which is bivalent and may manifest many of the same antibody characteristics as intact IgG molecules, such as antitoxic activity in neutralizing bacterial toxins. Cleaving the Fc region from an IgG molecule deprives it of its ability to fix complement and bind to

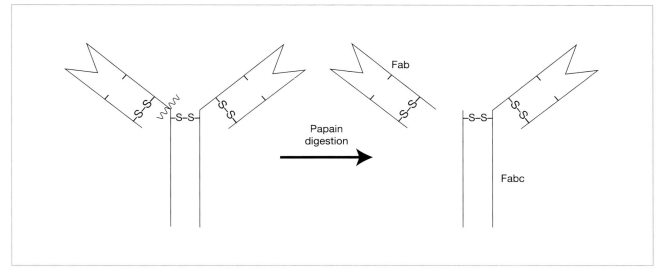

Figure 45 Generation of an Fabc fragment by papain digestion of IgG in which one Fab region is cleaved, leaving an Fabc fragment consisting of the Fc region and one Fab region of the molecule bearing a single antigen-binding site

Fc receptors on cell surfaces. Pepsin digestion is useful in diminishing the immunogenicity of antitoxins. It converts them to $F(ab')_2$ fragments which retain antitoxin activity.

pFc′ fragment is a fragment of pepsin digestion of IgG or of the Fc fragment. Pepsin digestion of IgG or of the Fc fragment yields low-molecular-weight peptides and a pFc′ fragment that is still capable of binding to an Fc receptor on a macrophage or monocyte. It is a 27-kDa dimer without a covalent bond comprising two C_H3 domains, the carboxy-terminal 116 residues of each chain. Unlike the Fc′ fragment, it has the basic N-terminal and C-terminal peptides of this immunoglobulin domain.

Papain (Figure 45) is a proteolytic enzyme extracted from *Carica papaya* that is used to digest each IgG immunoglobulin molecule into two Fab fragments and one crystallizable Fc fragment. This aids efforts to reveal the molecular structure of immunoglobulins. Papain cleaves the immunoglobulin G molecule on the opposite side of the central disulfide bond from pepsin, which cleaves the molecule to the C-terminus side leading to the formation of one $F(ab')_2$ fragment, which is bivalent, in contrast to the Fab fragments which are univalent. The Fc fragment of papain digestion has no antigen-binding capacity, although it does have complement-fixing functions and attaches

immunoglobulin molecules to Fc receptors on a cell membrane. The enzyme has also been used to render red blood cell surfaces susceptible to agglutination by incomplete antibody.

Immunoglobulin fragment is a term reserved for products that result from the action of proteolytic enzymes on immunoglobulin molecules. Intrachain disulfide bonds can be severed by reduction in the presence of denaturing agents such as urea, guanidine or detergents. Peptide bonds in intact domains are not easily split by proteolytic enzymes. Light chains can be cleaved at the V–C junction, giving rise to large segments that correspond to the V_L and C_L domains. Similar cleavage of the heavy chain is more difficult to achieve. Papain cleaves heavy chains at the N-terminus of the H–H disulfide bonds, giving two individual portions of the terminus of the molecule, called Fab, and the fragment of the C-terminus region, Fc, which is crystallizable. In contrast, pepsin cleaves heavy chains at the C-terminus of the H–H disulfide bonds. Thus, the two Fab fragments will remain joined and are called $F(ab')_2$. It degrades the C_H2 domains, but splits the C_H3 domains, which remain non-covalently bonded in dimeric form and are called pFc′. Further digestion of the pFc′ with papain results in smaller dimeric fragments called Fc′. Plasmin has been found to cleave the immunoglobulin molecule between C_H2 and C_H3 giving rise to a fragment designated as Facb. The heavy chain portion of the Fab, designated as Fd, and the heavy chain portion of the Fab' fragment, designated Fd', results from the breakdown of an F(ab')₂ fragment produced by pepsin digestion of the IgG molecule. The Fv fragment consists of the variable domain of heavy and light chains on an immunoglobulin molecule where antigen binding occurs.

A **Fab fragment** (Figure 45) is a product of papain digestion of an IgG molecule. It comprises one light chain and the segment of heavy chain on the N-terminal side of the central disulfide bond. The light and heavy chain segments are linked by interchain disulfide bonds. It is 47 kDa and has a sedimentation coefficient of 3.5S. The Fab fragment has a single antigen-binding site. There are two Fab regions in each IgG molecule.

Fd fragment is the heavy chain portion of a Fab fragment produced by papain digestion of an IgG molecule. It is on the N-terminal side of the papain digestion site.

The **Fv region** consists of the N-terminal variable segments of both the heavy and light chains in each Fab region of an immunoglobulin molecule with a four-chain unit structure.

The **Fc fragment (fragment crystallizable)** (Figure 28) is a product of papain digestion of an IgG molecule. It comprises two C-terminal heavy chain segments (C_H2, C_H3) and a portion of the hinge region linked by the central disulfide bond and non-covalent forces. This 50-kDa fragment is unable to bind antigen, but it has multiple other biological functions, including complement fixation, interaction with Fc receptors on the cell surfaces and placental transmission of IgG. One Fc fragment is produced by papain digestion of each IgG molecule. The Fc region of an intact IgG molecule mediates effector functions by binding to cell surface receptors or C1q complement protein.

Gm allotype is a genetic variant determinant of the human IgG heavy chain. Allelic genes that encode the γ1, γ2 and γ3 heavy chain constant regions encode the Gm allotypes. They were recognized by the ability of blood sera from rheumatoid arthritis patients, which contain anti-IgG rheumatoid factor, to react with them. Gm allotypic determinants are associated with specific amino acid substitution in different γ chain constant regions in man. IgG subclasses are associated with certain Gm determinants. For example, IgG1 is associated with G1m(1) and G1m(4), and IgG3 is associated with G3m(5). Although the great majority of Gm allotypes are restricted to the IgG-γ chain Fc region, a substitution at position 214 of C_H1 of arginine yields the G1m(4) allotype, and a substitution at this same site of lysine yields G1m(17). For Gm expression, the light chain part of the molecule must be intact.

The **Fc' fragment** is a product of papain digestion of IgG. It comprises two non-covalently bonded C_H3 domains that lack the terminal 13 amino acids. This 24-kDa dimer consists of the region between the heavy chain amino acid residues 14 through 105 from the carboxy-terminal end. Normal human urine contains minute quantities of Fc' fragment.

An **Fabc fragment** (Figure 45) is a 5S intermediate fragment produced by partial digestion of IgG by papain in which only one Fab fragment is cleaved from the parent molecule in the hinge region. This leaves the Fabc fragment, which comprises a Fab region bound covalently to an Fc region and is functionally univalent.

Fab' fragment is a product of reduction of an F(ab')₂ fragment that results from pepsin digestion of IgG. It comprises one light chain linked by disulfide bonds to the N-terminal segment of heavy chain. The Fab' fragment has a single antigen-binding site. There are two Fab' fragments in each F(ab')₂ fragment.

F(ab')₂ fragment is a product of pepsin digestion of an IgG molecule. This 95-kDa immunoglobulin fragment has a valence, or antigen-binding capacity, of two, which renders it capable of inducing agglutination or precipitation with homologous antigen. However, the functions associated with the intact IgG molecule's Fc region, such as complement fixation and attachment to Fc receptors on cell surfaces, are missing. Pepsin digestion occurs on the carboxy-terminal side of the central disulfide bond at the hinge region of the molecule, which leaves the central disulfide bond intact. The C_H2 domain is converted to minute peptides, yet the C_H3 domain is left whole, and the two C_H3 domains constitute the pFc' fragment.

An Fd' fragment is the heavy chain portion of an Fab' fragment produced by reduction of the $F(ab')_2$ fragment that results from pepsin digestion of IgG. It comprises V_H1, C_H1 and the heavy chain hinge region. Fd' contains 235 amino acid residues.

An Facb fragment (Figure 46) is a fragment that is both antigen- and complement-binding. The action of plasmin on IgG molecules denatured by acid cleaves C_H3 domains from both heavy chain constituents of the Fc region. This yields a bivalent fragment functionally capable of precipitation and agglutination with an Fc remnant still capable of fixing complement.

Fb fragment (Figure 47) is the product of subtilisin digestion. It comprises the Fab fragment's C_H1 and C_L (constant) domains.

An Fv fragment consists of the N-terminal variable segments of both heavy (V_H) and light (V_L) chain domains that are joined by non-covalent forces. The fragment has one antigen-binding site.

Isotype refers to the antigens that determine the class or subclass of heavy chains or the type and subtype of light chains of immunoglobulin molecules. Every normal member of a species expresses each isotype. An immunoglobulin subtype is found in all normal individuals. Among the immunoglobulin classes, IgG and IgA have subclasses that are designated with arabic numerals. They are distinguished according to domain number and size, as well as the constant region's number of both intrachain and interchain disulfide bonds. The four isotypes of IgG are designated IgG1, IgG2, IgG3 and IgG4. The two IgA isotypes are designated IgA1 and IgA2. The μ, δ, and ε heavy chains and the κ and λ light chains each have one isotype. Immunoglobulin isotypes are responsible for an antibody molecule's biological effector functions.

An allotype is a distinct antigenic form of a serum protein that results from allelic variations present on the immunoglobulin heavy chain constant region. Allotypes were originally defined by antisera which differentiated allelic variants of immunoglobulin subclasses. The allotype is due to the existence of different alleles at the genetic locus which determines the expression of a given determinant. Immunoglobulin allotypes have been extensively investigated in inbred rabbits. Currently, allotypes are usually defined by DNA techniques. To be designated as an official allotype, the polymorphism must be present in a reasonable subset of the population (approximately 1%) and follow Mendelian genetics. Allotype examples include the IgG3 Caucasian allotypes G3m[b] and

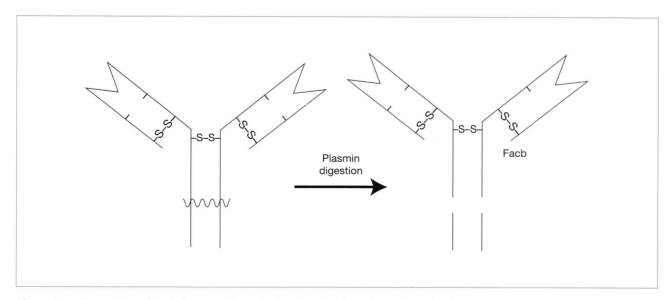

Figure 46   Generation of Facb fragment through plasmin digestion of an IgG molecule

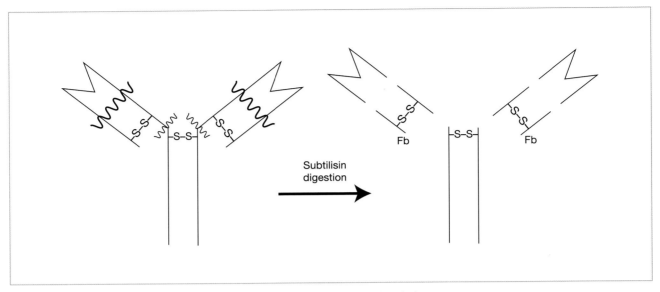

Figure 47   Formation of Fb fragments by digestion of IgG molecules with subtilisin

G3m^g. These two alleles vary at positions 291, 296 and 384. Another example is the allotype at the IgA2 locus. The IgA2m(1) allele is European/Near Eastern, while IgA2m(2) is African/East Asian. The allotypic differences are in Ca$_1$ and Ca$_3$, and the IgA2m(2) allele has a shorter hinge than the IgA2m(1) allele. An **allotope** is an allotype's antigenic determinant. Allotypic differences in immunoglobulin molecules have been important in solving the genetics of antibodies.

An **alloantibody** is an antibody that interacts with an alloantigen, such as the antibodies generated in the recipient of an organ allotransplant (such as kidney or heart) which then may react with the homologous alloantigen of the allograft. Alloantibodies interact with antigens that result from allelic variation at polymorphic genes. Examples include those that recognize blood group antigens and HLA class I and class II molecules.

Gm allotype refers to a genetic variant determinant of the human IgG heavy chain. Allelic genes that encode the γ1, γ2 and γ3 heavy chain constant regions encode the Gm allotypes. They were recognized by the ability of blood sera from rheumatoid arthritis patients, which contain anti-IgG rheumatoid factor, to react with them. Gm allotypic determinants are associated with specific amino acid substitution in different γ chain constant regions in man. IgG subclasses are associated with certain Gm determinants. For example, IgG is associated with Glm(1) and G1m(4), and IgG3 is associated with G3m(5). Although the great majority of Gm allotypes are restricted to the IgG γ chain Fc region, a substitution at position 214 of C$_H$1 of the arginine yields the G1m(4) allotype and a substitution at this same site of lysine yields G1m(17). For Gm expression, the light chain part of the molecule must be intact.

An **Am allotypic marker** is an allotypic antigenic determinant located on a heavy chain of the IgA molecule in man. Of the two IgA subclasses, the IgA1 subclass has no known allotypic determinant. The IgA2 subclass has two allotypic determinants designated A2m(1) and A2m(2) based on differences in α2 heavy chain primary structures. Allelic genes at the A2m locus encode these allotypes which are expressed on the α2 heavy chain constant regions.

Idiotype (Figure 48) refers to that segment of an immunoglobulin or antibody molecule that determines its specificity for antigen and is based upon the multiple combinations of variable (V), diversity (D) and joining (J) exons. The idiotype is located in the Fab region, and its expression usually requires participation of the variable regions of both heavy and light chains, namely the Fv fragment which contains the antigen-combining site. The antigen-binding specificity of the combining site may imply that all antibodies produced by an animal in response to a given

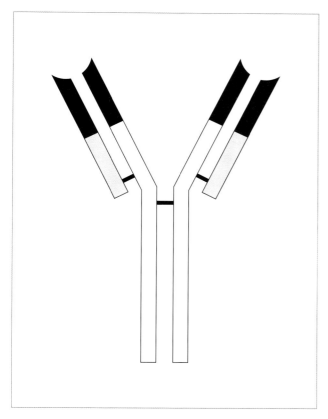

Figure 48 Idiotype which is determined by the variable regions of heavy and light chains of an immunoglobulin molecule

immunogen have the same idiotype. This is not true, since the antibody response is heterogeneous. There will usually be a major idiotype representing 20–70% of the specific antibody response. The remainder carry different idiotypes that may cross-react with the major idiotype. Cross-reacting idiotypy represents the extent of heterogeneity among the antibodies of a given specificity.

The unique antigenic determinants that govern the idiotype (Id) of an immunoglobulin molecule occur on the products of either a single or several clones of cells synthesizing immunoglobulins. This unique idiotypic determinant is sometimes called a private idiotype that appears in all V regions of immunoglobulin molecules whose amino acid sequences are the same. Shared idiotypes are also known as public idiotype determinants. These may appear in a relatively large number of immunoglobulin molecules produced by inbred strains of mice or other genetically identical animals in response to a specific antigen. The localization of idiotypes in the antigen-binding site of

the molecule's V region is illustrated by the ability of haptens to block or inhibit the interaction of anti-idiotypic antibodies with their homologous antigenic markers or determinants in the antigen-binding region of antibody molecules (Figure 49).

The **network theory** (Figure 50) is an hypothesis proposed by **Niels Jerne** which explains immunoregulation through a network of idiotype–anti-idiotype reactions involving T cell receptors and the antigen-binding regions of antibody molecules, i.e. the paratope regions. Jerne hypothesized that antibodies produced in response to a specific antigen would themselves induce a second group of antibodies which would in turn downregulate the original antibody-producing cells. The second antigen (Ab-2) would recognize epitopes of antibody 1's antibody-binding region. These would be anti-idiotypic antibodies. Such anti-idiotypic antibodies would also be reactive with the antigen-binding region of T cell receptors for which they were specific. Thus, a network of antiantibodies would produce a homeostatic effect on the immune response to a particular antigen. The antibody molecules' antigen-binding sites (paratopes), which are encoded by variable region genes, have idiotopes as phenotypic markers. Each paratope recognizes idiotopes on a different antibody molecule. Interaction of idiotypes with anti-idiotypes is physiologic idiotypy and is shared among immunoglobulin classes. This comprises antibodies produced in response to the same antigen. The idiotypic network consists of the interaction of idiotypes involving free molecules as well as B and T lymphocyte receptors. Idiotypes are considered central in immunoregulation involving autoantigens. Exposure to antigens interrupts the delicate balance of the idiotype–anti-idiotype network, leading to the increased synthesis of some idiotypes as well as of the corresponding anti-idiotypes, leading to modulation of the response. Anti-idiotypes occur following immunization against selected antigens and may prevent the response to the antigen. Selected anti-idiotypic antibodies have a binding site that is closely similar to the immunizing epitope. It is referred to as the internal image of the epitope. Other anti-idiotypic antibodies are directed to idiotopes of the antigen-binding region and are not internal images. Anti-idiotypic antibodies with an internal image may be substituted for an antigen, leading to specific antigen-binding antibodies.

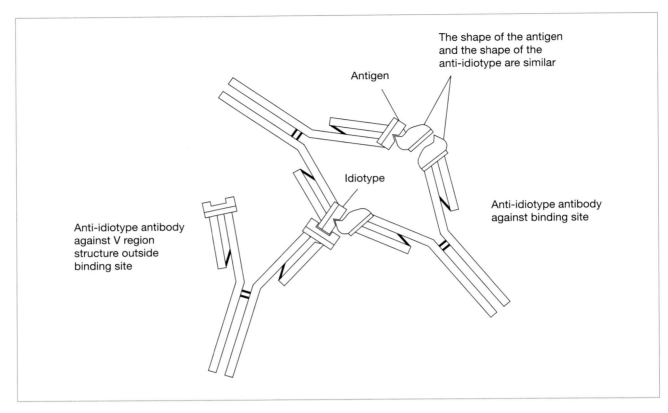

The shape of the antigen
and the shape of the
anti-idiotype are similar

Antigen

Idiotype

Anti-idiotype antibody
against V region
structure outside
binding site

Anti-idiotype antibody
against binding site

Figure 49 Idiotype network

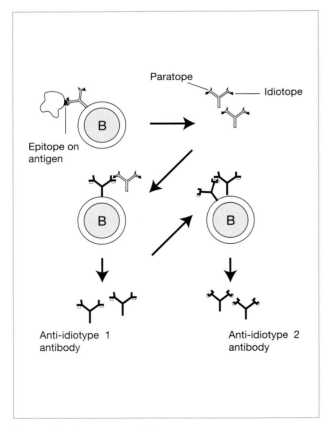

Paratope

Idiotope

Epitope on
antigen

B

B

B

Anti-idiotype 1
antibody

Anti-idiotype 2
antibody

Figure 50 Jerne network theory

These are the basis for so-called idiotypic vaccines in which the individual never has to be exposed to the infecting agent. Anti-idiotypes may also block T cell receptors for the corresponding antigen. Each new immune response stimulated in this network interrupts the finely tuned immune network balance as anti-idiotype antibodies are produced, eventually downregulating the response and bringing it back to homeostasis. This theory was subsequently proved and confirmed by numerous investigators.

The **unitarian hypothesis** was the view that one type of antibody produced in response to an injection of antigen could induce agglutination, complement fixation, precipitation and lysis based upon the type of ligand with which it interacted. This view was in contrast to the earlier belief that separate antibodies accounted for every type of serological reactivity described above. Usually, more than one class of immunoglobulin may manifest a particular serological reactivity such as precipitation.

Switch refers to the change within an immunologically competent B lymphocyte from synthesizing one isotype of a heavy polypeptide chain, such as μ, to another isotype, such as γ, during differentiation. The switch signal comes from T cells. Isotype switching does not alter the antigen-binding variable region of the chain at the N-terminus.

A **B lymphocyte hybridoma** is a hybrid cell produced by the fusion of a splenic antibody-secreting cell immunized against that particular antigen with a mutant myeloma cell from the same species that no longer secretes its own protein product. Polyethylene glycol is used to effect cell fusion. Antibody-synthesizing cells do not secrete hypoxanthine guanine phosphoribosyl transferase (HGPRT), an enzyme needed for DNA nucleotide synthesis, but do provide the ability to produce a specific monoclonal antibody. The mutant myeloma cell line confers immortality upon the hybridoma. If the nucleotide synthesis pathway is inhibited, the myeloma cells become HGPRT-dependent. The antibody synthesizing cells provide the HGPRT and the mutant myeloma cell enables endless reproduction. Once isolated through use of a selective medium such as hypoxanthine aminopterin thymidine (HAT), hybridoma cell lines can be maintained for relatively long periods. Hybridomas produce specific monoclonal antibodies that may be collected in great quantities for use in diagnosis and selected types of therapy.

Polyclonal antibodies are multiple immunoglobulins responding to different epitopes on an antigen molecule. This multiple stimulation leads to the expansion of several antibody-forming clones whose products represent a mixture of immunoglobulins, in contrast to proliferation of a single clone which would yield a homogeneous monoclonal antibody product. Thus, polyclonal antibodies represent the natural consequence of an immune response in contrast to monoclonal antibodies, which occur *in vivo* in pathologic conditions such as multiple myeloma or are produced artificially by hybridoma technology against one of a variety of antigens.

Doctrine of original antigenic sin The immune response against a virus, such as a parental strain, to which an individual was previously exposed may be greater than it is against the immunizing agent, such as type A influenza virus variant. This concept is known as the doctrine of original antigenic sin.

When an individual is exposed to an antigen that is similar to, but not identical to, an antigen to which he was previously exposed by either infection or immunization, the immune response to the second exposure is still directed against the first antigen. This was first noticed in influenza virus infection. Due to antigenic drift and antigenic shift in influenza virus, reinfection with an antigenically altered strain generates a secondary immune response that is specific for the influenza virus strain that produced an earlier infection. Other highly immunogenic epitopes on a second and subsequent viruses are ignored.

Maternal immunoglobulins (Figures 51 and 52) are passed to the offspring both *in utero* and in the neonatal period. In humans, immunoglobulin G is transferred by way of the placenta as early as at 38 days' gestation. Transfer remains stable until the 17th week and then increases until term. Only the IgG class of antibodies crosses the placenta. The SC portion of the immunoglobulin is bound to specific placental membrane receptors of the SC γ type III variety (CD16) that possess binding sites for the Fc region of IgG, in addition to epitopes that can be recognized by the antigen-binding site of IgG. The receptors have low affinity for aggregated or complex IgG and strongest affinity for IgG1 and IgG3, less for IgG4 and least for IgG2 and no affinity for IgM and IgA. The receptors are concentrated on the syncytiotrophoblast that makes direct contact with the mother's circulation (refer also to Brambell receptor below). Human colostrum and fresh breast milk contain numerous host-resistance factors that are both specific and non-specific. Secretory IgA is present in these fluids, with highest concentration in colostrom that peaks during the first 34 days postpartum. Breast-fed children receive 0.5 g of secretory IgA per day. Human milk also contains IgG and IgM as well as secretory IgA, but in lower concentrations. Factors other than immunoglobulins that protect against infections include lactoferrin that serves as a bacterial static agent depriving microbes of iron. Lysozyme is also present in milk. Breast milk also contains macrophages, T and B cells, neutrophils and epithelial cells and also contains immunomodulators. Diseases caused by maternal antibodies are listed in the separate diseases.

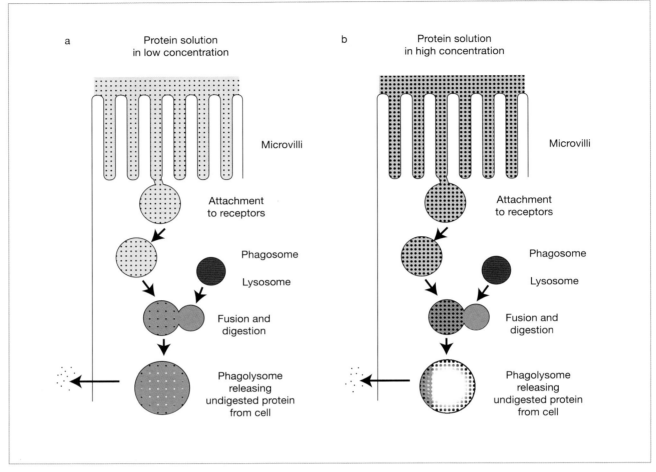

Figure 51 Mechanism of γ-globulin transmission by the cell. (a) Concentration of γ-globulin is only a little more than sufficient to saturate the receptors and the proportion degraded is < 40%. (b) Concentration is about four times that in (a), and hence over 80% is degraded. The amount released from the cell remains constant, irrespective of concentration

The **Brambell receptor (FcRB)**, named for F. W. R. Brambell (Figure 53), a pioneer in transmission of immunity, conserves IgG by binding to its Fc region and protects it from catabolism by lysosomes (Figure 54). It is an Fc receptor that transports IgG across epithelial surfaces. Its structure resembles that of an MHC class I molecule. The mechanism of binding is pH dependent. In the endosomes' low pH, the receptor FcRB binds to IgG. IgG is then transported to the luminal surface of the catabolic cell, where the neutral pH mediates release of the bound IgG.

Avidity refers to the strength of binding between an antibody and its specific antigen. The stability of this union is a reflection of the number of binding sites that they share. **Avidity** is the binding force or intensity between multivalent antigen and multivalent antibody. Multiple binding sites on both the antigen and

the antibody (e.g. IgM or multiple antibodies interacting with various epitopes on the antigen) and reactions of high affinity between each of the antigens and its homologous antibody all increase the avidity. Such non-specific factors as ionic and hydrophobic interactions also increase avidity. Whereas affinity is described in thermodynamic terms, avidity is not, as it is described according to the assay procedure employed. The sum of the forces contributing to the avidity of an antigen (Ag) and antibody (Ab) interaction may be greater than the strength of binding of the individual antibody–antigen combinations contributing to the overall avidity of a particular interaction. K_A, the association constant for the Ab + Ag = AbAg interaction, is frequently used to indicate avidity. Avidity may also describe the strength of cell-to-cell interactions which are mediated by numerous binding interactions between cell surface molecules. Avidity is

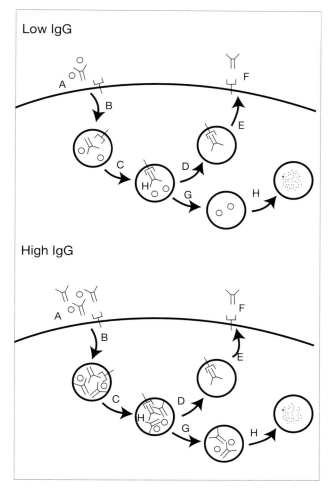

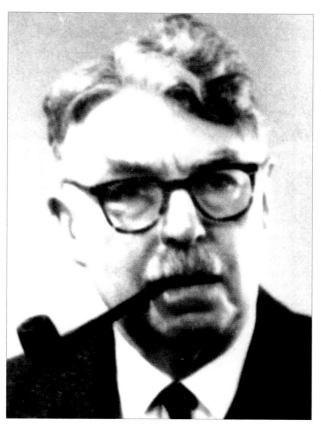

Figure 53   F. W. R. Brambell

Figure 52   Mechanism of γ globulin protection from catabolism. IgG (γ) and plasma proteins (o) (A) are internalized into endosomes of endothelium (B) without prior binding. In the low pH (H⁺) of the endosome (C), binding of IgG is promoted (D, E, F). IgG retained by receptor recycles to the cell surface and dissociates in the neutral pH of the extracellular fluid, returning to circulation (G, H). Unbound proteins are shunted to the lysosomes for degradation. With 'low IgG', receptor efficiently 'rescues' IgG from catabolism. With 'high IgG', receptor is saturated and excess IgG passes to catabolism for a net acceleration of IgG catabolism

distinct from affinity, which describes the strength of binding between a single molecular site and its ligand.

The **avidity hypothesis** was previously termed the affinity hypothesis of T cell selection in the thymus. The avidity hypothesis is based on the concept that T cells must have a measurable affinity for self-major histocompatibility complex (MHC) molecules to mature, but not an affinity sufficient to cause activation of the cell when it matures, as this would necessitate deletion of the cell to maintain self-tolerance.

Antibody affinity is the force of binding of one antibody molecule's paratope with its homologous epitope on the antigen molecule (Figure 55). It is a consequence of positive and negative portions affecting these molecular interactions.

Functional affinity is the association constant for a bivalent or multivalent antibody's interaction with a bivalent or multivalent ligand. The multivalent reactivity may enhance the affinity of multiple antigen–antibody reactions. Avidity has a similar connotation, but it is a less precise term than is functional affinity.

Affinity maturation refers to the sustained increase in affinity of antibodies for an antigen with time following immunization. The genes encoding the antibody variable regions undergo somatic hypermutation with the selection of B lymphocytes whose receptors express high affinity for the antigen. The IgG antibodies that form following the early, heterogeneous IgM response manifest greater specificity and less heterogeneity than do the IgM molecules.

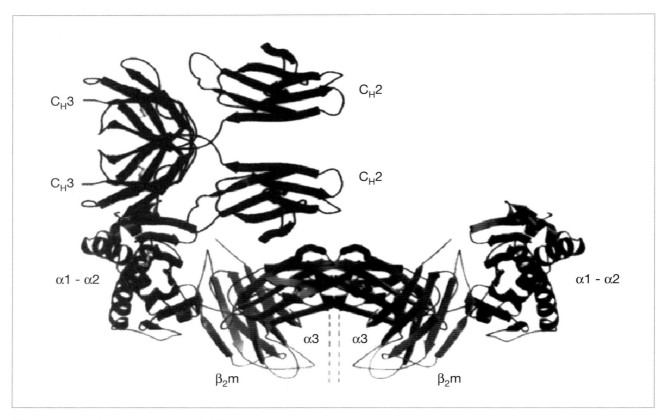

Figure 54   The Brambell receptor (FcRB)

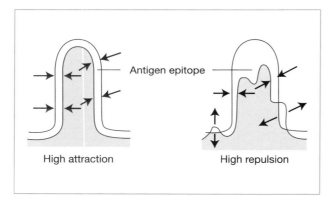

Figure 55   Antibody affinity

An **abzyme** is the union of antibody and enzyme molecules to form a hybrid catalytic molecule. Specificity for a target antigen is provided through the antibody portion and for a catalytic function through the enzyme portion. Thus, these molecules have numerous potential uses. These molecules are capable of catalyzing various chemical reactions and show great promise as protein-clearing antibodies, as in the dissolution of fibrin clots from occluded coronary arteries in myocardial infarction.

Designer antibody is a genetically engineered immunoglobulin needed for a specific purpose. The term has been used to refer to chimeric antibodies produced by linking mouse gene segments that encode the variable region of immunoglobulin with those that encode the constant region of a human immunoglobulin. This technique provides the antigen specificity obtained from the mouse antibody, while substituting the less immunogenic Fc region of the molecule from a human source. This greatly diminishes the likelihood of an immune response in humans receiving the hybrid immunoglobulin molecules, since most of the mouse immunoglobulin Fc region epitopes have been eliminated through the human Fc substitution.

Passive immunization describes the transfer of a specific antibody or of sensitized lymphoid cells from an immune to a previously non-immune recipient host. Unlike active immunity, which may be of relatively long duration, passive immunity is brief, lasting only until the injected immunoglobulin or lymphoid cells have disappeared. Examples of passive immunization include: the administration of γ-globulin to immunodeficient individuals; and the transfer of immunity from mother to young (antibodies across the placenta or the ingestion of colostrum-containing antibodies).

An **anti-idiotypic antibody** is an antibody that interacts with antigenic determinants (idiotopes) at the variable N-terminus of the heavy and light chains constituting the paratope region of an antibody molecule where the antigen-binding site is located. The idiotope antigenic determinants may be situated either within the cleft of the antigen-binding region or on the periphery or outer edge of the variable region of heavy and light chain components.

Blocking antibody is:

(1) An incomplete IgG antibody that, when diluted, may combine with red blood cell surface antigens and inhibit agglutination reactions used for erythrocyte antigen identification. This can lead to errors in blood grouping for Rh, K and k blood types. Pretreatment of red cells with enzymes may correct the problem.

(2) An IgG antibody specifically induced by exposure of allergic subjects to specific allergens, to which they are sensitive, in a form that favors IgG rather than IgE production. The IgG, specific for the allergens to which they are sensitized, compete within IgE molecules bound to mast cell surfaces, thereby preventing their degranulation and inhibiting a type I hypersensitivity response.

(3) A specific immunoglobulin molecule that may inhibit the combination of a competing antibody molecule with a particular epitope. Blocking antibodies may also interfere with the union of T cell receptors with an epitope for which they are specific, as occurs in some tumor-bearing patients with blocking antibodies which may inhibit the tumoricidal action of cytotoxic T lymphocytes.

Fc receptor is a structure on the surface of some lymphocytes, macrophages or mast cells that specifically binds the Fc region of immunoglobulin, often when the Fc is aggregated. Fc receptors are found on 95% of human peripheral blood T lymphocytes. On about 75% of the cells, the FcR are specific for IgM; the remaining 20% are specific for IgG.

The **polyimmunoglobulin receptor** is an attachment site for polymeric immunoglobulins located on epithelial cell and hepatocyte surfaces that facilitate polymeric IgA and IgM transcytosis to the secretions.

Class switching (isotype switching) is a change in the isotype or class of an immunoglobulin synthesized by a B lymphocyte undergoing differentiation. IgM is the main antibody produced first in a primary humoral response to thymus-dependent antigens, with IgG being produced later in the response.

A **variable region** is that segment of an immunoglobulin molecule or antibody formed by the variable domain of a light polypeptide chain (κ or λ) or of a heavy polypeptide chain (α, γ, μ, δ or ϵ). This is sometimes referred to as the Fv region and is encoded by the V gene. This antigen-binding region of the molecule is responsible for the specificity of the antigen bound. The antigen-binding variable sequences are present in the extended loop structures or hypervariable segment. This term refers also to the variable region (V) region of T cell receptor α, β, γ, δ chains that contain variable amino acid sequences.

Framework regions (FRs) These are relatively invariant regions within variable domains of immunoglobulins and T cell receptors that constitute a protein scaffold for hypervariable regions interacting with antigen. These are amino acid sequences in variable regions of heavy or light immunoglobulin chains other than the hypervariable sequences. There is much less variability in the framework region than in the hypervariable region. Two β-pleated sheets opposing one another constitute the structural features of an antibody domain's framework regions. Polypeptide chain loops join the β-pleated sheet strands. The framework regions contribute to the secondary and tertiary structure of the variable region domain, although they are less significant than the hypervariable regions for the antigen-binding site. The framework region forms the folding part of the immunoglobulin molecule. Light chain FRs are found at amino acid residues 1–28, 38–50, 56–89 and 97–107. Heavy chain FRs are present at amino acid residues 1–31, 35–49, 66–101 and 110–117.

A **haplotype** consists of those phenotypic characteristics encoded by closely linked genes on one chromosome inherited from one parent. It frequently describes several major histocompatibility complex (MHC) alleles on a single chromosome. Selected haplotypes are in strong linkage disequilibrium between alleles of different loci. According to Mendelian genetics, 25% of siblings will share both haplotypes.

REFERENCES

1. Arrhenius SA. *Immunochemie. Anwendungen der physicalischen Chemie auf die Lehre von den physiologischen Antikorpern.* Leipzig: Akademische Verlagsgesellschaft, 1907

2. Obermayer F, Pick EP. Über Veranderungen des Brechungsvermogens von Glykosiden und Eiweisskorpern durch Fermente, Sauren and Bakterien. *Beitr Z Chem Phys Path Brnschwg* 1903;VII:331

3. Landsteiner K. Über die Abhängigkeit der serologischen Spezifität von der chemischen Struktur. (Darstellung von Antigenen mit bekannter chemischer Konstitution der specifischen Gruppen) XII Mitteilung uber Antigene. *Biochem Z* 1918;86:343–94

4. Gene. In *New Encyclopedia Britannica,* 15th edn, Vol 7, *Macropaedia.* Chicago: Encyclopedia Britannica, 1978:981

5. Pauling L. A theory of the structure and process of formation of antibodies. *J Am Chem Soc* 1940;62:2643–57

6. Breinl F, Haurowitz F. Chemische Untersuchung des Prazipitäts aus Hämoglobin and Anti-Hämoglobin Serum und über die Natur der Antikorper. *Z F Physiol Chem* 1930;192:45

7. Mudd S. Hypothetical mechanism of antibody formation. *J Immunol* 1932;23:423–7

8. Heidelberger M, Kendall FE. A quantitative theory of the precipitin reaction. III. The reaction between crystalline egg albumin and its homologous antibody. *J Exp Med* 1935;62:697

9. Tiselius AWK, Kabat E. An electrophoretic study of immune sera and purified antibody preparations. *J Exp Med* 1929;69:119–31

10. Porter RR. Separation and isolation of fractions of rabbit gammaglobulin containing the antibody and antigenic combining sites. *Nature (London)* 1958;182:670–1

11. Edelman GM, Cunningham BA, Gall WE. The covalent structure of an entire gamma G immunoglobulin molecule. *Proc Natl Acad Sci USA* 1969;63:78–85

12. Valentine RC, Green NMJ. Electron microscopy of an antibody–hapten complex. *J Mol Biol* 1967;27:615-17

13. Putman FW, *et al.* Complete amino acid sequence of the Mu heavy chain of a human IgM immunoglobulin. *Science* 1973;182:287–91

14. Besredka A. *Local Immunization. Specific Dressings* (Plotz H, ed. and transl.). Baltimore: Williams and Wilkins, 1927:181

15. Tomasi TB Jr. *The Immune System of Secretions.* Englewood Cliffs, NJ: Prentice-Hall, 1976:161

CHAPTER 4

The complement system: chronology and mystique

'Blut ist ein ganz besonderer Saft'
                              Goethe

Throughout the ages, man has been fascinated and, at times, obsessed by the marvelous, mysterious and even baffling qualities of the blood. A ferment of research activity in the latter 1800s was designed to elucidate mechanisms of host immunity against infectious disease agents. Elie Metchnikoff's demonstration that blood cells could phagocytize (ingest) invading microorganisms led to the 'cellular theory', the first of two opposing concepts of bacteriolysis. The other, the 'humoral

theory' was based on Fodor, Nuttall and Buchner's detection of the heat-labile constituent of fresh, cell-free serum, which could include bacteriolysis. Hans Buchner named this principle 'alexin' (Greek *without a name*) (Figure 1). In 1889, Buchner[1] (Figure 2) described a heat-labile bactericidal principle in the blood, which he termed *alexine*. This was later identified as the complement system. In 1894, Pfeiffer discovered specific *in vivo* lysis of bacteria by observing that cholera vibrios injected

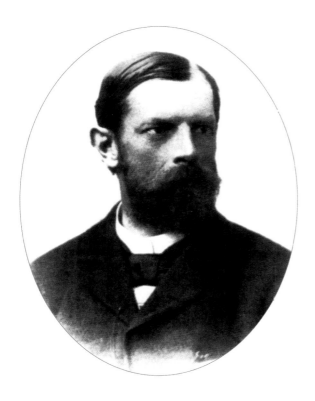

Figure 1 Portrait of Hans Buchner, who first described a lytic principle in serum that ultimately was known as the 'complement system'

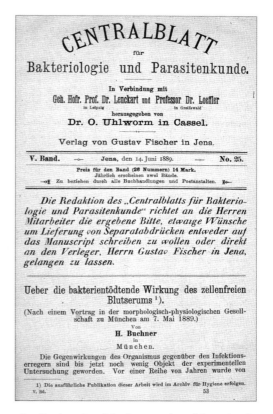

Figure 2 Buchner's original paper describing what became known as 'complement activity'

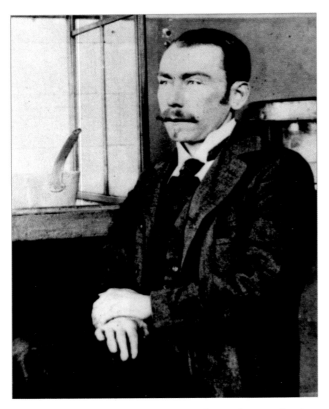

Figure 3   Jules Bordet, discoverer of complement fixation and Nobel Laureate in Medicine for immunology, 1919

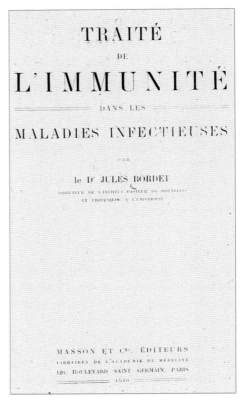

Figure 4   Bordet's first book on immunology published in 1920

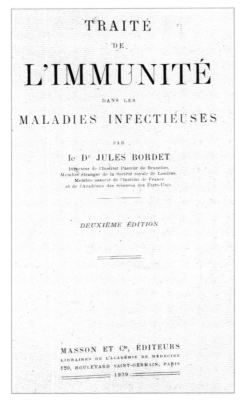

Figure 5   Bordet's second edition of his famous book on immunology published in 1939

into the peritoneum of immune guinea pigs were lysed. In 1895, Jules Bordet[2] (Figure 3), working at the Institut Pasteur in Metchnikoff's laboratory, extended this finding by demonstrating that the lytic or bactericidal action of freshly drawn blood, which had been destroyed by heating, was promptly restored by the addition of fresh, normal, unheated serum. Paul Ehrlich[3] called Bordet's alexine 'das Komplement'. In 1901, Bordet and Gengou[4] developed the complement fixation test to measure antigen–antibody reactions (Figures 4–6). von Wassermann applied this principle to the serologic diagnosis of syphilis.

Hans Buchner (1850–1902), German bacteriologist who was a professor of hygiene in Munich in 1894. He discovered complement. Through his studies of normal serum and its bactericidal effects, he became an advocate of the humoral theory of immunity.

Jules Jean Baptiste Vincent Bordet (1870–1961), Belgian bacteriologist and immunologist, who discovered *Bordetella pertussis*, the causative agent of

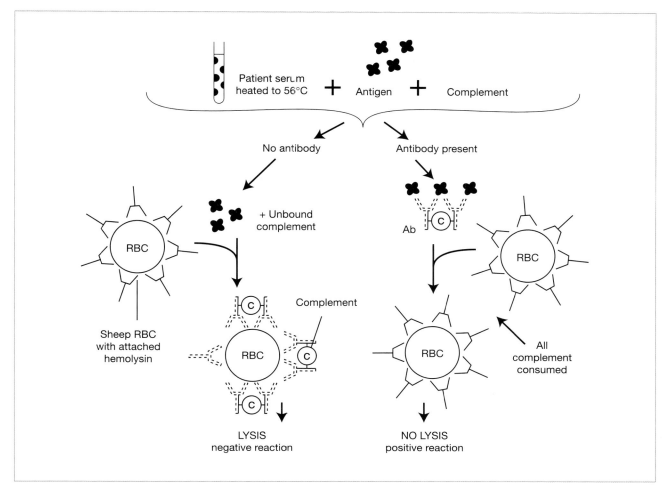

Figure 6   Complement fixation. RBC, red blood cell; Ab, antibody

whooping cough, immune hemolysis and complement fixation. He received the Nobel Prize in Medicine or Physiology in 1919 for his studies on complement.

Bordet was born at Soignies, Belgium, and at age 16 entered the University of Brussels, graduating as Doctor of Medicine in 1892. By 1890, Jules was enhancing the virulence of *Vibrio metschnikovii* by passage in immunized animals. He received a travel grant in 1894 and served as *preparateur* in Metchnikoff's laboratory at the Institut Pasteur in Paris from 1894 to 1901. In 1897 he traveled to the Transvaal to investigate rinderpest. He left the Institut Pasteur in 1901 to accept the post as Director of the Rabies and Bacteriology Institute of Brabant in Belgium. He received Madame Marie Pasteur's permission to rename the facility the Institut Pasteur de Bruxelles in 1903. In 1907, he was appointed Professor of Bacteriology in the Faculty of Medicine of the Free University of Brussels.

In addition to his discovery of *Bordetella pertussis*, the causative agent of whooping cough, Bordet also described the mycoplasma of bovine pleuropneumonia, bacteriophage lysogeny. He discovered the spirochete of syphilis but did not publish this finding. These are in addition to his legion of discoveries in immunology that include specific agglutination (1895), conglutination (1909), the antigenicity of antibodies and complement and, most important, his investigations of complement reactions. Noting the similarity of specific lysis of cholera vibrios by Richard Pfeiffer to the phenomenon of hemolysis described by Hans Buchner, Bordet decided to use the red blood cell system to illustrate complement activity rather than lysis of pathogenic bacteria as a model system. He investigated both bacterial lysis and the lysis of red blood cells. The lytic action of serum was sensitive to heat but could be restored by the addition of unheated normal serum. Bordet's experiment showed complement to be non-specific and able to function only when target cells were sensitized. He showed the similarities of bacterial lysis and hemolysis. In 1900, Bordet showed that complement action was non-specific by using the same source of complement for both hemolysis and bacterial lysis. He and Gengou described complement fixation, and pointed to its use in the diagnosis of infectious diseases. They showed that complement, specifically C1, is fixed by bacteria that resist lysis, providing the foundation for the highly sensitive complement fixation test to detect specific antibodies in serum. von Wassermann applied the complement fixation technique to the diagnosis of syphilis, which was used worldwide.

Bordet debated with Paul Ehrlich concerning his complex explanations of immune reactions. For example, Bordet believed toxin to be neutralized by antitoxin through adsorption, similar to a fabric interacting with a dye. He considered antitoxic sera to contain *substance sensibilisatrice*, i.e. antibody, which sensitized red blood cells or bacteria to the action of *alexine*, his term for complement. He postulated that this acts as a mordant does for a dyestuff. Thus, he disputed with Ehrlich about the nature and mechanism of action of antibodies and complement. This led to the publication in 1909–10 of competing volumes entitled *Studies on Immunity*, one by the 'Bordet school' and the other by Ehrlich and his colleagues. He received the Nobel Prize in Medicine or Physiology in 1919 for his studies on complement and its reactions. During his long and productive career, Bordet wrote a popular text entitled *Trait de l'Immunité dans les Maladies Infectieuses* and trained a spate of gifted investigators, including the prominent American bacteriologist/immunologist, Frederick P. Gay of Columbia University.

Further reading

Bordet J. *Trait de l'Immunité dans les Maladies Infectieuses*. Paris: Masson et Cie, 1920. De Kruif P. *Men Against Death*. New York: Harcourt Brace, 1932

Dictionary of Science Biography. 1970;2:300

Volume Jubilaire de Jules Bordet. *Ann Inst Pasteur, Paris*. 1950;79

Bordet J, obituary. *Ann Inst Pasteur, Paris* 1967:101(1)

The **complement fixation assay** is a serologic test based on the fixation of complement by antigen–antibody complexes. It has been applied to many antigen–antibody systems and was widely used earlier in the century as a serologic test for syphilis.

Complement fixing antibody is an antibody of the immunoglobulin IgG or IgM class that binds complement after reacting with its homologous antigen. This represents complement fixation by the classic pathway. Non-antibody mechanisms, as well as IgA, fix complement by the alternative pathway.

Complement fixation (Figure 7) is a primary union of an antigen with an antibody in the complement fixation reaction that takes place almost instantaneously and is invisible. A measured amount of complement present in the reaction mixture is taken up by complexes of antigen and antibody. Complement fixation is the consumption or binding of complement by antigen–antibody complexes. This serves as the basis for a serologic assay in which antigen is combined with a serum specimen suspected of containing the homologous antibody. Following the addition of a measured amount of complement, which is fixed or consumed only if antibody was present in the serum and has formed a complex with the antigen, sheep red blood cells sensitized (coated) with specific antibody are added to determine whether or not complement has been fixed in the first phase of the reaction. Failure of the sensitized sheep red blood cells to lyse constitutes a positive test since no complement is available. However, sheep red blood cell lysis indicates that complement was not consumed during the first phase of the reaction, implying that homologous antibody was not present in the serum and complement remains free to lyse the sheep red blood cells sensitized with antibody. Hemolysis constitutes a negative reaction. The sensitivity of the complement fixation test falls between those of agglutination and precipitation. Complement fixation tests may be carried out in microtiter plates that are designed for the use of relatively small volumes of reagents. The lysis of sheep red blood cells sensitized with rabbit antibody is measured either in a spectrophotometer at 413 nm or by the release of ^{51}Cr from red cells that have been previously labeled with the isotope. Complement fixation can detect either soluble or

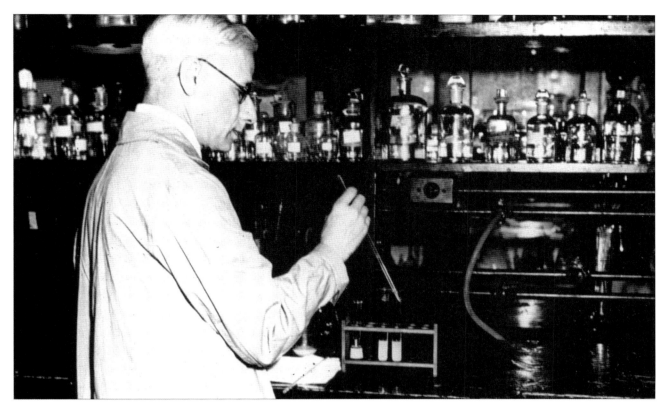

Figure 7 Michael Heidelberger, who purified the first component of complement and showed that complement was a real substance with real weight and a protein

insoluble antigen. Its ability to detect virus antigens in impure tissue preparations means that the test remains useful in the diagnosis of virus infections.

The **Wassermann reaction** is a complement fixation assay that was used extensively in the past to diagnose syphilis. Cardiolipin extracted from ox heart serves as antigen that reacts with antibodies that develop in patients with syphilis. Biologic false-positive reactions using this test require the use of such confirmatory tests as the fluorescent treponemal antibody absorption (FTA-ABS) test, the Reiter's complement fixation test or the *Treponema pallidum* immobilization (TPI) test. Both FTA and TPI tests use *T. pallidum* as antigen.

Heat inactivation is the loss of biological activity through heating. Heating a serum sample at 56°C in a water bath for 30 min destroys complement activity through inactivation of C1, C2 and factor B. By diminishing the heat to 52°C for 30 min, only factor B is destroyed, whereas C1 and C2 remain intact. This inactivates the alternative complement pathway but not the classical pathway. IgG, IgM and IgA are resistant to incubation in a 56°C water bath for 30 min, whereas IgE antibodies are destroyed by this temperature.

Complement deviation (Neisser–Wechsberg phenomenon) is the blocking of complement fixation or of complement-induced lysis when excess antibody is present. There is deviation of the complement by the antibody.

The **Neisser–Wechsberg phenomenon** is the deviation of complement by antibody. Although complement does not react with antigen alone, it demonstrates weak affinity for unreacted antibody.

Ferrata[5], in 1907, recognized complement to be a multiple component system, a complex of protein substances of mixed globulin composition present in normal sera of many animal species. When electrolytes were removed from serum by dialysis against distilled water, the euglobulin fraction of serum proteins precipitated. A portion of complement activity was present in this fraction and a part in the supernatant. Neither was active alone, but activity was present when the two were combined. Ferrata demonstrated that euglobulin and pseudoglobulin fractions were each hemolytically inactive. However, hemolytic activity could be restored when they were combined. The component present in the euglobulin portion was found to combine with antigen–antibody complexes and not produce lysis. The soluble fraction failed to combine with antigen–antibody complexes but did combine with antigen–antibody complex plus euglobulin fraction. Therefore, in the early literature, the euglobulin fraction was called the midpiece of complement, while the other pseudoglobulin was designated as the 'endpiece'. Current information reveals that what was referred to as the 'endpiece' did not contain C1 but did contain all of the C2 and some other complement components.

Bordet[6] believed alexine (i.e. complement) to be a transient colloidal state of the serum. By contrast, Ehrlich[7] hypothesized that complement represented a specific substance with the ability to induce lysis. Heidelberger[8] (Figure 7) at Columbia University designed investigations to determine whether complement was a distinct substance which could be measured with respect to weight and size. They showed that complement-containing sera added appreciable weight to specific precipitates formed with rabbit antipolysaccharide or antiprotein antibodies. Their classic experiments proved that complement was a real nitrogen-containing substance, or substances, with weight. Thus, the Ehrlich hypothesis rather than Bordet's theory of complement was substantiated. This discovery, and Pillemer and Ecker's[9] independent purification of the first component, enabled other investigators to purify and analyze the complement system.

The classical pathway of complement activation was described first by investigators using sheep red blood cells sensitized with specific antibody and lysed with guinea-pig or human complement. Coca[10] in 1914 described the third complement component and postulated an alternative pathway of complement activation by yeast cell walls, which should not involve C1 or C2.

The lack of advanced biochemical methods delayed demonstration that the complement system is protein and comprises multiple components. In the late 1920s, Ferrata, followed by Coca and Gordon, identified four complement components. By 1941, Pillemer and associates confirmed the protein nature of complement. In the

1960s, Nelson identified a minimum of six components in guinea pig serum that were requisite for hemolytic activity. Each of these was subsequently purified and characterized by Müller-Eberhard and colleagues. During this same period, Ueno and subsequently Mayer (Figures 8–12) elucidated the classical pathway's reaction sequence by combining partially purified components with antibody-sensitized sheep red blood cells.

Since these early studies, multiple (i.e. more than 20) complement proteins have been identified. These include C1qrs (Figure 13) C2, C3, C4, C5, C6, C7, C8 and C9. In addition to immune lysis, complement has many other functions, and is important in the biological amplification mechanism that is significant in resistance against infectious disease agents. Complement's mechanism of action in the various biological reactions in which it participates has occupied the attention of a host of investigators. In 1954, Pillemer et al.[11] (Figure 14) suggested the existence of a non-antibody-dependent protein in the serum that is significant for early defense of the host against bacteria and viruses. This protein was named 'properdin'. Pillemer et al.[11] first described properdin as a serum factor that activates complement without antibody. It was found to be a serum protein physiochemically, and immunologically distinct from the immunoglobulins. It participates in a non-specific manner in various types of immune reactions of normal serum. It acts in combination with certain inorganic ions and complement components that make up the so-called properdin system which constitutes a part of the natural defense mechanism of the blood. In later years, the properdin system came to be known as the alternative pathway of complement activation.

Complement (C) is a system of 20 soluble plasma and other body fluid proteins together with cellular receptors for many of them and regulatory proteins found on blood and other tissue cells. These proteins play a critical role in aiding phagocytosis of immune complexes, which activate the complement system. These molecules and their fragments, resulting from the activation process, are significant in the regulation of cellular immune responsiveness. Once complement proteins identify and combine with target substance, serine proteases are activated. This leads ultimately to the assembly of C3 convertase, a protease on the surface of the target substance. The enzyme cleaves C3, yielding a C3b fragment that is bound to the target

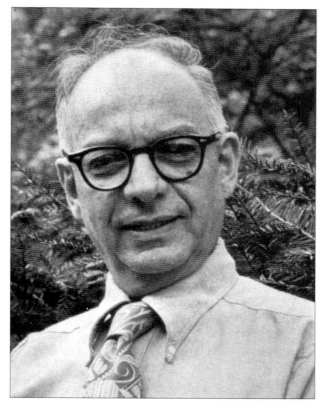

Figure 8 Manfred Mayer, student of Heidelberger and professor at Johns Hopkins University, who described the role of complement in immune lysis

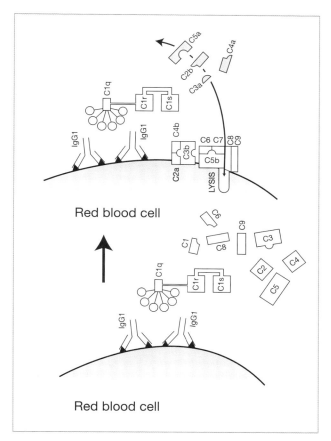

Figure 9 Classical pathway of complement activation

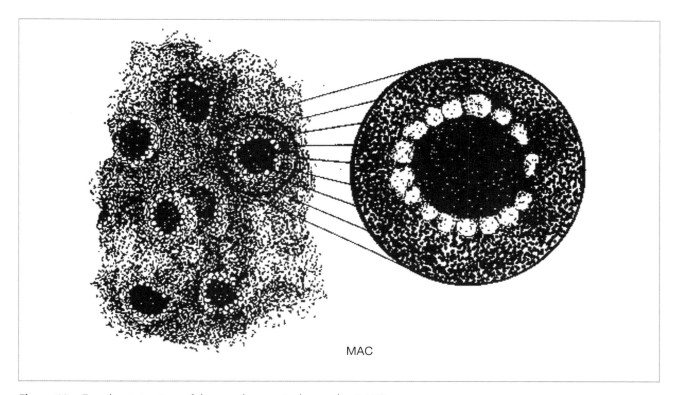

Figure 10 Doughnut structure of the membrane attack complex (MAC)

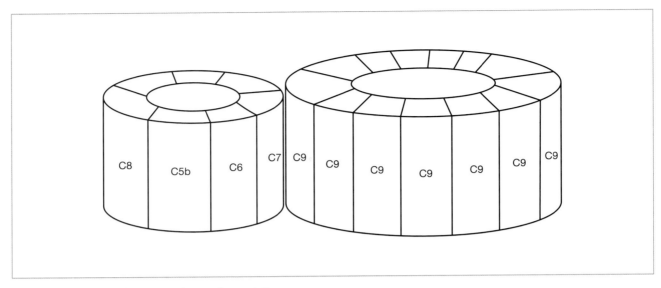

Figure 11 The membrane attack complex (MAC)

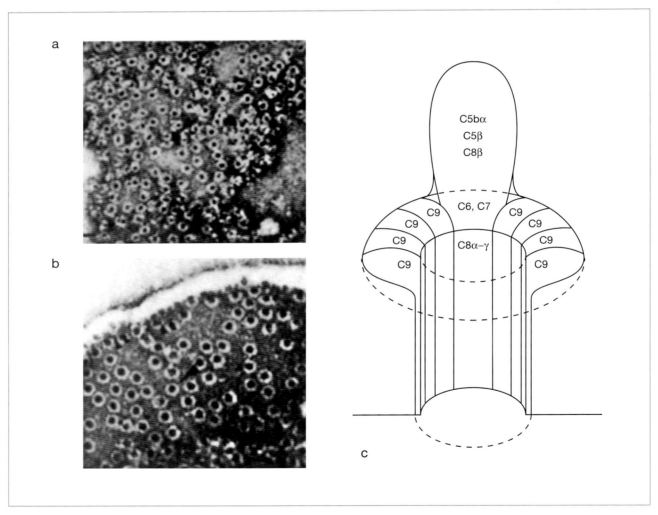

Figure 12 Perforations in a cell membrane (a) and (b) induced by complement (poly C9 tubular complexes). (c) Model of the membrane attack complex (MAC) subunit arrangement

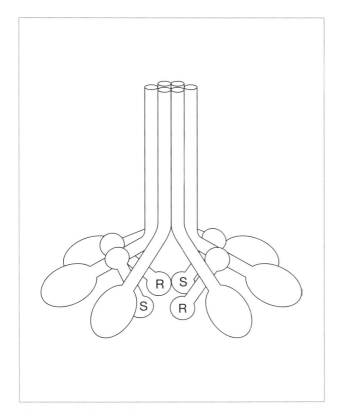

Figure 13 C1 complex

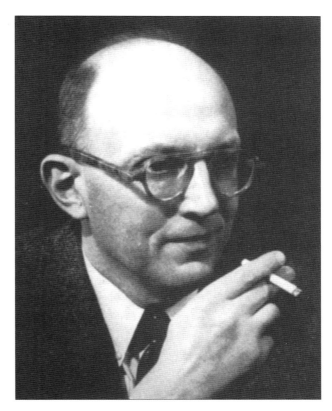

Figure 14 Louis Pillemer, who described properdin and the alternative pathway of complement activation

through a covalent linkage. C3b or C3bi bound to phagocytic cell surfaces become ligands for C3 receptors, as well as binding sites for C5. The union of C5b with C6, C7, C8 and C9 generates the membrane attack complex (MAC) which may associate with the cell's lipid bilayer membrane to produce lysis, which is critical in resistance against certain species of bacteria. The complement proteins are significant, non-specific mediators of humoral immunity. Multiple substances may trigger the complement system. There are two pathways of complement activation. The first is termed the classical pathway, in which an antigen, e.g. red blood cell, and antibody combine and fix the first subcomponent designated C1q. This is followed in sequence: C1qrs, 4, 2, 3, 5, 6, 7, 8, 9, to produce lysis. The alternative pathway does not utilize C1, 4 and 2 components. Bacterial products such as endotoxin and other agents may activate this pathway through C3. There are numerous biological activities associated with complement besides immune lysis. These include the formation of anaphylatoxin, chemotaxis, opsonization, phagocytosis, bacteriolysis, hemolysis and other amplification mechanisms.

The **classical pathway of complement** is a mechanism to activate C3 through participation by the serum proteins C1, C4 and C2. Either IgM or a doublet of IgG may bind the C1 subcomponent C1q. Following subsequent activation of C1r and C1s, the two C1s substrates, C4 and C2, are cleaved. This yields C4b and C2a fragments that produce C4b2a, known as C3 convertase. It activates opsonization, chemotaxis of leukocytes, increased permeability of vessels and cell lysis. Activators of the classical pathway include IgM, IgG, staphylococcal protein A, C-reactive protein and DNA. C1 inhibitor blocks the classical pathway by separating C1r and C1s from C1q. C4-binding protein also blocks the classical pathway by linking to C4b, separating it from C2a and permitting factor I to split the C4b heavy chain to yield C4bi, which is unable to unite with C2a, thereby inhibiting the classical pathway. The first complement component designated C1 consists of a complex of three separate proteins denoted by C1q, C1r and C1s. The formation of an active fragment following proteolysis of a component such as C3 is designated by a lower case letter such as C3a and C3b (Figures 11–13).

Active fragments degrade either spontaneously or by the action of serum proteases. Inactive fragments are designated by i, such as iC3b. The interaction of antibody with antigen forms antigen–antibody complexes that initiate the classical pathway. One molecule each of C1q and of C1s together with two molecules of C1r constitute the C1 complex or **recognition** unit. C1q facilitates recognition unit binding to cell surface antigen–antibody complexes. To launch the classical complement cascade, C1q must link to two IgG antibodies through their Fc regions. By contrast, one pentameric IgM molecule attached to a cell surface may interact with C1q to initiate the classical pathway. Binding of C1q activates C1r to become activated $C\overline{1}r$. This in turn activates C1s.

To create the **activation unit**, $C\overline{1}s$ splits C4 to produce C4a and C4b and C2 to form C2a and C2b. The ability of a single recognition unit to split numerous C2 and C4 molecules represents an amplification mechanism in the cascade. The union of C4b and C2a produces C4b2a which is known as **C3 convertase**. C4b2a binds to the cell membrane and splits C3 into C3a and C3b fragments. The ability of C4b2a to cleave multiple C3 molecules represents another amplification mechanism. The interaction of C3b with C4b2a bound to the cell membrane produces a complete activation unit, C4b2a3b, which is termed C5 convertase. It splits C5 into C5a and C5b fragments and represents yet another amplification mechanism because a single molecule of C5 convertase may cleave multiple C5 molecules.

Pillemer et al.[11] proposed an alternative mechanism of complement activation which they termed the 'properdin pathway' (Figures 15 and 16). Since antibody was not involved, they predicted that this alternative pathway was significant in non-specific immunity. They conceived this mechanism to have significance in resistance against infectious diseases and neoplasms. The alternative pathway hypothesis was challenged in the late 1950s but came to be accepted in the 1960s once C2 and C4 genetically deficient sera were described. When target cells stimulate the production of complement-fixing antibody of the IgG or IgM class, the classical complement pathway is activated. By contrast, antibody classes that do not fix complement by the classic

pathway, e.g. IgA, as well as selected non-antibody substances, may activate the alternative pathway. The separate complement proteins began to be isolated and identified immunologically and the biochemistry of their reactions determined. Further clarification of the alternative pathway evolved in the 1970s[12].

In 1953, Pillemer reported that zymosan depleted C3 from serum without affecting C1, C2 and C4 levels. He also described a properdin pathway of complement activation with properdin as the activating factor. Louis Pillemer was a professor of biochemistry at Case Western Reserve in Cleveland, Ohio when he identified a new protein, which he believed served as an alternative non-specific defense mechanism to trigger complement action without antibody. His theory was hailed at first, but then opinion turned against him. In 1958, Nelson challenged Pillemer's interpretation of these data and suggested that the properdin system was in fact the classical pathway activated by antibodies to zymosan. In later years, the properdin system came to be known as the 'alternative pathway of complement activation'.

The **doughnut structure** is the assembly and insertion of complement C9 protein monomers into a cell membrane to produce a transmembrane pore which leads to cell destruction through the cytolytic action of the complement cascade.

Complement multimer is a doughnut-shaped configuration as a part of the complement reaction sequence.

The **membrane attack complex (MAC)** consists of the five terminal proteins C5, C6, C7, C8 and C9 associated into MAC on a target cell membrane to mediate injury. Initiation of the MAC assembly begins with C5 cleavage into C5a and C5b fragments. A $(C5b678)_1(C9)_n$ complex then either forms on natural membranes or, in their absence, may combine with such plasma inhibitors as lipoproteins, antithrombin III and S protein. cDNA sequencing reveals the primary structure of all five related complement proteins. C9 and C8 α-proteins resemble each other not only structurally but also in sequence homologies. Both bind calcium and furnish domains that bind lipid, enabling MAC to attach to the membrane.

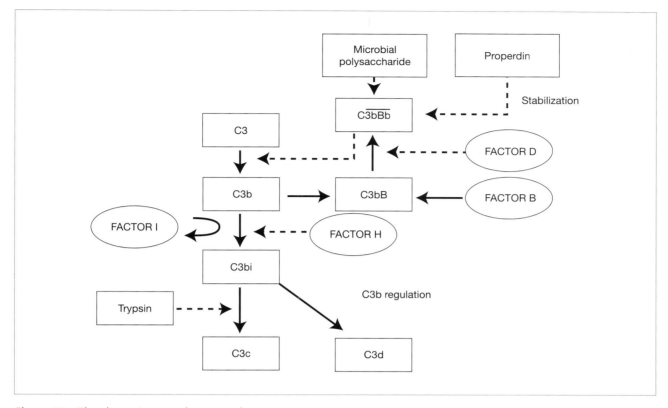

Figure 15 The alternative complement pathway

Mechanisms proposed for complement-mediated cytolysis include extrinsic protein channel incorporation into the plasma membrane or membrane deformation and destruction. Central regions of C6, C7, C8α, C8β and C9 have been postulated to contain amphiphilic structures that may be membrane anchors.

A single C9 molecule per C5b–8 leads to erythrocyte lysis. C8 polymerization is not required. Gram-negative bacteria, which have both outer and inner membranes, resist complement action by lengthening surface carbohydrate content, which interferes with MAC binding. MAC assembly and insertion into the outer membrane are requisite for lysis of bacteria. Nucleated cells may rid their surfaces of MAC through endocytosis or exocytosis. Platelets have provided much data concerning sublytic actions of C5b–9 proteins.

Control proteins acting at different levels may inhibit killing of homologous cells mediated by MAC. Besides C8-binding protein or homologous restriction factor (HRF) found on human erythrocyte membranes, the functionally similar but smaller phosphatidylinositol glycan (PIG)-tailed membrane

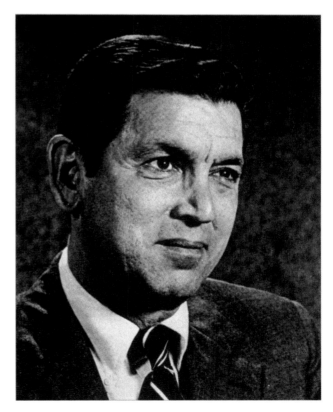

Figure 16 Irwin Lepow, co-worker of Pillemer, who was also instrumental in describing the alternative pathway

protein harnesses complement-induced cell lysis. Sublytic actions of MAC may be of greater consequence for host cells than are its cytotoxic effects.

C1 is a 750-kDa multimeric molecule comprising one C1q subcomponent, two C1r and two C1s subcomponents. The classical pathway of complement activation begins with the binding of C1q to IgM or IgG molecules. C1q, C1r and C1s form a macromolecular complex in a Ca^{2+}-dependent manner. The 400-kDa C1q molecule possesses three separate polypeptide chains that unite into a heterotrimeric structure resembling stems which contain an amino terminal in triple helix, and a globular structure at the carboxy terminus that resembles a tulip. Six of these tulip-like structures with globular heads and stems form a circular and symmetric molecular complex in the C1q molecule. There is a central core. The serine esterase molecules designated C1r and C1s are needed for the complement cascade to progress. These 85-kDa proteins that are single chains unite in the presence of calcium to produce a tetramer comprising two C1r and two C1s subcomponents to form a structure that is flexible and has a C1s–C1r–C1r–C1s sequence. When at least two C1q globular regions bind to IgM or IgG molecules, the C1r in a tetramer associated with the C1q molecule becomes activated, leading to splitting of the C1r molecules in the tetramer with the formation of a 57-kDa and a 28-kDa chain. The latter, termed C1r, functions as a serine esterase, splitting the C1s molecules into 57-kDa and 28-kDa chains. The 28-kDa chain derived from the cleavage of C1̄s molecules, designated C1s, also functions as a serine esterase, cleaving C4 and C2 and causing progression of the classical complement pathway cascade.

Properdin (factor P) is a globulin in normal serum that has a central role in activation of the alternative complement pathway activation. Additional factors such as magnesium ions are required for properdin activity. It is an alternative complement pathway protein that has a significant role in resistance against infection. It combines with and stabilizes the C3 convertase of the alternative pathway, which is designated C3bBb. It is a 441-amino acid residue polypeptide chain with two points where N-linked oligosaccharides may become attached. Electron microscopy

reveals it to have a cyclic oligomer conformation. Molecules are composed of six repeating 60-residue motifs which are homologous to 60 amino acids at C7, C8α and C8β amino- and carboxy-terminal ends and the C9 amino-terminal end.

The **properdin system** is an older term for the alternative complement pathway. It consists of several proteins that are significant in resistance against infection. The first protein to be discovered was properdin. The properdin system also consists of factor B, a 95-kDa β_2-globulin which is also termed C3 proactivator, glycine-rich β glycoprotein or β_2 glycoprotein II. Properdin factor D is a 25-kDa, α-globulin which is also termed C3 proactivator convertase or glycine-rich β glycoproteinase. The properdin system, or alternative pathway, does not require the participation of antibody to activate complement. It may be activated by endotoxin or other substances (see alternative complement pathway).

The **alternative complement pathway** (Figure 15) is a non-antibody dependent pathway for complement activation in which the early components C1, C2 and C4 are not required. It involves the protein properdin factor D, properdin factor B and C3b, leading to C3 activation and continuing to C9 in a manner identical to that which takes place in the activation of complement by the classical pathway. Substances such as endotoxin, human IgA, microbial polysaccharides and other agents may activate complement by the alternative pathway. The C3bB complex forms as C3b combines with factor B. Factor D splits factor B in the complex to yield the Bb active fragment that remains linked to C3b and Ba, which is inactive and is split off. C3bBb, the alternative pathway C3 convertase, splits C3 into C3b and C3a, thereby producing more C3bBb, which represents a positive feedback loop (Figures 11–15). Factor I, when accompanied by factor H, splits C3b's heavy chain to yield C3bi, which is unable to anchor Bb, thereby inhibiting the alternative pathway. Properdin and C3 nephritic factor stabilize C3bBb. C3 convertase stabilized by properdin activates complement's late components, resulting in opsonization, chemotaxis of leukocytes, enhanced permeability and cytolysis. Properdin, IgA, IgG, lipopolysaccharide and snake venom can initiate the alternaive pathway. Trypsin-related enzymes can activate both pathways. The alternative pathway is the activation of complement not by antibody but through the binding of complement protein C3b to the surface of a pathogenic microorganism. This innate immune mechanism amplifies complement activation through the classical pathway.

When target cells stimulate the production of complement-fixing antibodies of the IgG or IgM class, complement is fixed by the classical pathway. By contrast, when cells stimulate the production of antibody classes that do not fix complement by the classic pathway, e.g. IgA, or if lysis is required prior to expression of an antibody response, the alternative pathway is activated.

Müller-Eberhard's (Figure 17) subsequent purification of C3 proactivator and proposal that the C3 activator system is an alternative pathway of complement activation substantiated Pillemer's original concept. Regrettably, Pillemer's untimely death preceded the proof that his hypothesis was correct. His colleague and student, Irwin Lepow, prepared nine of his papers for posthumous publication. Lepow (Figure 16) and others published details of the characteristics of properdin in 1968, and in 1970 several laboratories correctly described its role as an alternative pathway to complement activation. Pillemer's theories were vindicated, the truth being a synthesis of the opposing points of view. Dr Lepow paid tribute to Pillemer in his presidential address to the American Association of Immunologists in 1980.

A century of investigations has revealed that more than 20 soluble plasma and other body fluid proteins, together with an equivalent number of cell receptors and control proteins found on blood and other tissue cells, constitute the complement system[13]. These proteins play a critical role in the phagocytosis of immune complexes, which activate the complement system. These molecules and their fragments resulting from the activation process are significant in the regulation of cellular immune responsiveness. Once complement proteins identify and combine with the target substance, serine proteases are activated. This leads ultimately to the assembly of C3 convertase, a protease on the surface of the target substance. The enzyme cleaves C3, yielding the C3b fragment that is bound to the

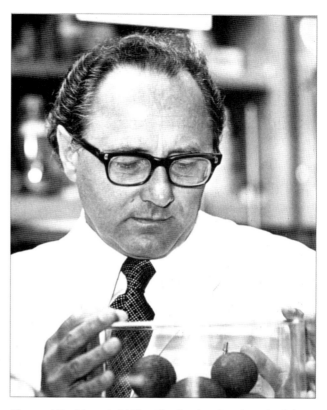

Figure 17 Hans J. Müller-Eberhard, who described later complement components

target through a covalent linkage. C3b or iC3b bound to phagocytic cell surfaces become ligands for C3 receptors as well as binding sites for C5. The union of C5b with C6, C7, C8 and C9 generates the membrane attack complex (MAC), which may associate with the cell's lipid bilayer membrane to produce lysis, which is critical in resistance against certain species of bacteria (Figures 18 and 19).

The **lectin pathway of complement activation** is a mechanism, not involving antibody, that is initiated by the binding of microbial polysaccharide to circulating lectins such as mannose-binding lectin (MBL) which structurally resembles C1q. Similar to C1q, it activates the C1r–C1s enzyme complex or another serine esterase, termed mannose-binding protein-associated serine esterase. Thereafter, all steps of the lectin pathway are the same as in the classical pathway following cleavage of C4.

Multiple plasma proteins may be activated during inflammation. Immune complexes activate the classical

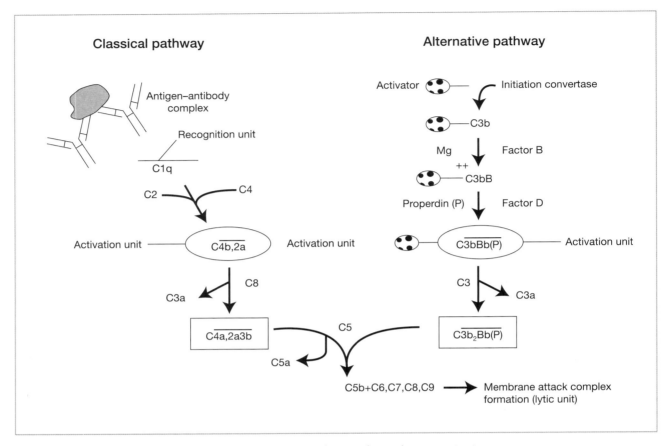

Figure 18 A comparison of the classical and alternative pathways of complement activation

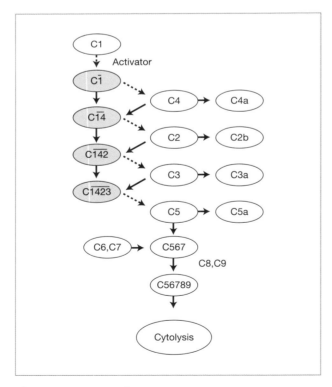

Figure 19 Immune lysis

pathway of complement whereas bacterial products activate the alternative pathway without participation by specific antibody. Many antimicrobial effects are produced by complement. C5a, C5b67 and C3a induce chemotaxis of leukocytes. C3b has opsonic properties. The membrane attack complex leads to lysis of bacterial cells. Complement also facilitates the antimicrobial effects of polymorphonuclear neutrophils (PMNs) and macrophages through the alternative pathway.

Thus, it is apparent that complement has captured the interest of an eclectic group of investigators from biochemists to internists. Indeed, the century-old science has emerged as the distinct and independent discipline of 'complementology', with its proponents often referring to themselves as 'complementologists'. The future holds bright prospects that should further elucidate the significant role that the complement system plays in molecular and cellular biology, as well as in health and disease (Table 1).

Table 1 Three pathways of complement system activation

	Classical pathway	Alternative pathway	Lectin pathway
Activated by	binding of antibody molecules (specifically IgM and IgG1, IgG2, IgG3) to a foreign particle	invading microorganisms	binding of MBP to the mannose groups of carbohydrates on microorganisms
Activation mechanism	antibody-dependent	antibody-independent	antibody-independent
Limb of immunity	adaptive immune response	innate immune response	innate immune response
Components	C1 (C1q, C1r, C1s) to C9	factors B, D, P, H, I	C1 (C1r, C1s) to C9
Components that initiate enzyme cascade	C1 (q,r,s), C4, C2	C3, B, D	Lectin, MASP1, MASP2, C4, C2
C3 convertase	C4bC2a, C2b	C3bBb	C2b, C4bC2a
C5 convertase	C4bC2aC3b	C3bBbC3b	C4bC2aC3b
Terminal components	C5–C9, MAC (C5b678[9]$_n$)	C5–C9, MAC (C5b678[9]$_n$)	C5–C9, (C5b678[9]$_n$)

B, plasma factor B; D, plasma protease factor D; P, properdin; H, protein H; I, factor I; MBP, mannose-binding protein; MASP, MBP-associated serine protease; MAC, membrane attack complex

REFERENCES

1. Buchner H. Über die bakterientötende Wirkung des zellenfreien Blutserums. *Zentralbl Bakteriol* 1889;5:817-23; 1889;6:1–11

2. Bordet J. Contribution à l'étude du serum chez les animaux vaccines. *Ann Soc R Sci Med Natl Brux* 1895;4:455–530

3. Ehrlich P. *Gesammelte Arbeiten zur Immunitätsforschung.* Berlin: August Hirschwald, 1904

4. Bordet J, Gengou O. Sur l'existence de substances sensibilisatrices dans la plupart des serums antimicrobiens. *Ann Inst Pasteur* 1901;15:289–302

5. Ferrata A. Die Unwirksamkeit der komplexen Hamolysine in salzfreien Lösungen und ihre Ursache. *Berl Klin Wochenschr* 1907;44:366

6. Bordet J. *Studies in Immunity* (collected and transl. by Gay FP). New York: Wiley, 1909:1–545

7. Ehrlich P. *Collected Studies on Immunity* (transl. by Bolduan C); with several new contributions including a chapter written expressly for this edition by Ehrlich P). New York: Wiley, 1906:1–586

8. Heidelberger M. *Lectures in Immunochemistry.* New York: Academic Press, 1956:1–150

9. Pillemer L, Ecker EE, Oncley JL, Cohn EJ. The preparation and physicochemical characterization of the serum protein components of human complement. *J Exp Med* 1941;74:297–308

10. Coca AF. A study of the anticomplementary action of yeast of certain bacteria and of cobra venom. *Z Immunitatsforsch Exp Ther* 1914;21:604

11. Pillemer L, Blum L, Lepow IH, *et al*. The properdin system and immunity: demonstration and isolation of a new serum protein, properdin, and its role in immune phenomena. *Science* 1954;120:279–85

12. Maves KK, Weiler J. Properdin: approaching four decades of research. *Immunol Res* 1993;12:233–43

13. Sim RB. Complement, classical pathway. In Roitt IM, Delves PJ, eds. *Encyclopedia of Immunology.* London: Academic Press

CHAPTER 5

Anaphylaxis

Charles Richet (1850–1935) and Paul Portier, in 1902, observed that the injection of toxic extracts from the tentacles of various sea anemones or eel serum into dogs, which had 3 weeks previously received a smaller injection of the same antigen, produced severe symptoms, and in some cases death[1]. These two physiologists from the University of Paris had been asked by the Prince of Monaco to study the toxic properties of the *Physalia* found in the South Seas. What had been intended to result in a state of protective immunity, had, much to their surprise, resulted in a state of hyper-susceptibility of the tissues of the animals receiving the injections. The administration of this same extract into normal animals produced no adverse effect.

In 1837, Magendie (Figure 1) noted the violent death of rabbits following repeated injections of egg albumin, and published his findings in 1839[2]. Charles Richet (Figures 2–6) and Paul Portier (Figure 7)

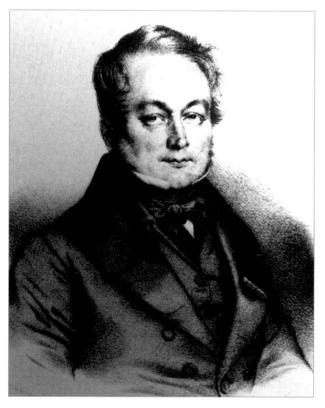

Figure 1 F. Magendie, who first observed anaphylaxis in rabbits in 1837

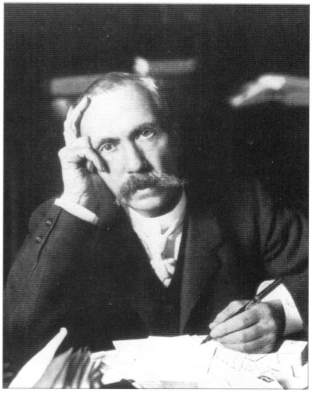

Figure 2 Charles Richet, Nobel Laureate, for his discoveries related to anaphylaxis

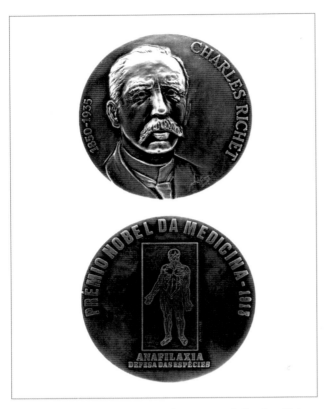

Figure 3 Medallion bearing the image of Charles Richet, commemorating his research on anaphylaxis

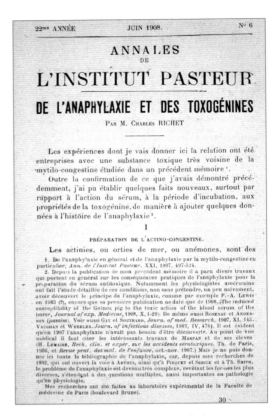

Figure 4 Richet's publication on anaphylaxis

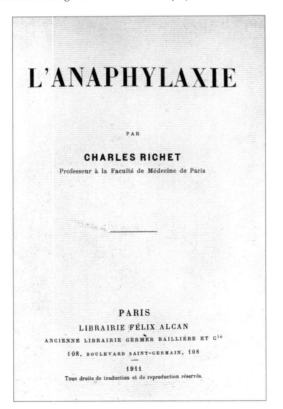

Figure 5 A monograph by Charles Richet on anaphylaxis

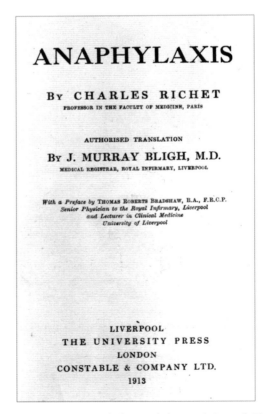

Figure 6 Dr Murray Bligh's English translation of Charles Richet's book on anaphylaxis

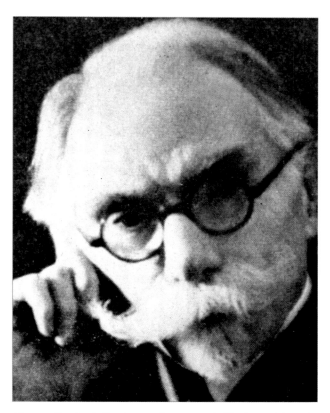

Figure 7 Paul Portier, colleague of Charles Richet in research on anaphylaxis

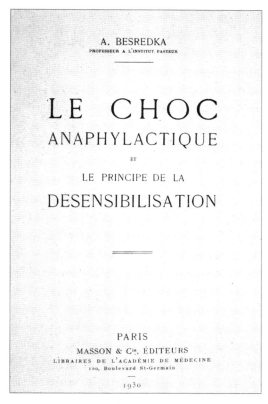

A. BESREDKA
PROFESSEUR A L'INSTITUT PASTEUR

LE CHOC
ANAPHYLACTIQUE
ET
LE PRINCIPE DE LA
DESENSIBILISATION

PARIS
MASSON & Cⁱᵉ, ÉDITEURS
LIBRAIRES DE L'ACADÉMIE DE MÉDECINE
120, Boulevard St-Germain
1930

Figure 8 Besredka's book on anaphylactic shock

decided to consider that state of hypersusceptibility as the opposite of protection or prophylaxis. They used the prefix 'ana', derived from the Greek, which does not mean against. Although chosen in error, its use became well established to imply antibody-mediated hypersensitivity in man and other animals. Richet continued to study the phenomenon and was awarded the Nobel Prize for his work in 1913. A. Besredka wrote extensively on anaphylaxis (Figures 8–10).

Henry Hallett Dale (1875–1968) (Figures 11 and 12), British investigator who made a wide range of scientific contributions including work on the chemistry of nerve impulse transmission, the discovery of histamine and the development of an *in vitro* assay for anaphylaxis termed 'the Schultz–Dale test for anaphylaxis'. He received a Nobel Prize in Medicine or Physiology in 1935. In the **Schultz–Dale test**, strong contraction of the isolated uterine horn muscle of a virgin guinea-pig that has been either actively or passively sensitized occurs following the addition of specific antigen to the 37°C tissue bath in which it is suspended. Muscle contraction is caused by the release of histamine and other pharmacological mediators of immediate hypersensitivity following antigen interaction with antibody fixed to tissue cells.

Following the demonstration of the three major classes of immunoglobulin, IgG, IgA and IgM, a patient with multiple myeloma was found to have significant quantities of antibody or immunoglobulin in the serum which did not cross-react with the antisera against the three known major immunoglobulin classes. Kimishige and Terako Ishizaka (Figure 13) described this newly discovered immunoglobulin as IgE[3]. It was found to occur in minute quantities in all normal human sera examined, and to be responsible for the mediation of anaphylaxis in man. Although certain IgG antibodies are associated with anaphylactic reactions in guinea pigs, human anaphylaxis is dependent upon these IgE antibodies which were formerly known as reagins, a group of antibodies with physical and biological characteristics different from those producing the classical serological reactions such as precipitation and agglutination. The IgE antibodies, which have the basic four-chain unit

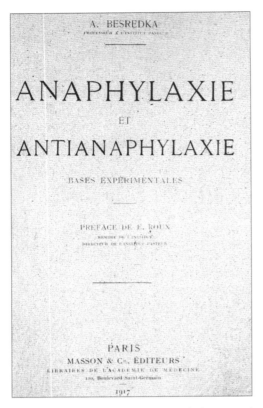

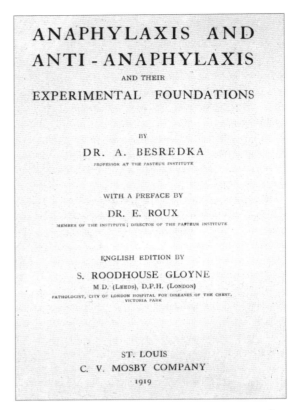

Figure 9 Besredka's book on anaphylaxis and anti-anaphylaxis

Figure 10 Besredka's book on anaphylaxis and anti-anaphylaxis in the English translation

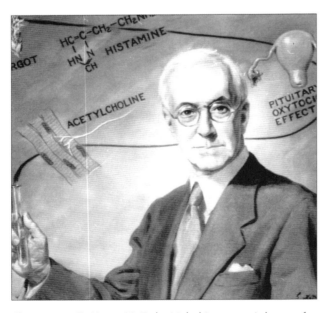

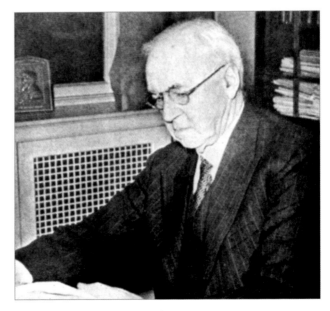

Figure 11 Sir Henry H. Dale, Nobel Laureate, is known for the *in vitro* anaphylaxis assay, the Shultz–Dale test

Figure 12 Sir Henry H. Dale

structure of immunoglobulin molecules, are bound through their Fc receptors to mast cells of the tissue or basophils of the blood. Following the combination of the antigen-binding receptors with antigen or allergen, the pharmacological mediators stored in granules in the cytoplasm of the cells are released, resulting in increased vascular permeability, smooth muscle contraction and vasomotor shock.

Kimishige Ishizaka (1925–) and Terako Ishizaka, discovered IgE and have contributed to elucidation of its function.

Among the many substances in clinical use that are known to induce hypersensitivity of the anaphylactic type, penicillin and related antibiotic substances are among the more notorious. This led to the search for many substitute drugs to circumvent allergic reactions.

Charles Robert Richet (1850–1935), Parisian physician who became professor of physiology at the University of Paris. He was interested in the physiology of toxins, and with Portier discovered anaphylaxis, for which he was awarded the Nobel Prize in Medicine or Physiology in 1913. He and Portier discovered anaphylaxis in dogs exposed to the toxins of murine invertebrates to which they had been previously sensitized. Thus, an immune type reaction that was harmful rather than protective was demonstrated. Experimental anaphylaxis was later shown to be similar to certain types which lent clinical as well as theoretical significance to the discovery. *L'Anaphylaxie*, 1911.

Paul Jules Portier (1866–1968), French physiologist who, with Richet, was among the first to describe anaphylaxis.

Hypersensitivity is increased reactivity or increased sensitivity by the animal body to an antigen to which it has been previously exposed. The term is often used as a synonym for allergy, which describes a state of altered reactivity to an antigen. Hypersensitivity has been divided into categories based upon whether it can be passively transferred by antibodies or by specifically immune lymphoid cells. The most widely adopted current classification is that of Coombs and Gell that designates immunoglobulin-mediated (immediate) hypersensitivity reactions as types I, II and III and lymphoid cell-mediated (delayed-type) hypersensitivity/cell-mediated immunity as a type IV reaction. 'Hypersensitivity' generally represents the 'dark side', signifying the undesirable aspects of an immune reaction, whereas the term 'immunity' implies a desirable effect.

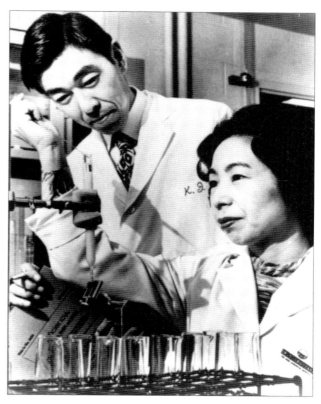

Figure 13 Kimishige and Terako Ishizaka, discoverers of immunoglobulin E. In 1939, Teselius, in Sweden, had discovered that antibody was immunoglobulin. Structures of the molecules were established for IgG and IgM, and IgA was investigated. Because it appears in such tiny amounts in serum, IgE was not described until 1967, when the Ishizakas, and Johansson and Bennich in Sweden, found myeloma proteins that were different from the three main classes and which, they discovered, had the reaginic antibody properties associated with anaphylaxis and atopic (type I hypersensitivity) allergic reactions. IgD was also discovered during the same decade

Sensitization refers to exposure of an animal to an antigen for the first time in order that subsequent or secondary exposure to the same antigen will lead to a greater response. The term has been used especially when the reaction induced is more of a hypersensitive or allergic nature than of an immune protective type of response. Thus, an allergic response may be induced in a host sensitized by prior exposure to the same allergen.

Passive transfer is the transfer of immunity or hypersensitivity from an immune or sensitized animal to a previously non-immune or unsensitized (and preferably syngeneic) recipient animal by serum containing specific antibodies or by specifically immune lymphoid cells. The transfer of immunity by lymphoid cells is referred to as adoptive immunization. Humoral immunity and antibody-mediated hypersensitivity reactions are transferred with serum, whereas delayed-type hypersensitivity, including contact hypersensitivity, is transferred with lymphoid cells. Passive transfer was used to help delineate which immune and hypersensitivity reactions were mediated by cells and which were mediated by serum.

Immediate hypersensitivity is an antibody-mediated hypersensitivity. In man, this homocytotrophic antibody is IgE and in certain other species IgG1. The IgE antibodies are attached to mast cells through their Fc receptors. Once the Fab regions of the mast cell-bound IgE molecules interact with specific antigen, vasoactive amines are released from the cytoplasmic granules as described under type I hypersensitivity reactions. The term 'immediate' is used to indicate that this type of reaction occurs within seconds to minutes following contact of a cell-fixed IgE antibody with antigen. Skin tests and the radioallergosorbent test (RAST) are useful to detect immediate hypersensitivity in humans, and passive cutaneous anaphylaxis reveals immediate hypersensitivity in selected other species. Examples of immediate hypersensitivity in humans include the classic anaphylactic reaction to penicillin administration, hay fever and environmental allergens such as tree and grass pollens, bee stings, etc.

The **triple response of Lewis** refers to skin changes in immediate hypersensitivity illustrated by striking the skin with a sharp object such as the side of a ruler. The first response termed the 'stroke response' is caused by the production of histamine and related mediators at the point of contact with the skin. The second response is a flare produced by vasodilatation, and resembles a red halo. The third response is a wheal characterized by swelling and blanching, induced by histamine from mast cell degranulation. The swelling is attributable to edema between the junctions of cells that become rich in protein and fluid.

Type I anaphylactic hypersensitivity is a reaction mediated by IgE antibodies reactive with specific allergens (antigens that induce allergy) attached to basophil or mast cell Fc receptors. Cross-linking of the cell-bound IgE antibodies by antigen is followed by mast cell or basophil degranulation, with release of pharmacological mediators. These mediators include vasoactive amines such as histamine, which causes increased vascular permeability, vasodilatation, bronchial spasm and mucus secretion (Figures 14 and 15). Secondary mediators of type I hypersensitivity include leukotrienes, prostaglandin D_2, platelet-activating factor and various cytokines. Systemic anaphylaxis is a serious clinical problem and can follow the injection of protein antigens, such as antitoxin, or of drugs, such as penicillin.

Skin-sensitizing antibody is an antibody, usually of the IgE class, that binds to the Fc receptors of mast cells in the skin, thereby conditioning this area of skin for a type I immediate hypersensitivity reaction following cross-linking of the IgE Fab regions by a specific allergen (antigen). In guinea pig skin, human IgG1 antibodies may be used to induce passive cutaneous anaphylaxis.

Dander antigen is a combination of debris such as desquamated epithelial cells, microorganisms, hair and other materials trapped in perspiration and sebum that are constantly deleted from the skin. Dander antigens may induce immediate, IgE-mediated, type I hypersensitivity reactions in atopic individuals.

Anaphylaxis is a shock reaction that occurs within seconds following the injection of an antigen or drug, or after a bee sting, to which the susceptible subject has IgE-specific antibodies. There is embarrassed respiration due to laryngeal and bronchial constriction, and shock associated with decreased blood pressure. Signs and symptoms differ among species based on the primary target organs or tissues. Whereas IgE is the anaphylactic antibody in man, IgG1 may mediate anaphylaxis in selected other species. Type I hypersensitivity occurs following the cross-linking of IgE antibodies by a specific antigen or allergen on the surfaces of basophils in the blood, or mast cells in the tissues. This causes the release of the pharmacological mediators of immediate hypersensitivity, with a reaction occurring within seconds of contact with antigen or allergen (Figures 14 and 15). Eosinophils, chemotactic factor, heparin, histamine and serotonin, together with selected other substances, are released during the primary response. Acute-phase reactants are formed

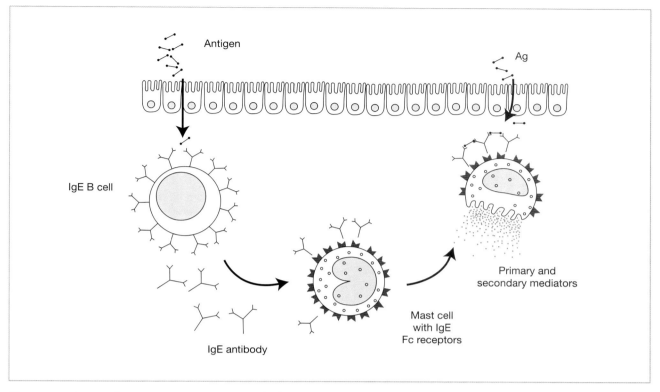

Figure 14 A type I hypersensitivity reaction in which antigen molecules cross-link IgE molecules on the surface of mast cells, resulting in their degranulation with the release of both primary and secondary mediators of anaphylaxis

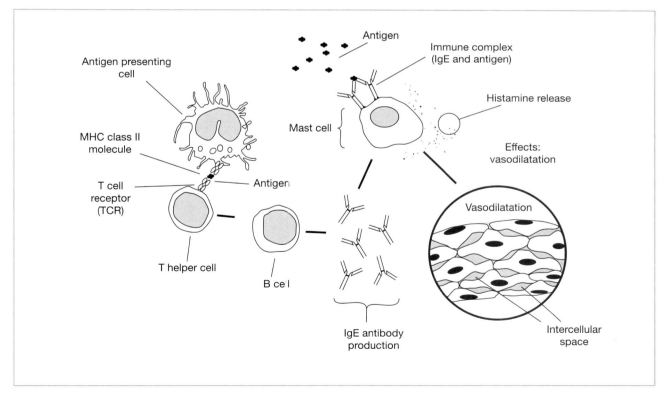

Figure 15 Schematic representation of events that follow degranulation of mast cells in tissues, resulting in vasodilatation of capillaries, leading to changes associated with type I hypersensitivity reactions in tissues

and released in the secondary response. Secondary mediators include slow-reacting substance of anaphylaxis (SRS-A), bradykinin and platelet-activating factor. In addition to systemic anaphylaxis described above, local anaphylaxis may occur in the skin, gut or nasal mucosa following contact with the antigen. The skin reaction, called urticaria, consists of a raised wheal surrounded by an area of erythema. Cytotoxic anaphylaxis follows the interaction of antibodies with cell surface antigens (see also aggregate anaphylaxis).

Anaphylactic shock is cardiovascular collapse and suffocation attributable to tracheal swelling that results from a systemic anaphylactic (immediate hypersensitivity) reaction following an antigen that has been systemically administered. This allergic reaction is a consequence of the binding of antigen to IgE antibodies on mast cells in the connective tissue throughout the body, resulting in a disseminated release of inflammatory mediators.

Arachidonic acid (AA) and leukotrienes are critical constituents of mammalian cell membranes. AA is released from membrane phospholipids as a consequence of membrane alterations or receptor-mediated signaling that leads to activation of phospholipase A_2 (PLA_2). Oxidative metabolism of AA through cyclooxygenase leads to the formation of various prostaglandins via the cytochrome P450 system or through one of the lipoxygenases. Molecules derived from the lipoxygenase pathway of arachidonic acid are termed leukotrienes (LTs). They are derived from the combined actions of 5-lipoxygenase (5-LOX) and 5-LOX-activating protein (FLAP). Initially, 5-hydroperoxyeicosatetraenoic (5-HPETE) acid is formed, followed by LTA_4. LTB_4 is an enzymatic, hydrolytic product of LTA_4. It differs from the other leukotrienes, LTC_4, LTD_4 and LTE_4, in that it does not have a peptide component. LTB_4 has powerful leukocytotropic effects. It is a powerful chemokinetic and chemotactic agent, with the ability to induce neutrophil aggregation, degranulation, hexose uptake and enhanced binding to endothelial cells. It can cause cation fluxes, augment cytoplasmic calcium concentrations, form intracellular pools and activate phosphatidylinositol hydrolysis. LTB_4 can act synergistically with prostaglandins E_1 (PGE_1) and PGE_2 to

induce macromolecule leakage in the skin through increased vascular permeability. When injected into the skin of a guinea pig, it can induce leukocytoclastic vasculitis. Human polymorphonuclear neutrophils have two sets of plasma membrane receptors. A high-affinity receptor set mediates aggregation, chemokinesis and increased surface adherence, whereas the low-affinity receptor set mediates degranulation and increased oxidative metabolism. A fraction of $CD4^+$ and $CD8^+$ T lymphocytes binds LTB_4, but LTB_4 receptors on lymphocytes remain to be characterized.

The **cyclooxygenase pathway** is the method whereby prostaglandins are produced by enzymatic metabolism of arachidonic acid derived from the cell membrane, as in type I (anaphylactic) hypersensitivity reactions.

The **lipoxygenase pathway** refers to the enzymatic metabolism of arachidonic acid derived from the cell membrane which is the source of leukotrienes.

Vasoactive amines are amino group-containing substances that include histamine and serotonin that cause dilatation of the peripheral vasculature and increase the permeability of capillaries and small vessels.

Hives is a wheal and flare reaction of the anaphylactic type produced in the skin as a consequence of histamine produced by activated mast cells. There is edema, erythema and pruritus. 'Hives' is a synonym for urticaria.

The **prick test** is an assay for immediate (IgE-mediated) hypersensitivity in humans. The epidermal surface of the skin on which drops of diluted antigen (allergen) are placed is pricked by a sterile needle passed through the allergen. The reaction produced is compared with one induced by histamine or another mast cell secretogogue. This test is convenient, simple and rapid, and produces little discomfort for the patient in comparison with the intradermal test. It may even be used for infants.

A **scratch test** is a skin test for the detection of IgE antibodies against a particular allergen that are anchored to mast cells in the skin. After scratching the skin with a needle, a minute amount of aqueous allergen is applied to the scratch site, and the area is observed for the development of urticaria manifested as a wheal and flare reaction. This signifies that the IgE antibodies are specific for the applied allergen and lead to the degranulation of mast cells with release of pharmacologic mediators of hypersensitivity, such as histamine.

Active anaphylaxis is an anaphylactic state induced by natural or experimental sensitization in atopic subjects or experimental animals.

Passive anaphylaxis is an anaphylactic reaction in an animal which has been administered an antigen after it has been conditioned by an inoculation of antibodies derived from an animal immunized against the antigen of interest.

Desensitization is a method of treatment used by allergists to diminish the effects of IgE-mediated type I hypersensitivity (Figure 16). The allergen to which an individual has been sensitized is repeatedly injected in a form that favors the generation of IgG (blocking) antibodies rather than IgE antibodies that mediate type I hypersensitivity in humans. This method has been used for many years to diminish the symptoms of atopy, such as asthma and allergic rhinitis, and to prevent anaphylaxis produced by bee venom. IgG antibodies are believed to prevent antigen interaction with IgE antibodies anchored to mast cell surfaces by intercepting the antigen molecules before they reach the cell-bound IgE. Thus, a type I hypersensitivity reaction of the anaphylactic type is prevented.

Systemic anaphylaxis is a type I, immediate, anaphylactic type of hypersensitivity mediated by IgE antibodies anchored to mast cells that become cross-linked by homologous antigen (allergen), causing release of the pharmacological mediators of immediate hypersensitivity, producing lesions in multiple organs and tissue sites. This is in contrast to local anaphylaxis, where the effects are produced in an isolated anatomical location. The intravenous administration of a serum product, antibiotic or other substance against which the patient has anaphylactic IgE-type hypersensitivity may lead to the symptoms of systemic anaphylaxis within seconds and may prove lethal.

Passive systemic anaphylaxis renders a normal, previously unsensitized animal susceptible to anaphy-

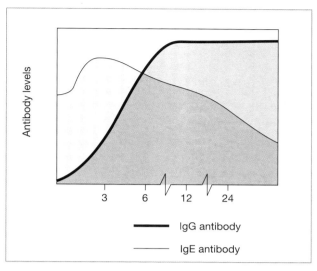

Figure 16 Desensitization

laxis by a passive injection, often intravenously, of homocytotrophic antibody derived from a sensitized animal, followed by antigen administration. Anaphylactic shock occurs soon after the passively transferred antibody and antigen interact *in vivo*, releasing the mediators of immediate hypersensitivity from mast cells of the host.

Generalized anaphylaxis occurs when the signs and symptoms of anaphylactic shock manifest within seconds to minutes following the administration of an antigen or allergen that interacts with specific IgE antibodies bound to mast cell or basophil surfaces, causing the release of pharmacologically active mediators that include vasoactive amines from their granules. Symptoms may vary from transient respiratory difficulties (due to contraction of the smooth muscle and terminal bronchioles) to even death.

Local anaphylaxis is a relatively common type I immediate hypersensitivity reaction. Local anaphylaxis is mediated by IgE cross-linked by allergen molecules at the surface of mast cells which then release histamines and other pharmacological mediators that produce signs and symptoms. The reaction occurs in a particular target organ such as the gastrointestinal tract, skin or nasal mucosa. Hay fever and asthma represent examples.

Basophils are polymorphonuclear leukocytes of the myeloid lineage with distinctive basophilic secondary granules in the cytoplasm that frequently overlie the nucleus. These granules are storage depots for heparin, histamine, platelet-activating factor and other pharmacological mediators of immediate hypersensitivity. Degranulation of the cells with release of these pharmacological mediators takes place following cross-linking by allergen or antigen of Fab regions of IgE receptor molecules bound through Fc receptors to the cell surface. They constitute less than 0.5% of peripheral blood leukocytes. Following cross-linking of surface-bound IgE molecules by specific allergen or antigen, granules are released by exocytosis. Substances liberated from the granules are pharmacological mediators of immediate (type I) anaphylactic hypersensitivity.

Aggregate anaphylaxis is a form of anaphylaxis caused by aggregates of antigen and antibody in the fluid phase. The aggregates bind complement-liberating complement fragments C3a, C5a and C4a, also called anaphylatoxins, which induce the release of mediators. Preformed aggregates of antigen–antibody complexes in the fluid phase fix complement. Fragments of complement components, the anaphylatoxins, may induce experimentally the release of mediators from mast cells. There is no evidence that these components play a role in anaphylactic reactions *in vivo*. Aggregates of antigen–IgG antibody, however, may induce anaphylaxis, whose manifestations are different in the various species.

Anaphylactoid reaction is a response resembling anaphylaxis, except that it is not attributable to an allergic reaction mediated by IgE antibody. It is due to the non-immunologic degranulation of mast cells such as that caused by drugs or chemical compounds like aspirin, radiocontrast media, chymopapain, bee or snake venom, and gum acacia, which cause release of the pharmacological mediators of immediate hypersensitivity including histamine and other vasoactive molecules.

An **eicosanoid** is an arachidonic acid-derived 20-carbon cyclic fatty acid. It is produced from membrane phospholipids. Eicosanoids, as well as other arachidonic acid metabolites, are elevated during shock and following injury and are site specific. They produce various effects, including bronchodilatation, bron-choconstriction, vasoconstriction and vasodilatation. Eicosanoids include leukotrienes, prostaglandins, thromboxanes and prostacyclin.

A **leukotriene** is a product of the enzymatic metabolism of arachidonic acid derived from the cell membrane. They are generated during an anaphylactic reaction by way of the lipoxygenase pathway. A leukotriene may include lipid mediators of inflammation and type 1 hypersensitivity. In the past they were referred to as slow-reacting substances of anaphylaxis (SRS-A). These lipid inflammatory mediators are produced by the lipoxygenase pathway in various types of cells. Most cells synthesize plentiful amounts of leukotriene C (LTC) and its breakdown products LTD and LTE that bind to smooth muscle cell receptors to produce prolonged bronchoconstruction. Leukotrienes play a significant role in the pathogenesis of bronchial asthma. Slow-reacting substance of anaphylaxis, used previously, represented the collective action of LTD and LTE (refer also to arachidonic acid (AA) and leukotrienes).

Anaphylatoxins are substances generated by the activation of complement that lead to increased vascular permeability as a consequence of the degranulation of mast cells, with the release of pharmacologically active mediators of immediate hypersensitivity. These biologically active peptides of low molecular weight are derived from C3, C4 and C5. They are generated in serum during fixation of complement by antigen–antibody complexes, immunoglobulin aggregates, etc. Small blood vessels, mast cells, smooth muscle and leukocytes in peripheral blood are targets of their action. Much is known about their primary structures. These complement fragments are designated C3a, C4a and C5a. They cause smooth muscle contraction, mast cell degranulation with histamine release, increased vascular permeability and the triple response in skin. They induce anaphylactic-like symptoms upon parenteral inoculation.

Cutaneous anaphylaxis is a local reaction specifically elicited in the skin of an actively or passively sensitized animal. Causes of cutaneous anaphylaxis include immediate wheal and flare response following prick tests with drugs or other substances; insect stings or bites; and contact urticaria in response to food substances such as nuts, fish or eggs or other substances such as rubber, dander or other environmental agents. The signs and symptoms of anaphylaxis are associated with the release of chemical mediators that include histamine and other substances from mast cell or basophil granules, following cross-linking of surface IgE by antigen or non-immunological degranulation of these cells. The pharmacological mediators act principally on the blood vessels and smooth muscle. The skin may be the site where an anaphylactic reaction is induced or it can be the target of a systemic anaphylactic reaction resulting in itching (pruritus), urticaria and angioedema.

Passive cutaneous anaphylaxis (PCA) is a skin test that involves the *in vivo* passive transfer of homocytotropic antibodies that mediate type I immediate hypersensitivity (e.g. IgE in man) from a sensitized to a previously non-sensitized individual by injecting the antibodies intradermally, which become anchored to mast cells through their Fc receptors (Figures 14 and 15). This is followed hours or even days later by intravenous injection of antigen mixed with a dye such as Evans Blue. Cross-linking of the cell-fixed (e.g. IgE) antibody receptors by the injected antigen induces a type I immediate hypersensitivity reaction in which histamine and other pharmacological mediators of immediate hypersensitivity are released. Vascular permeability factors act on the vessels to permit plasma and dye to leak into the extravascular space, forming a blue area which can be measured with calipers. In humans, this is called the Prausnitz–Küstner (PK) reaction. The PCA test was studied extensively by Zoltan Ovary, and will always be associated with his name (Figures 17 and 18).

Reverse passive cutaneous anaphylaxis (RPCA) is a passive cutaneous anaphylaxis assay in which the order of antigen and antibody administration is reversed, i.e. the antigen is first injected, followed by the antibody. In this case, the antigen must be an immunoglobulin that can fix to tissue cells.

Alexandre Besredka (1870–1940), Parisian immunologist who worked with Metchnikoff at the Institut Pasteur. He was born in Odessa. He contributed to studies of local immunity, anaphylaxis and

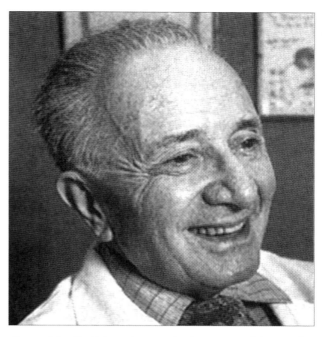

Figure 17 Dr Zoltan Ovary, who became well known for his research on passive cutaneous anaphylaxis

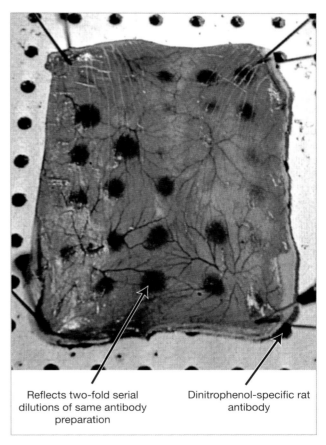

Reflects two-fold serial dilutions of same antibody preparation

Dinitrophenol-specific rat antibody

Figure 18 Passive cutaneous anaphylaxis in rats to dinitrophenol-specific rat reagin antibody. The diminished size of areas of increased capillary permeability is a consequence of two-fold serial dilutions of the antibody

119

antianaphylaxis. *Anaphylaxie et Antianaphylaxie*, 1918; *Histoire d'une Idee: L'Oeuvre de Metchnikoff*, 1921; *Etudes sur l'Immunité dans les Maladies Infectieuses*, 1928.

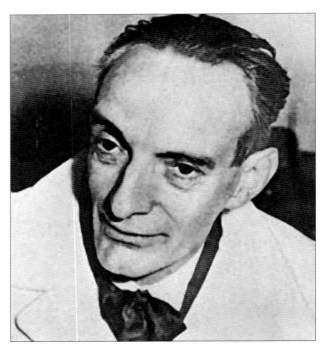

Figure 19   Daniel Bovet

Daniel Bovet (1907–92) (Figure 19), primarily a pharmacologist and physiologist, Bovet received the Nobel Prize in 1957 for his contributions to the understanding of the role histamine plays in allergic reactions and the development of antihistamines. *Structure Chimique et Activite Pharmacodynamique des Médicaments du Systeme Nerveux Vegetatif*, 1948; *Curare and Curare-Like Agents*, 1959.

REFERENCES

1. Portier P, Richet CR. De l'action anaphylactique de certains venins. *C R Soc Biol (Paris)* 1902;54:170–2

2. Magendie F. *Lectures of the Blood*. Philadelphia: Harrington Barrington & Haswell, 1839:244–9

3. Ishizaka K, Ishizaka T. Identification of gamma-E antibodies as a carrier of reaginic activity. *J Immunol* 1967;99:1187–98

4. Johansson SGO, Bennich H. Immunological studies of an atypical (myeloma) immunoglobulin. *Immunology* 1967;13:381–94

CHAPTER 6

Allergy, atopy, Arthus and Shwartzman reactions

The Jekyll and Hyde nature of the body's immune response mechanism was recognized early by Clemens von Pirquet (Figures 1 and 2), who introduced the term 'allergy' to denote a state of altered reactivity[1]. It was found that some types of allergy or hypersensitivity could be passively transferred to previously non-reactive individuals with serum, whereas others required lymphoid cells. Coca and Cooke introduced the term 'atopy', which means 'out of place' or 'strange disease',

to characterize certain hypersensitivity states which were considered to be heritable and to be limited in occurrence to the human being[2] (Figures 3–5). The atopic diseases include allergy to foods, hay fever and pollen, and constitute the so-called clinical allergies. Antibodies in the blood sera of atopic patients were described as being different from the precipitins and agglutinins involved in common serological reactions. The reagins, as these antibodies were called, are now known to

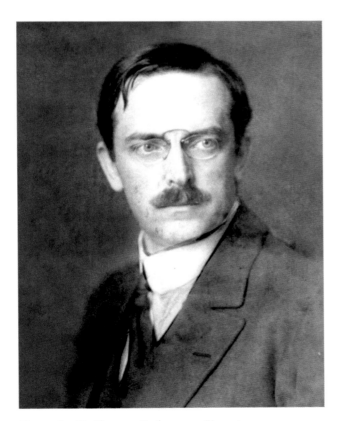

Figure 1   Dr Clemens Freiherr von Pirquet

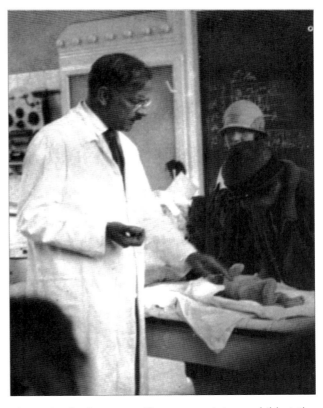

Figure 2   Professor von Pirquet examining a child at the Vienna Children's Clinic

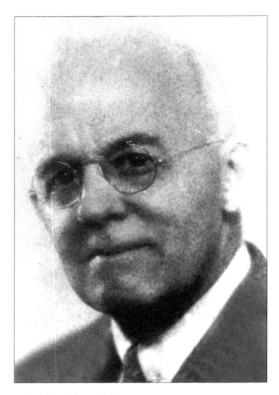

Figure 3   Dr Arthur F. Coca

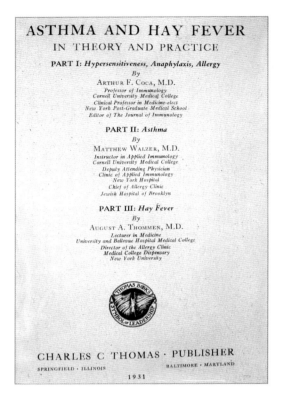

Figure 4   Title page of Dr Coca's book on asthma and hay fever

belong to the IgE class of immunoglobulin. Two physicians, Prausnitz (Figure 6) and Küstner, transmitted sensitivity to fish from one of them to the other by the injection of serum[3]. They were the first to demonstrate the passive transfer of specific reactivity with serum from atopic individuals to local skin sites in normal recipients, who subsequently demonstrate a wheal and flare response following injection of specific antigen into the same site. In studies on the relationship of hypersensitivity to immunity, Arthus, in 1903, observed that repeated injections of protein antigen into the same skin site of rabbits led to a hemorrhagic and necrotic reaction[4] (Figure 7). This local hypersensitivity reaction was subsequently demonstrated to be caused by immune complexes, classified by Coombs and Gell as type III hypersensitivity (Figures 8 and 9). This phenomenon, known since that time as the Arthus reaction, is proven by its specificity and dependence upon immune complexes to be immunologic in nature. By contrast, the Shwartzman phenomenon, which is remarkably similar to the Arthus reaction in many respects, is not immunologic. In 1928, Gregory Shwartzman found that a hemorrhagic and necrotic reaction could be produced at a local site 4h following a provocative intravenous injection of a small amount of *Salmonella typhi* culture filtrate

in rabbits treated 24h previously by an intradermal injection of an agar culture washing of the microorganisms (Figures 10–13). This led to the localized Shwartzman reaction. If both injections were administered intravenously, the generalized Shwartzman reaction took place with features closely resembling disseminated intravascular coagulation (DIC)[5].

Clemens Freiherr von Pirquet (1874–1929), Viennese physician who coined the term 'allergy' and described serum sickness and its pathogenesis. He also developed a skin test for tuberculosis. He held academic appointments at Vienna, Johns Hopkins and Breslau, and returned to Vienna in 1911 as Director of the University Children's Clinic. *Die Serumkrankheit* (with Schick), 1905; *Klinische Studien über vakzination und Vakzinale Allergie*, 1907; *Allergy*, 1911.

Arthur Fernandez Coca (1875–1959), American allergist and immunologist. He was a major force in allergy and immunology. He named atopic antibodies and was a pioneer in the isolation of allergens. Together with Robert A. Cooke, Coca classified allergies in humans.

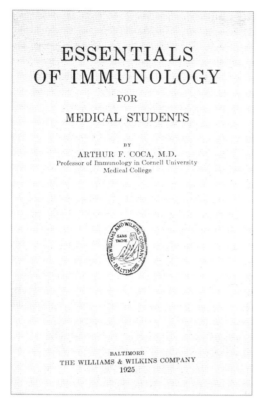

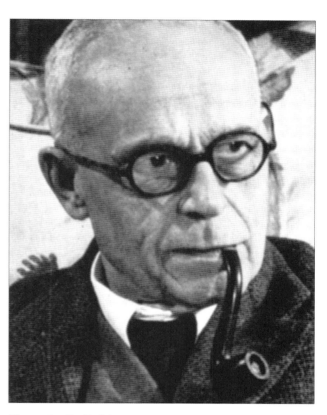

Figure 5 Title page of Dr Coca's immunology textbook for medical students

Figure 6 Dr Carl Prausnitz

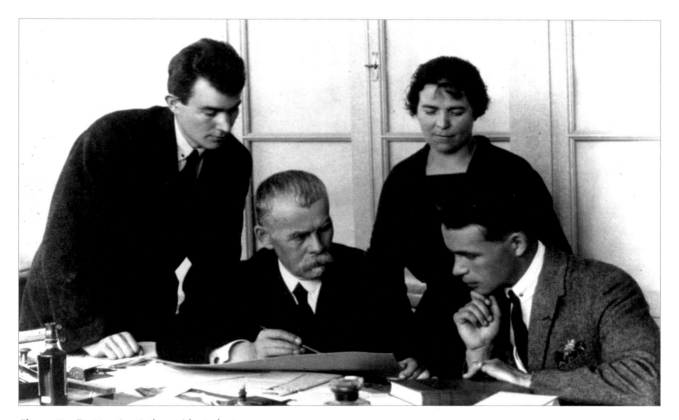

Figure 7 Dr Maurice Arthus with students

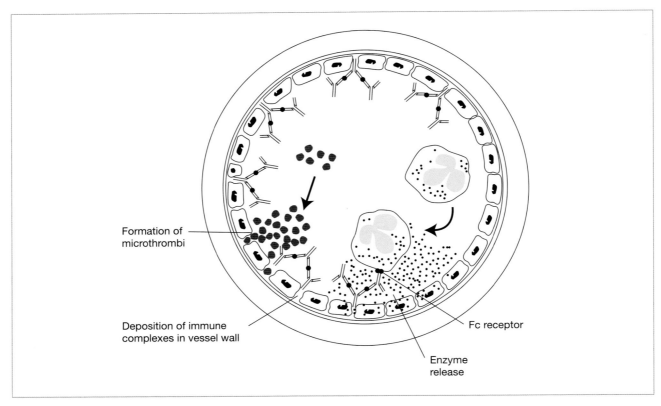

Figure 8 Schematic representation of the formation and deposition of immune complexes in vessel walls in type III hypersensitivity

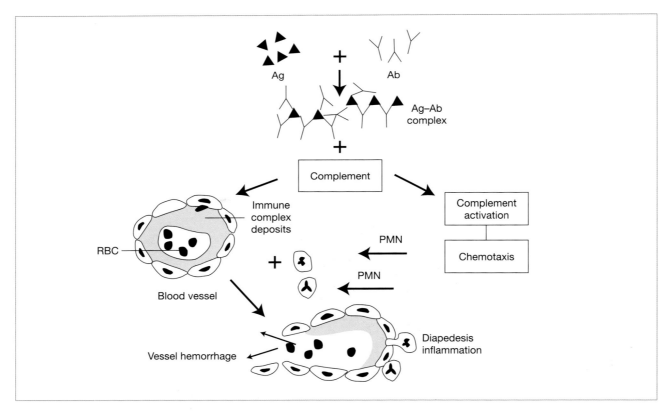

Figure 9 Schematic representation of molecular, cellular and tissue interactions in the Arthus reaction. RBC, red blood cell; PMN, polymorphonuclear neutrophil; Ag–Ab, antigen–antibody

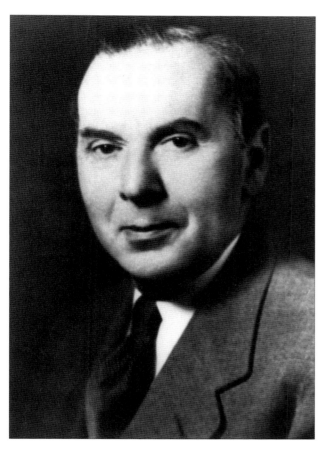

Figure 10 Dr Gregory Shwartzman

PHENOMENON
OF LOCAL TISSUE
REACTIVITY

*AND ITS IMMUNOLOGICAL, PATHO-
LOGICAL AND CLINICAL SIGNIFICANCE*

by

GREGORY SHWARTZMAN, M.D.
Bacteriologist, Mount Sinai Hospital, New York

Foreword by
JULES BORDET, M.D.
Paris

WITH 67 ILLUSTRATIONS
AND ONE COLOR PLATE

PAUL B. HOEBER, Iɴᴄ
MEDICAL BOOK DEPARTMENT OF HARPER & BROTHERS
NEW YORK   MCMXXXVII

Figure 11 Title page of Dr Shwartzman's famous monograph describing the reaction that bears his name

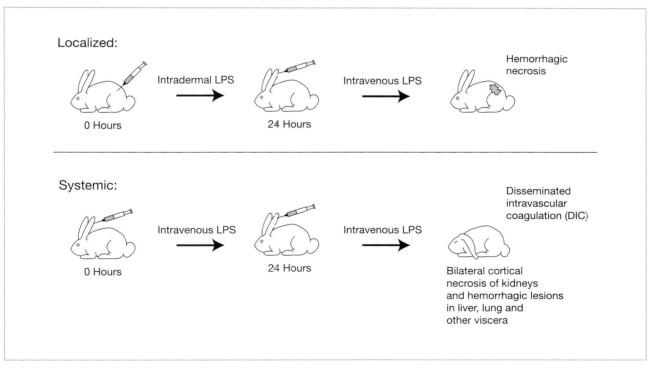

Figure 12 Schematic representation of the localized and systemic Shwartzman reaction. LPS, lipopolysaccharide

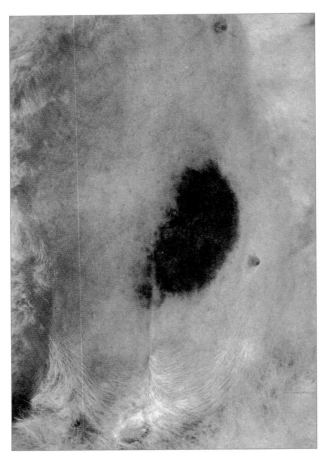

Figure 13 The ventral surface of a rabbit in which the localized Shwartzman reaction has been induced with endotoxin shows hemorrhage and necrosis

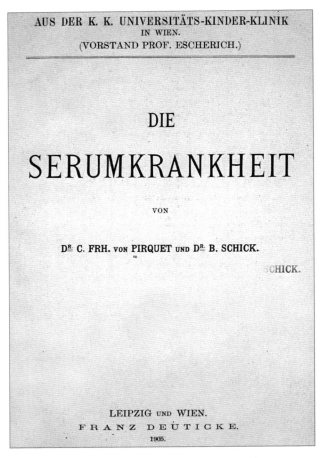

Figure 14 Dr von Pirquet's famous monograph on serum sickness

Robert Anderson Cooke (1880–1960), American immunologist and allergist who was instrumental in the founding of several allergy societies. With Coca, he classified allergies in humans. Cooke also pioneered skin test methods and desensitization techniques.

Carl Prausnitz-Giles (1876–1963), German physician from Breslau who conducted extensive research on allergies. He and Küstner successfully transferred food allergy with serum. This became the basis for the Prausnitz–Küstner test. He worked at the State Institute for Hygiene in Breslau and spent time at the Royal Institute for Public Health in London earlier in the century. In 1933, he left Germany and practiced medicine on the Isle of Wight.

Nicolas Maurice Arthus (1862–1945), Paris physician. He studied venoms and their physiological

effects, and was the first to describe local anaphylaxis, or the Arthus reaction, in 1903. Arthus investigated the local necrotic lesion resulting from a local antigen–antibody reaction in an immunized animal. *De l'Anaphylaxie a l'Immunité*, 1921.

Gregory Shwartzman (1896–1965), Russian-American microbiologist who described systemic and local reactions that follow the injection of bacterial endotoxins. The systemic Shwartzman reaction, a non-immunologic phenomenon, is related to disseminated intravascular coagulation. The local Shwartzman reaction in skin resembles the immunologically based Arthus reaction in appearance. *Phenomenon of Local Tissue Reactivity and Its Immunological and Clinical Significance*, 1937.

Following the development of antitoxin for the treatment of diphtheria, clinicians noted an adverse

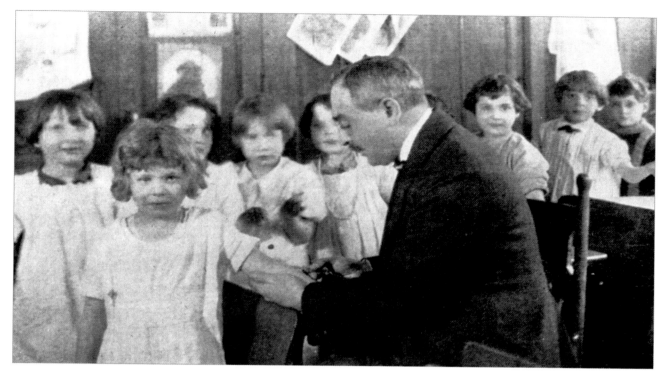

Figure 15   Dr Bela Schick, Austro–Hungarian pediatrician, coauthor with von Pirquet of the monograph *Serum Sickness*, which they discovered and described. He developed the test for diphtheria that bears his name

side-effect of the injection of the horse serum antitoxin. Within 8–12 days following the administration of a single large dose of diphtheria antitoxin, children began to develop signs and symptoms of serum sickness. von Pirquet and Schick reported their observations in a book entitled *Die Serumkrankheit* (Serum Sickness)[6] (Figures 14 and 15). The signs and symptoms they observed were caused by the formation of immune complexes which fixed complement, attracted polymorphonuclear neutrophils and led to inflammation in anatomical sites where the complexes were deposited, including the vessels, kidneys and joints.

As discussed in the chapter on 'Cellular immunity and delayed-type hypersensitivity', Hans Zinsser (Chapter 7, Figure 4), famous American bacteriologist and immunologist, in 1925 pointed to the differences between immediate and delayed-type hypersensitivity[7]. Thus, these early investigators had observed two main features associated with allergy or hypersensitivity. They found that it was important to know whether the reaction occurred within seconds to minutes following the administration of antigen, in which case it was referred to as immediate hypersensitivity, or whether it occurred hours to days after the administration of antigen, in which case it was termed delayed-type hypersensitivity.

Besides the significance of this temporal relationship with respect to antigen administration, they observed what was necessary to transfer the hypersensitivity passively, whether serum or specifically sensitized lymphoid cells.

Frank J. Dixon and associates developed an experimental model for serum sickness in the 1950s[8]. As antigen, they chose iodinated bovine serum albumin and injected it into rabbits. They followed the elimination of the antigen in three phases, one of which was immune elimination, and studied the development of experimentally induced pathological lesions in the vessels, kidneys and joints of the animals correlating with the immune complex content of the blood serum. As a result of studies by these and numerous other investigators, immune complex disorders have been demonstrated to be dynamic processes implicated in the pathogenesis of a host of immunological diseases (Figure 16). The pathological alterations which they induce are governed by their molar ratios in the deposition sites. The British immunopathologists, Gell and Coombs, developed a simplified classification of immunopathological phenomena that fall within the realm of hypersensitivity (type I, anaphylaxis; type II, cytotoxicity; type III, immune complex disease; type IV, delayed-type

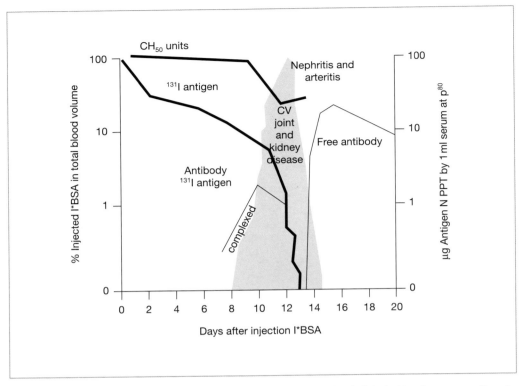

Figure 16   Experimental serum sickness induced by injection of radiolabeled bovine serum albumin (I*BSA) into rabbits by Frank J. Dixon and associates. CH$_{50}$ units, complement activity

hypersensitivity). Immune complex disorders of the serum sickness variety are called type III hypersensitivity in the Gell and Coombs classification[9]. The Scripps Clinic and Research Foundation directed by Dixon became a center for immunology research. By applying modern techniques such as radiolabeling of serum proteins to a disease process which had been described almost half a century earlier, they were able to shed light on some of the more important basic mechanisms of immunologically mediated human diseases. Cochrane and associates at Scripps carried out fundamental studies on the uptake of immune complexes by polymorphonuclear neutrophils (PMNs) and the role of complement in this phenomenon[10]. Other investigators have contributed much to our understanding of alterations in complement during the course of disease processes.

Frank James Dixon (1920–), American physician and researcher noted for his fundamental contributions to immunopathology that include the role of immune complexes in the production of disease. He is also known for his work on antibody formation. Dixon was the founding Director of the Research Institute of Scripps Clinic, La Jolla, CA.

Allergy is a term coined by Clemens von Pirquet in 1906 to describe the altered reactivity of the animal body to antigen. Currently, the term allergy refers to altered immune reactivity to a spectrum of environmental antigens, which include pollen, insect venom and food. Allergy is also referred to as hypersensitivity, and usually describes type I immediate hypersensitivity of the atopic/anaphylactic type. Some allergies, especially the delayed T-cell type, develop in subjects infected with certain microorganisms such as *Mycobacterium tuberculosis* or certain pathogenic fungi. Allergy is a consequence of the interaction between antigen (or allergen) and antibody or T lymphocytes produced by previous exposure to the same antigen or allergen.

An **allergic reaction** is a response to antigens or allergens in the environment as a consequence of either preformed antibodies or effector T cells. Allergic reactions are mediated by a number of immune mechanisms, the most common of which is type I hypersensitivity in which IgE antibody specific for an allergen is carried on the surface of mast cells. Combining with specific antigen leads to the release of pharmacological mediators, resulting in clinical symptoms of asthma, hay fever and other manifestations of allergic reactions.

The **Wheal and flare reaction** is an immediate hypersensitivity, IgE-mediated (in man) reaction to an antigen. Application of antigen by a scratch test in a hypersensitive individual may be followed by erythema, which is the red flare, and edema, which is the wheal. Atopic subjects who have a hereditary component to their allergy experience the effects of histamine and other vasoactive amines released from mast cell granules following cross-linking of surface IgE molecules by antigen or allergen.

Atopy is a type of immediate (type I) hypersensitivity to common environmental allergens in man mediated by humoral antibodies of the IgE class formerly termed reagins, which are able to transfer the effect passively. Atopic hypersensitivity states include hay fever, asthma, eczema, urticaria and certain gastrointestinal disorders. There is a genetic predisposition to atopic hypersensitivities, which affect more than 10% of the human population. Antigens that sensitize atopic individuals are termed allergens. They include: grass and tree pollens; dander, feathers and hair; eggs, milk and chocolate; and house dust, bacteria and fungi. IgE antibody is a skin-sensitizing homocytotropic antibody that occurs spontaneously in the sera of human subjects with atopic hypersensitivity. IgE antibodies are non-precipitating (*in vitro*), are heat sensitive (destroyed by heating to 60°C for 30–60 min), are not able to pass across the placenta, remain attached to local skin sites for weeks after injection and fail to induce passive cutaneous anaphylaxis (PCA) in guinea pigs.

Hay fever   This is allergic rhinitis, recurrent asthma, rhinitis and conjunctivitis in atopic individuals who inhale allergenic (antigenic) materials such as pollens, animal dander, house dust, etc. These substances do not induce allergic reactions in non-atopic (normal) individuals. Hay fever is a type I immediate hypersensitivity reaction mediated by homocytotrophic IgE antibodies specific for the allergen for which the individual is hypersensitive. Hay fever is worse during seasons when airborne environmental allergens are most concentrated.

Atopic allergy or atopy is an increased tendency of some members of the population to develop immediate hypersensitivity reactions, often mediated by IgE antibodies, against innocuous substances.

A **food allergy** is a type I (anaphylactic) or type III (antigen–antibody complex) hypersensitivity mechanism response to allergens or antigens in foods that have been ingested, which may lead to intestinal distress, producing nausea, vomiting and diarrhea. There may be edema of the buccal mucosa, generalized urticaria or eczema. Food categories associated with food allergy in some individuals include eggs, fish or nuts. Atopic sensitization to cow's milk is the most common food allergy; casein is the major allergenic and antigenic protein in cow's milk. Both skin tests and radioallergosorbent test (RAST) using the appropriate allergen or antigen may identify individuals with a particular food allergy.

The **Prausnitz–Küstner (PK) reaction (historical)** (Figure 17) is a skin test for hypersensitivity in which serum containing IgE antibodies specific for a particular allergen is transferred from an allergic individual to a non-allergic recipient by intradermal injection. This is followed by injection of the antigen or allergen in question into the same site as the serum injection. Fixation of the IgE antibodies in the 'allergic' serum to mast cells in the recipient results in local release of the pharmacological mediators of immediate hypersensitivity that include histamine. It results in a local anaphylactic reaction with a wheal and flare response. This is no longer used because of the risk of transmitting hepatitis or acquired immune deficiency syndrome (AIDS).

House dust allergy is a type I immediate hypersensitivity reaction in atopic individuals exposed to house dust, in which the principal allergen is *Dermatophagoides pteronyssinus*, the house dust mite. The condition is expressed as a respiratory allergy, with the atopic subject manifesting either asthma or allergic rhinitis.

Horse serum sensitivity is an allergic or hypersensitive reaction in a human or other animal receiving antitoxin or antithymocyte globulin generated by immunization of horses whose immune serum is used for therapeutic purposes. Classic serum sickness is an

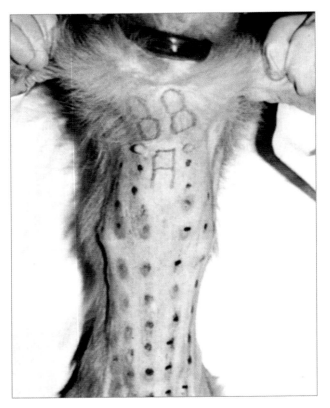

Figure 17 Prausnitz–Küstner reaction to ragweed antigen E in rhesus monkey. Skin sensitized 2 days before with human serum from a ragweed-sensitive atopic patient

example of this type of hypersensitivity that first appeared in children receiving diphtheria antitoxin early in the 20th century.

A **pollen hypersensitivity** is an immediate (type I) hypersensitivity which atopic individuals experience following inhalation of pollens such as ragweed in the USA. This is an IgE-mediated reaction that results in respiratory symptoms expressed as hay fever or asthma. Sensitivity to certain pollens can be detected through skin tests with pollen extracts.

Drug allergy is an immunopathologic or hypersensitivity reaction to a drug. Some drugs are notorious for acting as haptens that bind to proteins in the skin or other tissues that act as carriers. This hapten–carrier complex elicits an immune response manifested as either antibodies or T lymphocytes. Any of the four types of hypersensitivity in the Coombs and Gell classification may be mediated by drug allergy. One of the best known allergies is hypersensitivity to penicillin. Antibodies to a drug linked to carrier molecules

in the host may occur in autoimmune hemolytic anemia or thrombocytopenia, anaphylaxis, urticaria and serum sickness. Skin eruptions are frequent manifestations of a T cell-mediated drug allergy.

Allergen is an antigen that induces an allergic or hypersensitivity response in contrast to a classic immune response produced by the recipient host in response to most immunogens. Allergens include such environmental substances as pollens, i.e. their globular proteins, from trees, grasses and ragweed, as well as certain food substances, animal danders and insect venom. Selected subjects are predisposed to synthesizing IgE antibodies in response to allergens and are said to be atopic. The cross-linking of IgE molecules anchored to the surfaces of mast cells or basophils through their Fc regions results in the release of histamine and other pharmacological mediators of immediate hypersensitivity from mast cells/basophils.

Allergoids are allergens that have been chemically altered to favor the induction of IgG rather than IgE antibodies to diminish allergic manifestations in the hypersensitive individual. These formaldehyde-modified allergens are analogous to toxoids prepared from bacterial exotoxins. Some of the physical and chemical characteristics of allergens are similar to those of other antigens. However, the molecular weight of allergens is lower.

Asthma is a disease of the lungs characterized by reversible airway obstruction (in most cases), inflammation of the airway with prominent eosinophil participation and increased responsiveness by the airway to various stimuli. There is bronchospasm associated with recurrent paroxysmal dyspnea and wheezing. Some cases of asthma are allergic, i.e. bronchial allergy, mediated by IgE antibody to environmental allergens. Other cases are provoked by non-allergic factors that are not discussed here.

Type II antibody-mediated hypersensitivity is mediated by antibodies against antigens on cell surfaces or extracellular matrix.

Most type II hypersensitivity reactions involve the complement system and phagocytes, the effector mechanisms used by antibodies. Three different antibody-dependent mechanisms that mediate this reaction include:

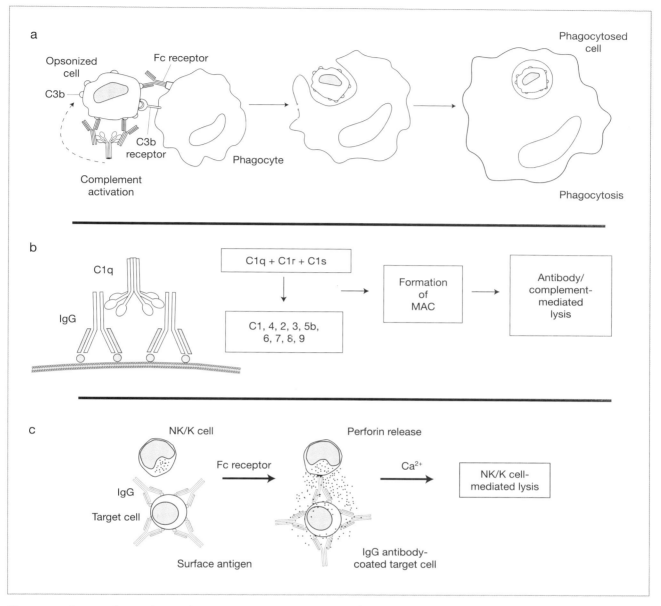

Figure 18 Separate forms of type II hypersensitivity. (a) Opsonization of cells by antibody and complement components and ingestion by phagocytes. (b) Depicts antibody- and complement-mediated lysis of a nucleated cell as a consequence of formation of the membrane attack complex (MAC). (c) Shows antibody-dependent cell-mediated cytotoxicity through the action of either a natural killer (NK) or a killer (K) cell with surface antibody specific for a target cell

(1) Opsonization and complement – and Fc receptor-mediated phagocytosis;

(2) Complement and Fc receptor-mediated inflammation;

(3) Antibody-mediated cellular dysfunction (Figures 18–22).

IgG- or IgM-coated (opsonized) cells may activate the complement system, leading to generation of the byproducts C3b and C4b, which are deposited on cell surfaces. Phagocytes recognize these proteins through specific receptors. This results in phagocytosis and destruction of the phagocytized cells. Complement activation on cells results in generation of the membrane attack complex (MAC) that disrupts the integrity of cell membranes by the formation of holes in the lipid bilayer causing osmotic lysis (Figure 18b).

Examples of type II hypersensitivity include the antiglomerular basement membrane antibody that develops in Goodpasture's syndrome (Figures 23–26),

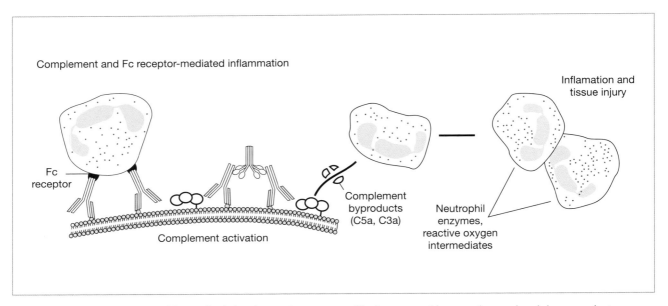

Complement and Fc receptor-mediated inflammation

Fc receptor

Complement activation

Complement byproducts (C5a, C3a)

Neutrophil enzymes, reactive oxygen intermediates

Inflamation and tissue injury

Figure 19   Inflamation induced by antibody binding to Fc receptors of leukocytes and by complement breakdown products

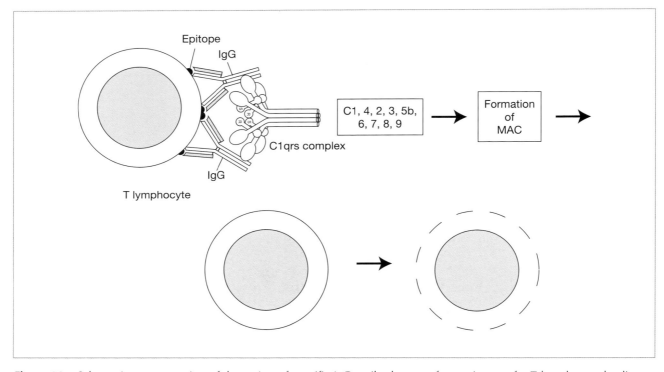

Epitope

IgG

C1, 4, 2, 3, 5b, 6, 7, 8, 9

Formation of MAC

C1qrs complex

IgG

T lymphocyte

Figure 20   Schematic representation of the action of specific IgG antibody on surface epitopes of a T lymphocyte leading to antibody–complement-mediated lysis of that cell. MAC, membrane attack complex

and antibodies that develop against erythrocytes in Rh incompatibility leading to erythroblastosis fetalis or autoimmune hemolytic anemia.

Goodpasture's syndrome (Figures 24–26) is a disease with pulmonary hemorrhage (with coughing up blood) and glomerulonephritis (with blood in the urine), induced by antiglomerular basement membrane autoantibodies that also interact with alveolar basement membrane antigens. A linear pattern of immunofluorescent staining confirms interaction of the IgG antibodies with basement membrane antigens in the kidney and lung, leading to membrane injury with pulmonary hemorrhage and acute

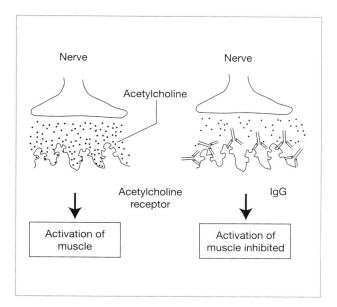

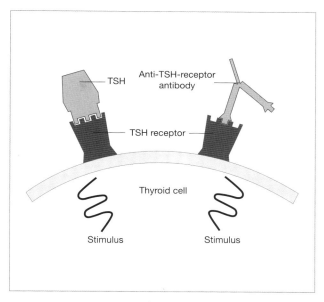

Figure 21 Schematic representation of the interference by acetylcholine receptor antibodies with chemical transmission of the nerve impulse. Acetylcholine receptor antibodies are IgG autoantibodies that cause loss of function of acetylcholine receptors, which are critical to chemical transmission of the nerve impulse at the neuromuscular junction. This represents a type II mechanism of hypersensitivity

Figure 22 Schematic representation of the third form of type II hypersensitivity in which long-acting thyroid stimulator (LATS), an IgG antibody specific for the thyroid stimulating hormone (TSH) receptor, leads to continuous stimulation of thyroid parenchymal cells, causing hyperthyroidism. The IgG antibody mimics the action of TSH

(rapidly progressive or crescentic) proliferative glomerulonephritis. Pulmonary hemorrhage may precede hematuria. In addition to linear IgG, membranes may reveal linear staining for C3 (Figure 26).

Goodpasture's antigen is an antigen found in the non-collagenous part of type IV collagen. This is present in human glomerular (and alveolar) basement membranes (GBM), making it a target for injury-inducing anti-GBM antibodies in blood sera of Goodpasture's syndrome patients. Interestingly, individuals with Alport's (hereditary) nephritis do not have the Goodpasture antigen in their basement membranes. Thus, renal transplants stimulate anti-GBM antibodies in Alport's patients.

A second variety of type II hypersensitivity is antibody-dependent cell-mediated cytotoxicity (ADCC). Killer (K) cells or natural killer (NK) cells, which have Fc receptors on their surfaces, may bind to the Fc region of IgG molecules. They may react with surface antigens on target cells to produce lysis of the antibody-coated cell. Complement fixation is not required and does not participate in this reaction. In addition to

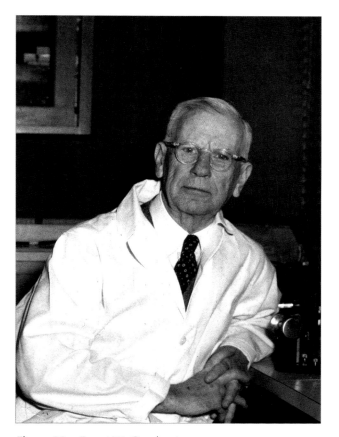

Figure 23 Ernest W. Goodpasture

133

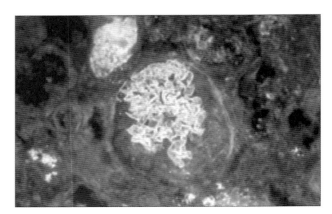

Figure 24 Goodpasture's syndrome. Kidney section. Stained with antiglomerular basement membrane (anti-GBM) antibody (immunofluorescence)

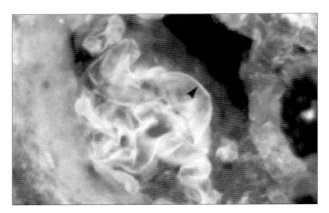

Figure 25 Goodpasture's syndrome. Kidney section. Stained with anti-GBM antibody (immunofluorescence)

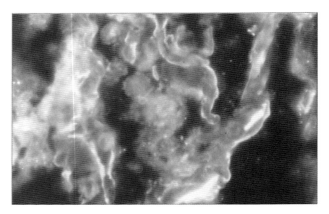

Figure 26 Goodpasture's syndrome. Lung section. Stained with anti-lung (alveolar) basement membrane antibody (immunofluorescence)

K and NK cells, neutrophils, eosinophils and macrophages may participate in ADCC.

Inflammation, rather than phagocytosis or cell lysis, is the cause of injury following deposition of antibodies in extracellular tissues including basement membranes and matrix. This leads to complement activation with the generation of C5a, C4a and C3a that attract neutrophils and monocytes, which bind to deposited antibodies via their Fc receptors. This results in activation with the release of enzymes, reactive oxygen intermediates and other injurious substances which result in tissue injury. Examples of antibody-mediated inflammation include the tissue injury mechanism in certain forms of glomerulonephritis and vascular rejection in organ grafts.

A third form of type II hypersensitivity is antibody against cell surface receptors that interferes with function, as in the case of antibodies against acetylcholine

receptors in motor endplates of skeletal muscle in myasthenia gravis. This interference with neuromuscular transmission results in muscular weakness, ultimately affecting the muscles of respiration and producing death. By contrast, stimulatory antibodies develop in hyperthyroidism (Graves' disease). They react with thyroid-stimulating hormone receptors on thyroid epithelial cells to produce hyperthyroidism.

Antibody-dependent cell-mediated cyotoxicity (ADCC) is a reaction in which T lymphocytes; NK cells, including large granular lymphocytes; neutrophils; and macrophages may lyse tumor cells, infectious agents and allogeneic cells by combining through their Fc receptors with the Fc region of IgG antibodies bound through their Fab regions to target cell surface antigens. Following linkage of Fc receptors with Fc regions, destruction of the target is accomplished through released cytokines. It represents an example of participation between antibody molecules and immune system cells to produce an effector function. NK cells mediate most ADCC through the Fc receptor FcγRIII or CD16 on their surface.

Type III immune complex-mediated hypersensitivity is a type of hypersensitivity mediated by antigen–antibody–complement complexes. Antigen–antibody complexes can stimulate an acute inflammatory response that leads to complement activation and polymorphonuclear (PMN) leukocyte infiltration. The immune complexes are formed either by exogenous antigens such as those from microbes or by endogenous antigens such as DNA, a target for antibodies produced in systemic lupus erythematosus. Immune complex-mediated injury may be either systemic or localized. In the systemic variety, antigen–antibody complexes are produced in the circulation, deposited in the tissues and initiate inflammation. Acute serum sickness occurred in children treated with diphtheria antitoxin earlier in the 20th century as a consequence of antibody produced against the horse serum protein. When immune complexes are deposited in tissues, complement is fixed, and PMNs are attracted to the site. Their lysosomal enzymes are released, resulting in tissue injury. Localized immune complex disease, sometimes called the Arthus reaction, is characterized by an acute immune complex vasculitis with fibrinoid necrosis occurring in the walls of small vessels.

Serum sickness is a systemic reaction that follows the injection of a relatively large, single dose of serum (e.g. antitoxin) into humans or other animals. It is characterized by systemic vasculitis (arteritis), glomerulonephritis and arthritis. The lesions follow the deposition in tissues, such as the microvasculature, of immune complexes that form after antibody appears in the circulation between the 5th and 14th day following antigen administration. The antigen–antibody complexes fix complement and initiate a classic type III hypersensitivity reaction resulting in immune-mediated tissue injury. Patients may develop fever, lymphadenopathy, urticaria and sometimes arthritis. The pathogenesis of serum sickness is that of a classic type III reaction. Antigen escaping into the circulation from the site of injection forms immune complexes that damage the small vessels. The antibodies involved in the classic type of serum sickness are of the precipitating variety, usually IgG. They may be detected by passive hemagglutination. Pathologically, serum sickness is a systemic immune complex disease characterized by vasculitis, glomerulonephritis and arthritis due to the intravascular formation and deposition of immune complexes that subsequently fix complement and attract polymorphonuclear neutrophils to the site through the chemotactic effects of C5a, thereby initiating inflammation. The classic reaction which occurs 7–15 days after the triggering injection is called the primary form of serum sickness. Similar manifestations appearing only 1–3 days following the injection represent the accelerated form of serum sickness and

occur in subjects who are presumably already sensitized. A third form, called the anaphylactic form, develops immediately after injection. This latter form is apparently due to reaginic IgE antibodies and usually occurs in atopic subjects sensitized by horse dander or by previous exposure to serum treatment. The serum sickness-like syndromes seen in drug allergy have a similar clinical picture and similar pathogenesis.

The **Arthus reaction** is induced by repeated intradermal injections of antigen into the same skin site. It is dependent upon the development of humoral antibodies of the precipitin type, which react *in vivo* with specific antigen at a local site. It may also be induced by the inoculation of antigen into a local skin site of an animal possessing preformed IgG antibodies specific for the antigen. Immune complexes comprise antigen, antibody and complement formed in vessels. The chemotactic complement fragment C5a and other chemotactic peptides produced attract neutrophils to antigen–antibody–complement complexes. This is followed by lysosomal enzyme release, which induces injury to vessel walls with the development of thrombi, hemorrhage, edema and necrosis. Events leading to vascular necrosis include: blood stasis; thrombosis; capillary compression in vascular injury, which causes extravasation; venule rupture; hemorrhage and local ischemia. There is extensive infiltration of polymorphonuclear cells, especially neutrophils, into the connective tissue. Grossly, edema, erythema, central blanching, induration and petechiae appear. Petechiae develop within 2 h, reach a maximum between 4 and 6 h, and then may diminish or persist for 24 h or longer with associated central necrosis, depending on the severity of the reaction. If the reaction is more prolonged, macrophages replace neutrophils; histiocytes and plasma cells may also be demonstrated. The Arthus reaction is considered a form of immediate-type hypersensitivity, but it does not occur as rapidly as does anaphylaxis. It takes place during a 4-h period and diminishes after 12 h. Thereafter, the area is cleared by mononuclear phagocytes. The passive cutaneous Arthus reaction consists of the inoculation of antibodies intravenously into a non-immune host, followed by local cutaneous injection of antigen. The reverse passive cutaneous Arthus reaction requires the intracutaneous injection of antibodies, followed by the intravenous or incutaneous (at the same site) administration of antigen. The Arthus reaction is a form of type III hypersensitivity since it is based upon the formation of immune complexes with complement fixation. Clinical situations for which it serves as an animal model include serum sickness, glomerulonephritis and farmer's lung.

A **passive Arthus reaction** is an inflammatory vasculitis produced in experimental animals by the passive intravenous injection of significant amounts of precipitating IgG antibody, followed by the intracutaneous or subcutaneous injection of the homologous antigen for which the antibodies are specific. This permits microprecipitates to occur in the intercellular spaces between the intravascular precipitating antibody and antigen in the extravascular space. This is followed by interaction with complement, attraction of polymorphonuclear leukocytes and an inflammatory response as described above under Arthus reaction.

The **Shwartzman (or Shwartzman–Sanarelli) reaction** is a non-immunologic phenomenon in which endotoxin (lipopolysaccharides) induces local and systemic reactions. Following the initial or preparatory injection of endotoxin into the skin, polymorphonuclear leukocytes accumulate and are then thought to release lysosomal acid hydrolases that injure the walls of small vessels, preparing them for the second provocative injection of endotoxin. The intradermal injection of endotoxin into the skin of a rabbit followed within 24 h by the intravenous injection of the same or a different endotoxin leads to hemorrhage at the local site of the initial injection. Although the local Shwartzman reaction may resemble an Arthus reaction in appearance, the Arthus reaction is immunological, whereas the Shwartzman reaction is not. In the Shwartzman reaction, there is insufficient time between the first and second injections to induce an immune reaction in a previously unsensitized host. There is also a lack of specificity since even a different endotoxin may be used for the first and second injections.

The generalized or systemic Shwartzman reaction again involves two injections of endotoxin. However,

both are administered intravenously, one 24 h following the first. The generalized Shwartzman reaction is the experimental equivalent of disseminated intravascular coagulation that occurs in a number of human diseases. Following the first injection, sparse fibrin thrombi are formed in the vasculature of the lungs, kidney, liver and capillaries of the spleen. There is blockade of the reticuloendothelial system as its mononuclear phagocytes proceed to clear thromboplastin and fibrin. Administration of the second dose of endotoxin while the reticuloendothelial system is blocked leads to profound intravascular coagulation since the mononuclear phagocytes are unable to remove the thromboplastin and fibrin. There is bilateral cortical necrosis of the kidneys and splenic hemorrhage and necrosis. Neither platelets nor leukocytes are present in the fibrin thrombi that are formed.

REFERENCES

1. von Pirquet C. Allergie. *Münch Med Wochr* 1906;53:1457–8

2. Coca AF, Cooke RA. On the classification of the phenomena of hypersensitiveness. *J Immunol* 1923;8:163–82

3. Prausnitz OCW, Kustner H. Studien uber die Ueberempfindlichkeit. *Zentralbl Bakteriol (I Abt Orig)* 1921;86:160–9

4. Arthus NM. Injections repetées de serum de cheval chez le lapin. *C R Soc Biol (Paris)* 1903;55:817–20

5. Shwartzman G. Studies on *Bacillus typhosus* toxic substances. I. Phenomenon of local skin reactivity to *B. typhosus* culture filtrate. *J Exp Med* 1928;48:247–68

6. von Pirquet CP, Schick B. *Die Serumkrankheit*. Vienna: F Deuticke, 1905

7. Zinsser H. Studies on tuberculin reaction and on specific hypersensitiveness in bacterial infection. *J Exp Med* 1921;34:495

8. Dixon FJ, Vasquez JJ, Weigle WO, *et al.* Pathogenesis of serum sickness. *Arch Pathol* 1958;65:18

9. Coombs RRA, Gell PGH. Classification of allergic reactions responsible for clinical hypersensitivity and disease. In Gell PGH, Coombs RRA, Lackman PJ, eds. *Clinical Aspects of Immunology*. Oxford: Blackwell, 1975:761

10. Cochrane CG. A role of polymorphonuclear leucocytes in nephrotoxic nephritis. *J Exp Med* 1965;122:99–116

CHAPTER 7

Cellular immunity and delayed-type hypersensitivity

Metchnikoff was among the first investigators to appreciate the role of cells in the immune response. He attempted to explain immunity to infectious diseases on the basis of the capabilities of phagocytes to destroy infecting microorganisms *in vivo* by absorption phenomena.

This was attributed to the action of two digestive ferments, one of which was released to the plasma and body fluids. The component referred to as *cytase*, compromising *macrocytase* and *microcytase*, by Metchnikoff (Figure 1) was the same substance Ehrlich called *das Komplement*. Metchnikoff's term 'fixateur'

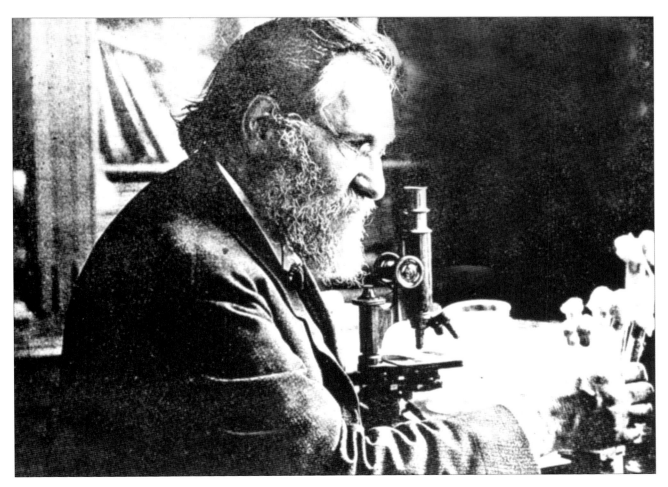

Figure 1   Elie Metchnikoff

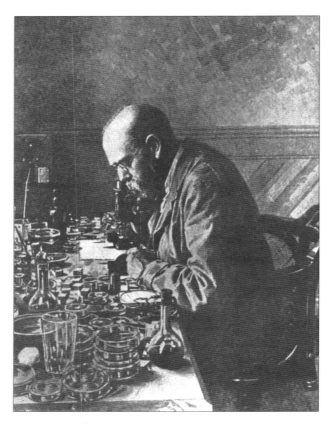

Figure 2   Robert Koch

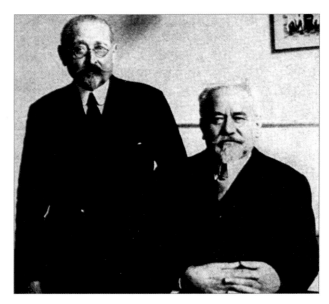

Figure 3   Albert Calmette (right) and C. Guérin (left)

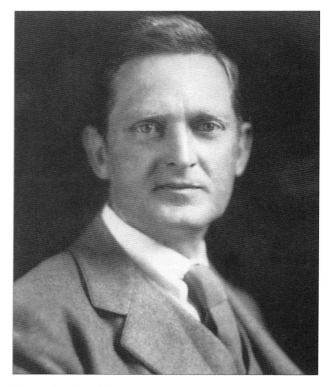

Figure 4   Hans Zinsser

meant the same as Ehrlich's 'Amboceptor'. Thus, this represented the first cellular theory of immunity which is quite different from our modern concept of the role that cells play in the immune response. In his extensive studies on tuberculosis, Robert Koch (Figure 2), Director of the Institute for Infectious Diseases in Berlin, discovered that an extract which he termed 'old tuberculin' was able to induce delayed hypersensitivity skin reactions in guinea pigs as well as in humans. Histological studies of these local sites of reactivity in the skin revealed accumulations of lymphocytes[1]. Delayed skin reactivity was found to be manifest within 24 h of the inoculation and to reach maximum reactivity at about 48 h after injection.

Albert Calmette (1863–1933) (Figure 3), French physician who was Subdirector of the Institut Pasteur in Paris. In a popular book published in 1920, *Bacillary Infection and Tuberculosis*, he emphasized the necessity of separating tuberculin reactivity from anaphylaxis. Together with Guérin, he perfected bacillus Calmette–Guérin (BCG) vaccine and also investigated snake venom and plague serum.

Hans Zinsser (1878–1940) (Figure 4), a leading American bacteriologist and immunologist who was a Columbia, Stanford and Harvard educator, whose work in immunology included hypersensitivity research, plague immunology, formulation of the unitarian theory of antibodies and demonstration of differences between tuberculin and anaphylactic hypersensitivity. His famous text, *Microbiology* (with Hiss), 1911, has been through two dozen editions since its first appearance.

From the turn of the century until approximately the early 1960s, *in vivo* reactivity manifested as skin lesions was essentially the only means to test for cell-mediated immune reactivity. However, Rich and Lewis, in 1928, developed a technique for the demonstration of delayed-type hypersensitivity (DTH) *in vitro*, which involved the immobilization of cells migrating from the edges of small fragments of lymphoid tissue in culture in the presence of specific antigens[2]. Of course, this was the predecessor of the migration inhibition factor (MIF) assay, which was widely employed in both clinial and research immunology laboratories.

In the early 1940s, Landsteiner and Merril W. Chase, and Battisto, performed extensive investigations into delayed-type hypersensitivity reactions to simple chemical haptens and described the successful transfer of reactivity to previously non-reactive animals by suspensions of lymphoid cells[3]. H. S. Lawrence, in 1949, described transfer factor, which was an extract of leukocytes from tuberculin positive-reacting patients that was released upon freezing and thawing the cells, spinning down the cellular debris and transferring the cell-free supernatant into tuberculin-negative individuals. These recipients became tuberculin positive. Thus, a cell-free extract proved capable of conferring specific delayed-type hypersensitive reactivity on individuals not previously contacted by the antigen[4]. Transfer factor has been extensively studied biochemically, biologically and by other methods[5].

Henry Sherwood Lawrence (1916–), American immunologist. While studying type IV hypersensitivity and contact dermatitis, he discovered transfer factor. *Cellular and Humoral Aspects of Delayed Hypersensitivity*, 1959.

A real breakthrough in cell-mediated immunity came with the demonstration that lymphocytes exposed to phytohemagglutinin or other plant mitogens could be successfully cultured *in vitro* over extended periods of time. This came about by serendipity. In blood-banking procedures where a plant extract called phytohemagglutinin (PHA) was added to agglutinate red cells, it was found that, upon centrifugation, the buffy-coat lymphocytes underwent blast transformation and developed the ability to survive over extended periods, a property not shared by lymphocytes untreated with phytohemagglutinin[6]. Besides the plant lectin's hemagglutinating property, it also had a mitogenic principle that induced blast transformation and division of lymphocytes in culture. These findings secured the lymphocyte as the central cell in the immune response. With this wealth of new information, lymphocytes were demonstrated to release a variety of soluble mediator substances termed lymphokines. Some of these were demonstrated to have effects on other cells such as MIF produced by lymphocytes, which actually prevents the migration of macrophages from the sites where they are needed.

John R. David and Barry R. Bloom[7,8], working independently, showed that immune lymphoid cells activated by their corresponding antigen secrete a substance that inhibits macrophage migration, a feature of delayed hypersensitivity. They termed this soluble factor migration inhibitory factor (MIF). David found that MIF had a molecular weight greater than 10 000 Da and was not preformed. Bloom and associates proved that lymphocytes synthesized MIF and macrophages were the target. Stimulation of lymphocytes was not antigen-specific, as mitogens or purified protein derivative (PPD) from tubercle bacilli could induce MIF synthesis and release. MIF was not species-specific. The description of MIF and its properties was the first demonstration that soluble factors regulate immune responses and play a significant role in intercellular communication.

Billingham and Simonsen, working independently, discovered the graft-versus-host reaction (GVHR) in 1957[9,10]. They demonstrated that the inoculation of immunocompetent lymphoid cells into an immuno-suppressed host from whatever cause could lead to a reaction of the lymphoid cell graft against the host on the basis of allogeneic differences between the two. This graft-versus-host disease is very significant in bone marrow transplantation, or can occur following the administration of a unit a blood containing as few as 1.0×10^6 lymphocytes to a child with T-cell immuno-deficiency.

Cell-mediated immunity (CMI) is the limb of the immune response that is mediated by specifically sensitized T lymphocytes that produce their effect through direct action, in contrast to the indirect effect mediated by antibodies of the humoral limb produced by B lymphocytes. The development of cell-mediated immunity to an exogenous antigen first involves processing of the antigen by an antigen-presenting cell such as a dendritic cell or a macrophage. Processed antigen is presented in the context of major histocompatibility complex (MHC) class II molecules to a CD4$^+$ T lymphocyte. Interleukin (IL)-1β is also released from the antigen-presenting cell to induce IL-2 synthesis in CD4$^+$ lymphocytes. The IL-2 has an autocrine effect on the cells producing it, causing their proliferation and also causing proliferation of other lymphocyte subsets including CD8$^+$ suppressor/cytotoxic T cells, B lymphocytes that form antibody and natural killer (NK) cells. Cell-mediated immunity is of critical importance in the defense against mycobacterial and fungal infections and resistance to tumors, and has a significant role in allograft rejection.

Type IV cell-mediated hypersensitivity is a form of hypersensitivity mediated by specifically sensitized cells (Figure 5). Whereas antibodies participate in types I, II and III reactions, T lymphocytes activated by antigen mediate type IV hypersensitivity. Two types of reactions, mediated by separate T cell subsets, are observed. Delayed-type hypersensitivity (DTH) is mediated by CD4$^+$ T cells, and direct cellular cytotoxicity is mediated principally by CD8$^+$ T cells.

A classic delayed hypersensitivity reaction is the tuberculin or Mantoux reaction. Following exposure to *Mycobacterium tuberculosis*, CD4$^+$ lymphocytes recognize the microbe's antigens complexed with class II MHC molecules on the surface of antigen-presenting cells that process the mycobacterial antigens. Memory T cells develop and remain in the circulation for prolonged periods. When tuberculin antigen is injected intradermally, sensitized T cells react with the antigen on the antigen-presenting cell's surface, undergo transformation and secrete lymphokines that lead to the manifestations of hypersensitivity. Unlike an antibody-mediated hypersensitivity, lymphokines are not antigen specific.

In T cell-mediated cytotoxicity, CD8$^+$ T lymphocytes kill antigen-bearing target cells. The cytotoxic T lymphocytes play a significant role in resistance to viral infections. Class I MHC molecules present viral antigens to CD8$^+$ T lymphocytes as a viral peptide–class I molecular complex, which is transported to the infected cell's surface. Cytotoxic CD8$^+$ cells recognize this and lyse the target before the virus can replicate, thereby stopping the infection.

In 1801, Jenner described the 'disposition to sudden cuticular inflammation' that occurred after cowpox had been re-inoculated into the skin of individuals vaccinated previously by cowpox or infected with smallpox virus. Thus, delayed, or cellular hypersensitivity was one of the earliest immunologic reactions reported.

Delayed-type hypersensitivity (DTH) is a cell-mediated immunity, or hypersensitivity mediated by sensitized T lymphocytes (Figures 6 and 7). Although originally described as a skin reaction that requires 24–48 h to develop following challenge with antigen, current usage emphasizes the mechanism, which is T cell-mediated, as opposed to emphasis on the temporal relationship of antigen injection and host response. The CD4$^+$ T lymphocyte is the principal cell that mediates DTH reactions. To induce a DTH reaction, antigen is injected intradermally in a primed individual. If the reaction is positive, an area of erythema and induration develops 24–48 h following antigen challenge. Edema and infiltration by lymphocytes and macrophages occurs at the local site. The CD4$^+$ T lymphocytes identify antigen on Ia-positive macrophages and release lymphokines, which entice more macrophages to enter the area where they become activated.

Skin tests are used clinically to reveal DTH to infectious disease agents. Skin test antigens include such substances as tuberculin, histoplasmin, candidin, etc. Tuberculin or purified protein derivative (PPD), which are extracts of the tubercle bacillus, have long been used to determine whether or not a patient has had previous contact with the organism from which the test antigen was derived. DTH reactions are always cell-mediated. Thus, they have a mechanism strikingly different from anaphylaxis or the Arthus reaction, which occur within minutes to hours following exposure of the host to antigen and are examples of antibody-mediated reactions. DTH is classified as type IV hypersensitivity (Coombs and Gell classification). A T$_{DTH}$ lymphocyte is a DTH T lymphocyte. DTH may be either permanent, persisting from months to years after sensitization, as occurs in classic tuberculin-type

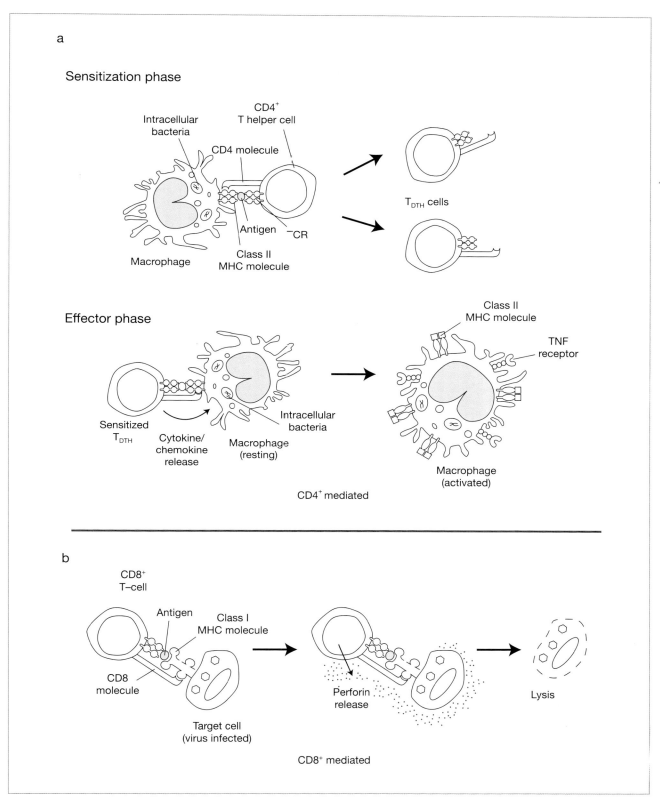

Figure 5 Schematic representation of type IV (cell-mediated) hypersensitivity. (a) Illustrates tuberculin reactivity in the skin that is mediated by CD4+ helper/inducer T cells and represents a form of bacterial allergy. (b) Illustrates the cytotoxic action of CD8+ T cells against a virus-infected target cell that presents antigen via class I major histocompatibility complex (MHC) molecules to its T cell receptor (TCR), resulting in the release of perforin and granzyme molecules that lead to target cell lysis. TNF, tumor necrosis factor

feron (IFN)-γ, IL-2, tumor necrosis factor (TNF)-β, TNF-α, granulocyte macrophage-colony stimulating factor (GM-CSF) and IL-3. Cytokines involved in a T_H2 CD4$^+$ cellular response include IL-3, IL-4, IL-5, IL-6, IL-10, IL-13, TNF-α and GM-CSF. T_H2 type immediate IgE-mediated hypersensitivity immune responses are induced by allergens such as animal dander, dust mites and pollens, which underly asthma. Positive tuberculin reactions induce T_H1 type DTH responses associated with T_H1 cytokines. T_H1 immunity might possibly inhibit atopic allergies by repressing T_H2 immune responses.

An **infection allergy** is a T cell-mediated DTH associated with infection by selected microorganisms such as *Mycobacterium tuberculosis*. This represents type IV hypersensitivity to antigenic products of microorganisms inducing a particular infection. It also develops in brucellosis, lymphogranuloma venereum, mumps and vaccinia. It is also called infection hypersensitivity.

A **bacterial allergy** is delayed-type hypersensitivity of infection, such as in tuberculosis.

Infection hypersensitivity is a tuberculin-type sensitivity that is more evident in some infections than others. It develops with great facility in tuberculosis, brucellosis, lymphogranuloma venereum, mumps and vaccinia. The sensitizing component of the antigen molecule is usually protein, although polysaccharides may induce delayed reactivity in cases of systemic fungal infections such as those caused by *Blastomyces*, *Histoplasma* and *Coccidioides*.

The **Koch phenomenon** is a delayed hypersensitivity reaction in the skin of a guinea pig after it has been infected with *Mycobacterium tuberculosis* (Figure 8). Robert Koch described the phenomenon in 1891 following the injection of either living or dead *M. tuberculosis* microorganisms into guinea pigs previously infected with the same microbes. He observed a severe necrotic reaction at the site of inoculation, which occasionally became generalized and induced death. The injection of killed *M. tuberculosis* microorganisms into healthy guinea pigs caused no ill effects. This is a demonstration of cell-mediated immunity and is the basis for the tuberculin test.

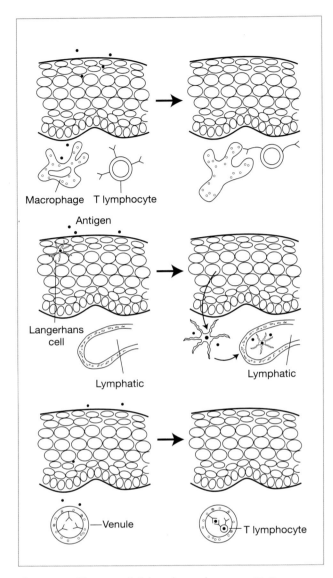

Figure 6 Diagram of delayed-type hypersensitivity

hypersensitivity, or transient, which resembles the permanent type morphologically but disappears 1–2 weeks following induction of sensitization. In the permanent type the inflammatory reaction remains prominent 72–96 h following intradermal injection of antigen, but the inflammatory reaction disappears 1–2 weeks after induction of sensitization in the transient type, in which the inflammatory lesion peaks at 24 h but disappears by 48–72 h (Jones–Mote hypersensitivity). The activation of T cells in DTH is associated with the secretion of cytokines. Activation of different subsets of T helper (T_H) cells leads to secretion of different types of cytokines. Those associated with a T_H1 CD4$^+$ cellular response profile include inter-

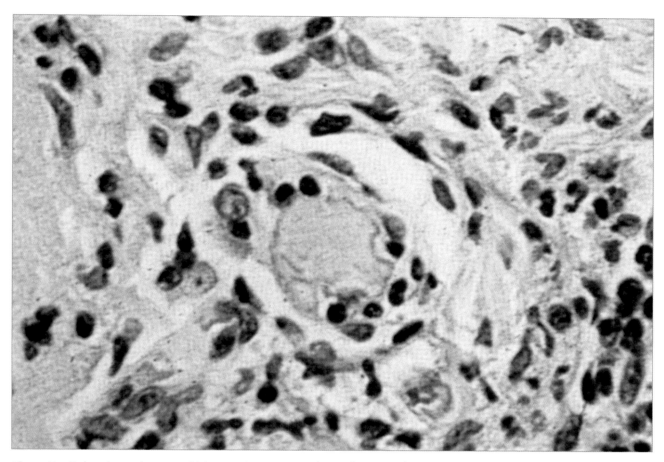

Figure 7 Delayed-type hypersensitivity reaction. Mononuclear cells accumulate around a small blood vessel

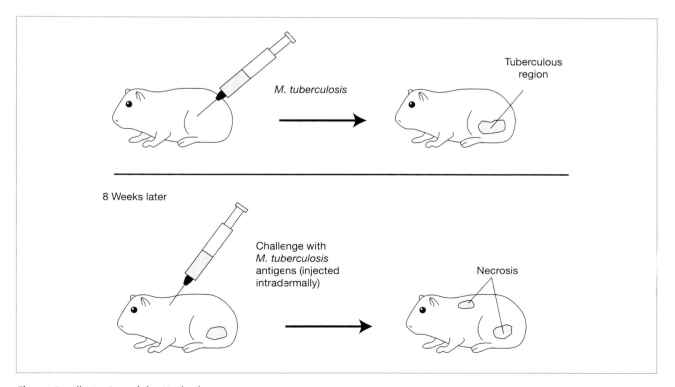

Figure 8 Illustration of the Koch phenomenon

Tuberculin is a sterile solution containing a group of proteins derived from culture medium where *Mycobacterium tuberculosis* microorganisms have been grown. It has been used for almost a century as a skin test preparation to detect delayed-type (type IV) hypersensitivity to infection with *M. tuberculosis*. Many tuberculin preparations have been used in the past, but only old tuberculin (OT) and purified protein derivative (PPD) are still used. Whereas OT is a heat-concentrated filtrate of the culture medium in which *M. tuberculosis* was grown, PPD of tuberculin is a trichloroacetic acid precipitate of the growth medium. Tuberculin is a mitogen for murine B lymphocytes, as well as a T lymphocyte mitogen.

Tuberculin hypersensitivity is a form of bacterial allergy specific for a product in culture filtrates of *Mycobacterium tuberculosis* which, when injected into the skin, elicits a cell-mediated delayed-type hypersensitivity (type IV) response. Tuberculin-type hypersensitivity is mediated by CD4$^+$ T lymphocytes. Following the intracutaneous inoculation of tuberculin extract or purified protein derivative (PPD), an area of redness and induration develops at the site within 24–48 h in individuals who have present or past interaction with *M. tuberculosis*.

PPD is an abbreviation for purified protein derivative of tuberculin.

Tuberculin reaction is a test of *in vivo* cell-mediated immunity. Robert Koch observed a localized lesion in the skin of tuberculous guinea pigs inoculated intradermally with broth from a culture of tubercle bacilli. The body's immune response to infection with the tubercle bacillus is signaled by the appearance of agglutinins, precipitins, opsonins and complement-fixing antibodies in the serum. This humoral response is, however, not marked, and such antibodies are present in low titer. The most striking response is the development of delayed-type hypersensitivity (DTH), which has a protective role in preventing reinfection with the same organism. Subcutaneous inoculation of tubercle bacilli in a normal animal produces no immediate response, but in 10–14 days a nodule develops at the site of inoculation. The nodule then becomes a typical tuberculous ulcer. The regional lymph nodes become swollen and caseous. In contrast, a similar inoculation in a tuberculous animal induces an indurated area at the site of injection within 1–2 days. This becomes a shallow ulcer which heals promptly. No swelling of the adjacent lymphatics is noted. The tubercle bacillus antigen responsible for DTH is wax D, a lipopolysaccharide–protein complex of the bacterial cell wall. The active peptide comprises diaminopimelic acid, glutamic acid and alanine. Testing for DTH to the tubercle bacillus is done with tuberculin, a heat-inactivated culture extract containing a mixture of bacterial proteins, or with PPD, a purified protein derivative of culture in non-proteinaceous media. Both these compounds are capable of sensitizing the recipient themselves. The protective role of DTH is supported by the observation that in positive reactors, living cells are usually free of tubercle bacilli and the bacteria are present in necrotic areas, separated by an avascular barrier. By contrast, in infected individuals giving a negative reaction, the tubercle bacilli are found in great numbers in living tissues. The reaction is permanently or transiently negative in individuals whose cell-mediated immune responses are transiently or permanently impaired.

Tuberculin test is the 24–48-h response to intradermal injection of tuberculin. If positive, it signifies delayed-type hypersensitivity (type IV) to tuberculin and implies cell-mediated immunity to *Mycobacterium tuberculosis*. The intradermal inoculation of tuberculin or of purified protein derivative (PPD) leads to an area of erythema and induration within 24–48 h in positive individuals. A positive reaction signifies the presence of cell-mediated immunity to *M. tuberculosis* as a consequence of past or current exposure to this microorganism. However, it is not a test for the diagnosis of active tuberculosis.

A **tuberculin-type reaction** is a cell-mediated delayed-type hypersensitivity skin response to an extract such as candidin, brucellin or histoplasmin. Individuals who have positive reactions have developed delayed-type hypersensitivity or cell-mediated immunity mediated by T lymphocytes following contact with the microorganism in question.

Tuberculosis immunization is the induction of protective immunity through injection of an attenuated vaccine containing bacillus Calmette–Guérin (BCG). This vaccine was more widely used in Europe than in the USA in an attempt to provide protection against development of tuberculosis. A local papule develops several weeks after injection in individuals who were previously tuberculin negative, as it is not administered to positive individuals. It is claimed to protect against development of tuberculosis, although not all authorities agree on its efficacy for this purpose. In recent years, oncologists have used BCG vaccine to reactivate the cellular immune system of patients bearing neoplasms in the hope of facilitating antitumor immunity.

Anergy is a diminished or absent delayed-type hypersensitivity, i.e. type IV hypersensitivity, as revealed by lack of responsiveness to commonly used skin test antigens, including purified protein derivative (PPD), histoplasmin, candidin, etc. Decreased skin test reactivity may be associated with uncontrolled infection, tumor, Hodgkin's disease, sarcoidosis, etc. (Figure 9). There is decreased capacity of T lymphocytes to secrete lymphokines when their T cell receptors interact with specific antigen.

Macrophage/monocyte inhibitory factor (MIF) is a substance synthesized by T lymphocytes in response to immunogenic challenge that inhibits the migration of macrophages. MIF is a 25-kDa lymphokine. Its mechanism of action is by elevating intracellular cyclic adenosine monophosphate (cAMP), polymerizing microtubules and stopping macrophage migration. MIF may increase the adhesive properties of macrophages, thereby inhibiting their migration. The two types of the protein MIF include one that is 65-kDa with an isoelectric point (pI) of 3–4 and another that is 25-kDa with a pI of approximately 5.

The **macrophage migration test** is an *in vitro* assay of cell-mediated immunity. Macrophages and lymphocytes from the individual to be tested are placed into segments of capillary tubes about the size of microhematocrit tubes and incubated in tissue culture medium containing the soluble antigen of interest, with maintenance of appropriate controls incubated in the same medium not containing the antigen. Lymphocytes, from an animal or human sensitized to the antigen, release a lymphokine called migration inhibitory factor that will block migration of macrophages from the end

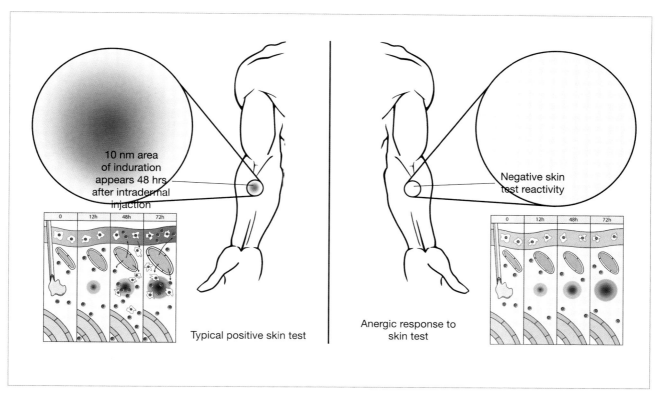

10 nm area of induration appears 48 hrs after intradermal injection

Negative skin test reactivity

Typical positive skin test

Anergic response to skin test

Figure 9 Representation of anergy

	No antigen	Ovalbumin	Toxoid
Normal cells	A	B	C
Ovalbumin–sensitive cells	D	E	F
Toxoid–sensitive cells	G	H	I

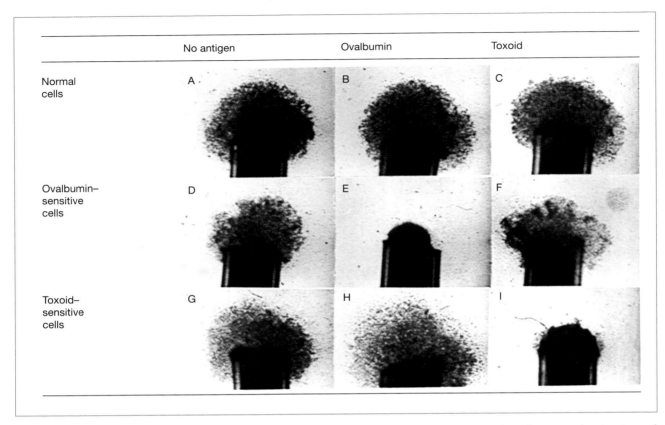

Figure 10 The macrophage/monocyte inhibitory factor (MIF) assay. Specific antigen inhibits the normal migration of macrophages from capillary tubes

of the tube where the cells form an aggregated mass. The macrophages in the control preparation (that does not contain antigen) will migrate out of the tube into a fan-like pattern (Figures 10 and 11).

Contact hypersensitivity is a type IV delayed-type hypersensitivity reaction in the skin characterized by a delayed-type hypersensitivity (cell-mediated) immune reaction produced by cytotoxic T lymphocytes invading the epidermis. It is often induced by applying a skin-sensitizing simple chemical such as dinitrochloroben-zene (DNCB) that acts as a hapten uniting with proteins in the skin, leading to the delayed-type hyper-sensitivity response mediated by CD4$^+$ T cells. Although substances such as DNCB alone are not anti-genic, they may combine with epidermal proteins which serve as carriers for these simple chemicals acting as haptens. Contact hypersensitivity may follow sensiti-zation by topical drugs, cosmetics or other types of contact chemicals. The causative agents, usually simple, low-molecular-weight compounds (mostly aromatic molecules), may also behave as haptens. The develop-

ment of sensitization depends on the penetrability of the agent and its ability to form covalent bonds with protein. Part of the sensitizing antigen molecule is thus represented by protein, usually the fibrous protein of the skin. Local skin conditions that alter local proteins, such as inflammation, stasis and others, facilitate the development of contact hypersensitivity, but some chemicals such as penicillin, picric acid or sulfonamides are unable to conjugate to proteins, but their degrada-tion products may have this property.

Contact sensitivity (CS) (or allergic contact dermatitis) is a form of delayed-type hypersensitivity (DTH) reaction limited to the skin and consisting of eczematous changes. It follows sensitization by topical drugs, cosmetics or other types of contact chemicals. The causative agents, usually simple, low-molecular-weight compounds (mostly aromatic molecules), behave as haptens. The development of sensitization depends on the penetrability of the agent and its ability to form covalent bonds with protein. Part of the sensi-tizing antigen molecule is thus represented by protein,

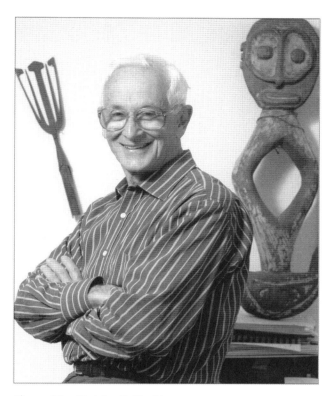

Figure 11 Dr John R. David

usually the fibrous protein of the skin. Local skin conditions that alter local proteins, such as inflammation, stasis and others, facilitate the development of CS, but some chemicals such as penicillin, picric acid or sulfonamides are unable to conjugate to proteins. It is believed that in this case the degradation products of such chemicals have this property. CS may also be induced by hapten conjugates given by other routes in adjuvant. The actual immunogen in CS remains unidentified. CS may also have a toxic, non-immunologic component, and frequently both toxic and sensitizing effects can be produced by the same compound. With exposure to industrial compounds, an initial period of increased sensitivity is followed by a gradual decrease in reactivity. This phenomenon is called hardening, and could represent a process of spontaneous desensitization. The histologic changes in CS are characteristic. Vascular endothelial cells in skin lesions produce cytokine-regulated surface molecules such as IL-2. IL-4 mRNA is strongly expressed in allergic contact dermatitis lesions. IFN-γ mRNA is the predominant cytokine in tuberculin reactions. IL-10 mRNA overexpression in atopic dermatitis might facilitate upregulation of humoral responses and downregulation of T_H1 responses. Selected allergic subjects manifest several types of autoantibodies including IgE and β-adrenergic receptor autoantibodies.

Poison ivy hypersensitivity is principally type IV contact hypersensitivity induced by urushiols, which are chemical constituents of poison ivy (*Rhus toxicodendron*), when poison ivy plants containing this chemical come into contact with the skin. The urushiol acts as a hapten by complexing with skin proteins to induce cellular (type IV) hypersensitivity on contact, also called delayed-type hypersensitivity.

Urushiols are catechols in poisoning (*Rhus toxicodendron*) plants that act as allergens to produce contact hypersensitivity, i.e. contact dermatitis at skin sites touched by the urushiol-bearing plant. The cutaneous lesion is T cell mediated and is classified as type IV hypersensitivity. There are four *Rhus* catechols that differ according to pentadecyl side-chain saturation. They induce type IV delayed hypersensitivity. These substances are present in such plants as poison oak, poison sumac and poison ivy.

Pentadecacatechol is the chemical constituent of the leaves of poison ivy plants that induces cell-mediated immunity associated with hypersensitivity to poison ivy.

A **patch test** is an assay to determine the cause of skin allergy, especially contact allergic (type IV) hypersensitivity. A small square of cotton, linen or paper impregnated with the suspected allergen is applied to the skin for 24–48 h. The test is read by examining the site 1–2 days after applying the patch. The development of redness (erythema) and edema and formation of vesicles constitutes a positive test. The impregnation of tuberculin into a patch was used by Vollmer for a modified tuberculin test. There are multiple chemicals, toxins and other allergens that may induce allergic contact dermatitis in exposed members of the population.

The **Jones–Mote reaction** is a delayed-type (type IV) hypersensitivity to protein antigens associated with prominent basophil infiltration of the skin immediately beneath the dermis, which gives the reaction the additional name 'cutaneous basophil hypersensitivity'. Compared with the other forms of delayed-type hypersensitivity, it is relatively weak, and appears on challenge several days following sensitization with minute quantities of protein antigens in aqueous medium or in incomplete Freund's adjuvant. No necrosis is produced. Jones–Mote hypersensitivity can be produced in laboratory animals such as guinea pigs appropriately exposed to protein antigens in aqueous media or in incomplete Freund's adjuvant. It can be induced by the intradermal injection of a soluble antigen such as ovalbumin incorporated into Freund's incomplete adjuvant. Swelling of the skin reaches a maximum between 7 and 10 days following induction, and vanishes when antibody is formed. Histologically, basophils predominate, but lymphocytes and mononuclear cells are also present. Jones–Mote hypersensitivity is greatly influenced by lymphocytes that are sensitive to cyclophosphamide (suppressor lymphocytes). It can be passively transferred by T lymphocytes.

REFERENCES

1. Koch R. *Dtsch Med Wschr* 1890;16:1029, 1891;17:101, 1189. ('old tuberculin', cited by Topley WWC. In Wilson GS, Miles AA, rev. *Topley and Wilson's Principles of Bacteriology and Immunity*, 3rd edn. Baltimore: Williams & Wilkins, 1946:1326–30)

2. Rich AR, Lewis MR. Nature of allergy in tuberculosis as revealed by tissue culture studies. *Johns Hopkins Hosp Bull* 1932;50:115–31

3. Landsteiner K, Chase MW. Experiments on transfer of cutaneous sensitivity to simple compounds. *Proc Soc Exp Biol Med* 1942;49:688–90

4. Lawrence HS. The cellular transfer of cutaneous hypersensitivity to tuberculin in man. *Proc Soc Exp Biol Med* 1949;71:516–22

5. Khan A, Kirkpatrick CH, Hill NO, eds. *International Symposium on Transfer Factor, 3rd Wadley Institutes of Molecular Medicine, 1978. Immune regulators in transfer factor.* New York: Academic Press, 1979

6. Nowell PC. Phytohemagglutinin: an initiator of mitosis in cultures of normal human leukocytes. *Cancer Res* 1960;20:462–6

7. David JR. Delayed hypersensitivity *in vitro*: its mediation by cell-free substances formed by lymphoid cell antigen interaction. *Proc Natl Acad Sci USA* 1966;56:72–7

8. Bloom BR. *In vitro* approaches to the mechanism of cell mediated immune reactions. *Adv Immunol* 1971; 13:101–208

9. Billingham RE, Brent L. A simple method for inducing tolerance of skin homografts in mice. *Transplant Bull* 1957;4:67–71

10. Simonsen M. The impact on a developing embryo and newborn animals of adult homologous cells. *Acta Pathol Microbiol Scand* 1957;40:480–500

CHAPTER 8

Immunobiology, cellular immunology and tumor immunity

IMMUNOBIOLOGY AND CELLULAR IMMUNOLOGY

There was a renaissance of interest in cellular immunology from 1942 through 1952. In 1942, Coons (Chapter 13, Figure 1a) perfected immunofluorescence to demonstrate antigens and antibodies in cells[1]. That same year, Landsteiner and Chase (Chapter 2, Figures 39 and 42) reported the transfer of delayed-type hypersensitivity with lymphoid cells but not with serum[2].

To speak of cellular immunity apart from humoral immunity could be considered unwarranted, because in actuality all of immunology is cellular. The renewed interest in cellular immunology is reminiscent of the revolution brought about by Virchow when he published his lectures on cellular pathology in 1858[3]. Nevertheless, it is important for us to trace the main events relating cells of the lymphoid system to antibody production and cell-mediated immunity. Even in the 1920s, Murphy, of the Rockefeller Institute for Medical Research, wrote a monograph on the lymphocyte[4]. In 1945, Harris and associates discussed the role of the lymphocyte in antibody formation[5], and in 1948, Astrid Fagraeus (Figure 1a–e) wrote her doctoral thesis on the role of the plasma cell in antibody formation[6]. While attempting to immunize chickens in which the bursa of Fabricius had been removed, Glick (Figure 2) and associates (1956) noted that antibody production did not take place[7]. This important discovery, which appeared in the journal *Poultry Science*, subsequently permitted the demonstration that the immune system of the chicken is divisible into a thymic-dependent T-cell system and a bursa-dependent B-lymphocyte limb.

Glick correctly interpreted a laboratory mistake to show the role of the bursa of Fabricius in the production of antibody and the division of labor in lymphocyte populations. H. Wolfe, University of Wisconsin, and Robert Good (Figures 3 and 4), University of Minnesota, immediately realized the significance of this finding for childhood immunodeficiencies. Good and his colleagues in Minneapolis[8,9] and J. F. A. P. Miller (Figure 5) in Melbourne[10] went on to show the role of

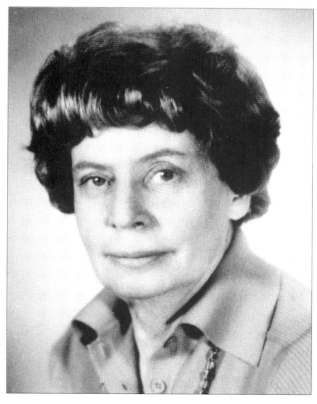

Figure 1a Astrid Fagraeus

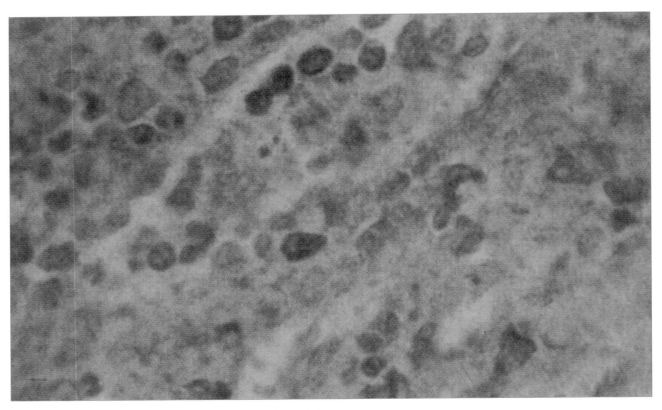

Figure 1b   Plasma cells (from Dr Astrid Fagraeus' doctoral thesis)

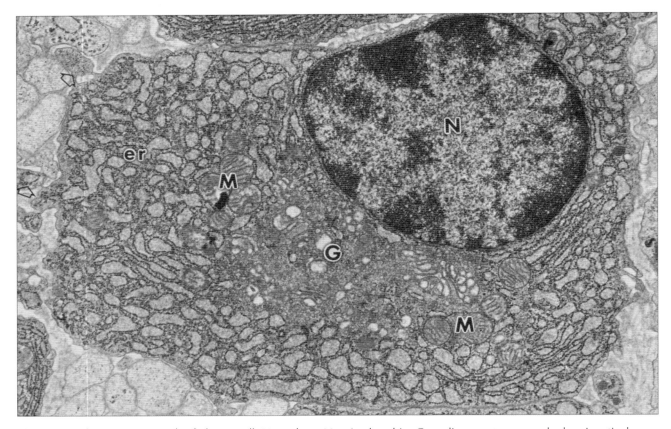

Figure 1c   Electron micrograph of plasma cell. N, nucleus; M, mitochondria; G, gogli apparatus; er, endoplasmic reticulum

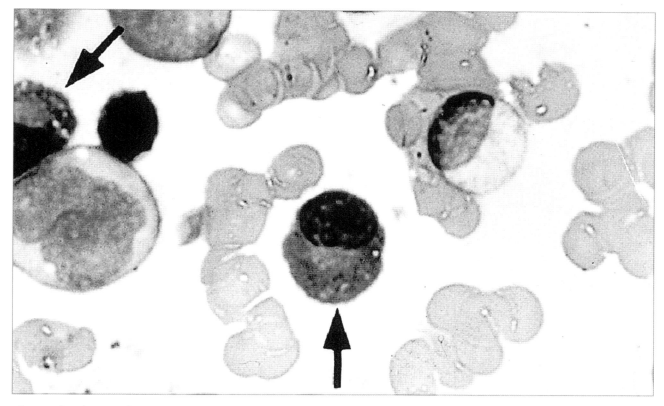

Figure 1d Plasma cells

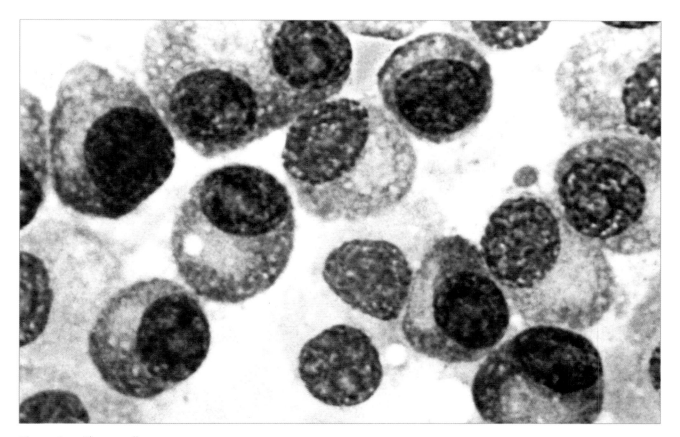

Figure 1e Plasma cells

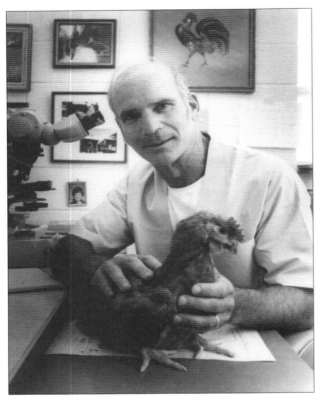

Figure 2   Bruce Glick

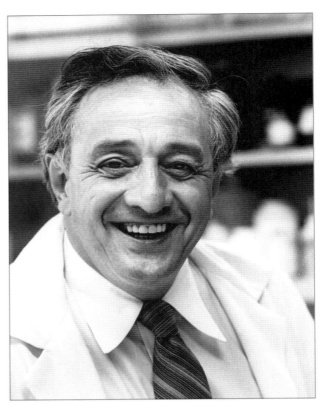

Figure 3   Robert A. Good

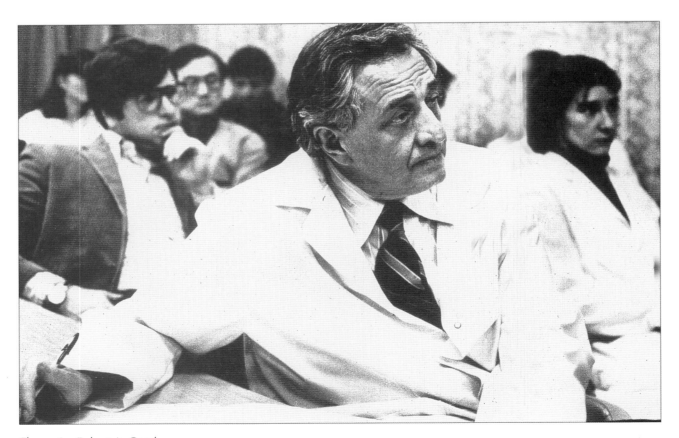

Figure 4   Robert A. Good

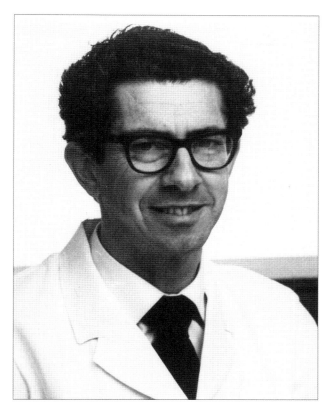

Figure 5   J. F. A. P. Miller

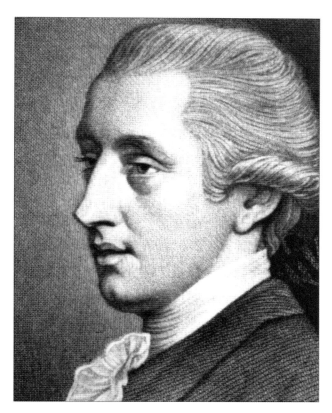

Figure 6   William Hewson (1739–74)

the thymus in the immune response, and various investigators began to search for bursa equivalents in many other animals. Interestingly, William Hewson's (1739–74) early concepts on the thymus were remarkably correct (Figure 6). J. F. A. P. Miller demonstrated the role of the thymus in immunity while in pursuit of gross leukemia virus in neonatal mice. Dr Robert Good and associates helped establish the role of the thymus in the education of lymphocytes, and made fundamental contributions to understanding the ontogeny and phylogeny of immunity. Hasek, studying parabiosis in chick embryos made fundamental contributions to immunologic tolerance and transplantation biology (Figure 7). In 1959, Gowans (Figure 8) proved that lymphocytes actually recirculate[11]. His insight that the lymphocytes recirculate via the thoracic duct made radical changes in the understanding of the role of lymphocytes. In 1966, Harris, Hummeler and Harris clearly demonstrated that lymphocytes could form antibodies[12]. In 1966 and 1967, Claman (Figure 9)[12], Davies[14] and Mitchison[15] showed that T and B lymphocytes cooperate with one another in the production of an immune response. Henry N. Claman (1930–)

produced some of the first evidence that T and B cells act synergistically in the humoral response. Various phenomena, such as the switch from forming one class of immunoglobulin to another by B cells was demonstrated to be dependent upon a signal from T cells, which could induce B cells to change from immunoglobulin IgM to IgG or IgA production. B cells stimulated by antigen in which no cell signal was given continued to produce IgM antibody. Such antigens were referred to as thymic-independent antigens, and others requiring T cell participation as thymic-dependent antigens. In 1971, Gershon (Figure 10) and Kondo demonstrated that among the T lymphocyte subsets were suppressor T cells[16]. This was one of the first demonstrations of the suppressive role of the T cell. They were the subject of much investigation, and were postulated to play an important role in immunoregulation and in various autoimmune disease states of man and animals. Thus, immune regulation was considered to depend in part upon a delicate balance between helper T lymphocytes and these T-suppressor cells. Later advances in molecular biology cast some doubt on the suppressor concept. Jerne

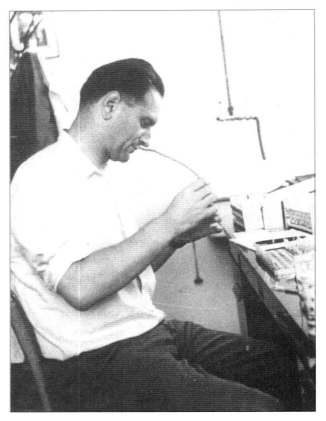

Figure 7   Milan Hasek

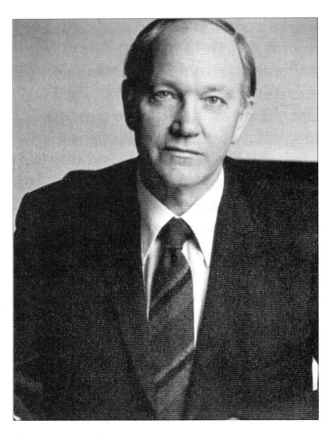

Figure 8   J. L. Gowans

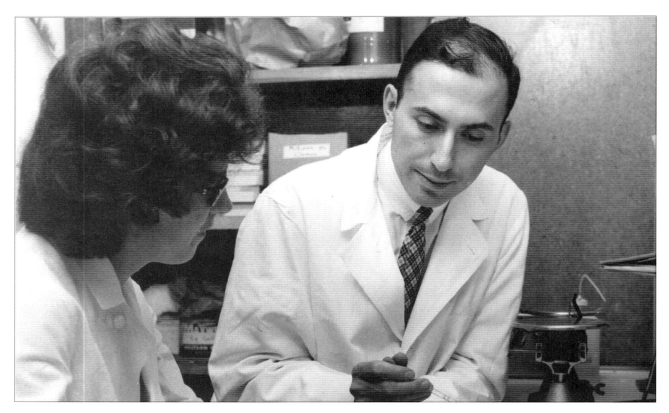

Figure 9   Henry Claman

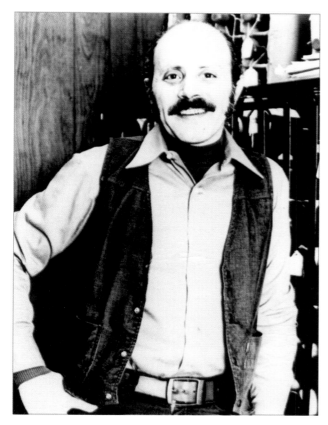

Figure 10 R. Gershon

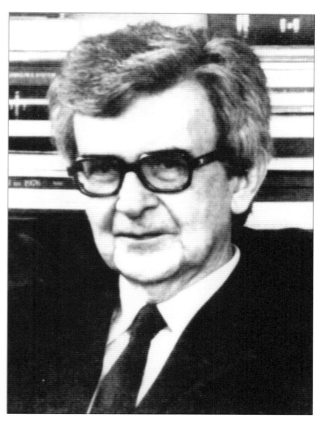

Figure 11 Niels Jerne

(Figure 11) (1974) proposed a network theory of immune regulation[17], and Cantor and Boyse (1975) described T-cell subclasses that were distinguished by their Ly antigens[18]. They also investigated cell cooperation in the cell-mediated lympholysis (CML) reaction[19].

Astrid Elsa Fagraeus–Wallbom (1913–), Swedish investigator noted for her doctoral thesis which provided the first clear evidence that immunoglobulins are made in plasma cells. In 1962, she became Chief of the Virus Department of the National Bacteriological Laboratory, and in 1965, Professor of Immunology at the Karolinska Institute in Stockholm. She also investigated cell membrane antigens and contributed to the field of clinical immunology. *Antibody Production in Relation to the Development of Plasma Cells*, Stockholm, 1948.

Milan Hasek (1925–85), Czechoslovakian scientist whose contributions to immunology include investigations of immunologic tolerance and the development of chick embryo parabiosis. Hasek also made fundamental contributions to transplantation biology.

Bruce Glick, as a graduate student at Ohio State University, became interested in the bursa of the chicken and removed the organ from the cloacas of some test animals for study. Some of the bursectomized chicks happened to be used for a class demonstration of antibody formation and failed to produce antibody. Glick and associates sent an article to *Science*, which was refused, so they published their finding in *Poultry Science*. Harold Wolfe, at the University of Wisconsin, Madison, understood the importance of this fact, and the hunt began to identify the two big classes of lymphocytes, T and B cells, the latter being so called because they are 'bursa derived'.

Henry Claman in Denver and A. J. S. Davies in London conducted studies with lethally irradiated

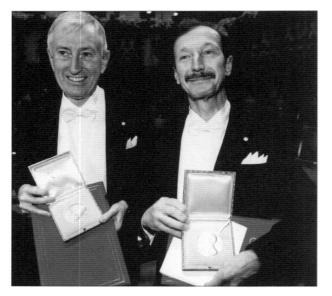

Figure 12 Peter Doherty and Rolf Zinkernagel

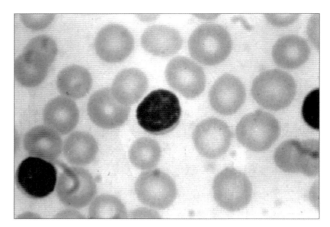

Figure 13 Lymphocytes

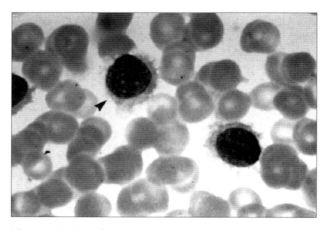

Figure 14 Lymphocytes

mice, which proved that both bursa-derived and thymus-derived lymphocytes were needed to produce an immune response, T and B cooperation.

Robert Alan Good (1922–2003), American immunologist and pediatrician who has made major contributions to studies on the ontogeny and phylogeny of the immune response. Much of his work focused on immunodeficiency diseases and the role of the thymus and the bursa of Fabricius in immunity. He and his colleagues demonstrated the role of the thymus in the education of lymphocytes. *The Thymus in Immunobiology*, 1964; *Phylogeny of Immunity*, 1966.

J. F. A. P. Miller (1931–), proved the role of the thymus in immunity while investigating gross leukemia in neonatal mice.

James Gowans (1924–), British physician and investigator whose principal contribution to immunology was the demonstration that lymphocytes recirculate via the thoracic duct, which radically changed understanding of the role lymphocytes play in immune reactions. He also investigated lymphocyte function. He served as Director of the Medical Research Council (MRC) Cellular Immunobiology Unit, Oxford, 1963.

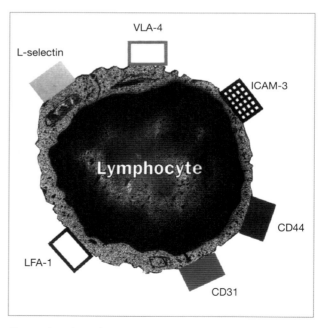

Figure 15 Lymphocyte

Richard K. Gershon (1932–83), one of the first to demonstrate the suppressor role of the T cell. The suppressor T cell was described as a subpopulation of lymphocytes that diminish or suppress antibody formation by B cells or downregulate the ability of T lymphocytes to mount a cellular immune response. The inability to confirm the presence of receptor molecules on their surface has cast a cloud over the suppressor cell; however, functional suppressor-cell effects are indisputable.

In 1975, Köhler (Chaper 13, Figure 8) and Milstein (Chaper 13, Figure 9) successfully fused splenic lymphocytes from mice forming antibody with tumor cells to produce what they called a 'hybridoma'[20]. The spleen cells conferred the antibody-forming capacity, while the tumor cells provided the capability for immortality or endless reproduction. This important technique permitted the formation of a homogeneous antibody population of a desired specificity by taking the spleen cells from animals specifically immunized with a certain antigen. At the 1980 International Congress of Immunology held in Paris, Henry Kaplan and Lennart Olsson of Stanford University reported a hybridoma formed with human cells[21]. Zinkernagel and Doherty (Figure 12) (1975) proposed an altered-self concept and dual recognition by T cells[22]. They proved major histocompatibility complex (MHC) restriction in the reaction of T cells with antigen. Further investigations of T cells have proceeded at an unprecedented pace.

A **lymphocyte** (Figures 13–15) is a round cell that measures 7–12 µm and contains a round to ovoid nucleus that may be indented. The chromatin is densely packed and stains dark blue with Romanowsky stain. Small lymphocytes contain a thin rim of robin's egg blue cytoplasm, and a few azurophilic granules may be present. Large lymphocytes have more cytoplasm and a similar nucleus. Electron microscopy reveals villi that cover most of the cell surface. Lymphocytes are divided into two principal groups, termed B and T lymphocytes. They are distinguished not on morphology, but on the expression of distinctive surface molecules that have precise roles in immune reaction. In addition, natural killer cells, which are large granular lymphocytes, constitute a small percentage of the lymphocyte population. Lymphocytes express variable cell surface receptors for antigen.

T cell development Stem cells in the bone marrow that are destined to develop into T cells migrate to the thymus where they undergo maturation and development. These precursors of T cells possess unrearranged T cell receptor (TCR) genes and express neither CD4 nor CD8 markers. Thymocytes, the developing T cells, are found first in the outer cortex where their numbers increase, the TCR genes are rearranged and CD3, CD4, CD8 and T cell receptor molecules are expressed on the surface. During maturation, these cells pass from the cortex to the medulla. As maturation proceeds, CD4$^-$CD8$^-$ (double negative) T cells develop into CD4$^+$CD8$^+$ cells that become either CD4$^+$CD8$^-$ or CD4$^-$CD8$^+$ single positive T cells. Somatic rearrangement of variable, diversity (β) and joining gene segments in the area of constant (C) gene segments lead to the production of functional genes that encode TCR α and β polypeptides. Many T cell specificities result from the numerous combinations possible for joining of separate gene segments in addition to various mechanisms for junctional diversity. Somatic rearrangement of germ line genes is also responsible for the functional genes that encode TCR γ and δ polypeptides. Even though there are fewer variable (V) genes in the γ and δ loci and greater junction diversity, the mechanisms to produce γδ diversity resemble those for the αβ receptor. A few cortical thymocytes express γδ receptors. Thereafter, a line of developing T lymphocytes express numerous αβ TCRs. Beta chains appear first followed by α chains of TCR. The β chain associates itself with an invariant pre-T α surrogate alpha chain. Signals transduced by the pTαβ receptor facilitate expression of CD4 and CD8 and facilitate expansion of immature thymocytes. CD4$^+$CD8$^+$ cortical thymocytes first express αβ receptors. Self-MHC restriction and self-tolerance develop as a consequence of the interaction between cortical epithelial cells and non-lymphoid cells derived from the bone marrow that both express MHC. This leads to selection of those T cells that are to be saved. During positive selection, CD4$^+$CD8$^+$ TCR αβ thymocytes recognize peptide–MHC complexes on thymic epithelial cells with low avidity. This saves them from programmed cell death or apoptosis. Recognition of self-peptide–MHC complexes on thymic antigen-presenting cells with avidity by CD4$^+$CD8$^+$ TCR αβ thymocytes leads to apoptosis. The majority of cortical thymocyes are killed during selection processes. Those αβ thymocytes that remain undergo maturation and proceed to the medulla, where they become single positive cells that are either CD4$^+$CD8$^-$ or CD4$^-$CD8$^+$. During residence in the medulla, these cells become either helper or cytolytic cells prior to their journey to the peripheral lymphoid tissues, where they function as self-MHC-restricted helper T cells or pre-cytotoxic T lymphocytes, capable of responding to foreign antigen.

A **T lymphocyte (T cell)** (Figures 16 and 17) is a thymus-derived lymphocyte that confers cell-mediated immunity. They cooperate with B lymphocytes, enabling them to synthesize antibody specific for thymus-dependent antigens, including switching from IgM to IgG and/or IgA production. T lymphocytes exiting the thymus recirculate in the blood and lymph and in the peripheral lymphoid organs. They migrate to the deep cortex of lymph nodes. Those in the blood may attach to postcapillary venule endothelial cells of lymph nodes and to the marginal sinus in the spleen. After passing across the venules into the splenic white pulp or lymph node cortex, they reside there for 12–24 h and exit by the efferent lymphatics. They proceed to the thoracic duct, and from there proceed to the left subclavian vein where they enter the blood circulation. Mature T cells are classified on the basis of their surface markers, such as CD4 and CD8. CD4$^+$ T lymphocytes recognize antigens in the context of MHC class II histocompatibility molecules, whereas CD8$^+$ T lymphocytes recognize antigen in the context of class I MHC histocompatibility molecules. The CD4$^+$ T cells participate in the afferent limb of the immune response to exogenous antigen, which is presented to them by antigen-presenting cells. This stimulates the synthesis of interleukin (IL)-2, which activates CD8$^+$ T cells, natural killer (NK) cells and B cells, thereby orchestrating an immune response to the antigen. Thus, they are termed helper T lymphocytes. They also mediate delayed-type hypersensitivity reactions. CD8$^+$ T lymphocytes include cytotoxic and suppressor cell populations. They react to endogenous antigen and often express their effector function by a cytotoxic mechanism, e.g. against a virus-infected cell. Other molecules on mature T cells in humans include the E rosette receptor CD2 molecule, the T cell receptor, the pan-T cell marker termed CD3 and transferrin receptors.

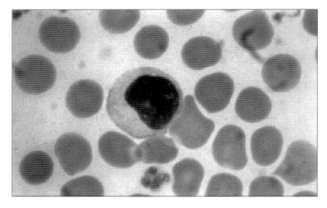

Figure 16   T lymphocyte

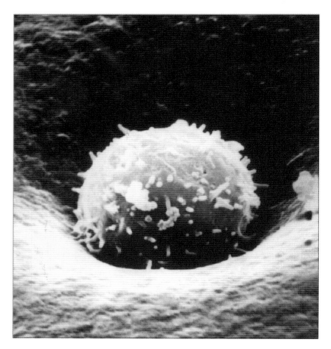

Figure 17   T lymphocyte

T lymphocytes are T cells. T lymphocyte precursors are detectable in the human fetus at 7 weeks of gestation. Between 7 and 14 weeks of gestation, thymic changes begin to imprint thymic lymphocytes as T cells. The maturation (mediated by hormones such as thymosin, thymulin and thymopoietin II) can be followed by identification of surface (cluster of differentiation (CD)) markers detectable by immunophenotyping methods. CD3, a widespread T cell marker, serves as a signal transducer from the antigen receptor to the cell interior. Thus, the CD3 molecule is intermittently associated with the T cell receptor for antigen. T lymphocytes in the medulla initially express both CD4 and CD8 class markers; however, these cells will later differentiate into either CD4$^+$ helper cells or CD8$^+$ suppressor cells. The CD4$^+$ cells, characterized by a 55-kDa surface marker, communicate with macrophages and B cells bearing MHC class II molecules during antigen presentation. The CD8$^+$ suppressor/cytotoxic cells interact with antigen-presenting cells bearing MHC class I molecules.

Helper T cells are CD4$^+$ helper/inducer T lymphocytes. They represent a subset of T cells which are critical for induction of an immune response to a foreign antigen. Antigen is presented by an antigen-presenting cell such as the macrophage in the context of self-MHC class II antigen and IL-1. Once activated, the CD4$^-$ T cells express IL-2 receptors and produce IL-2 molecules which can act in an autocrine fashion by combining with the IL-2 receptors and stimulating the CD4$^-$ cells to proliferate. Differentiated CD4$^-$ lymphocytes synthesize and secrete lymphokines that affect the function of other cells of the immune system, such as CD8$^-$ cells, B cells and NK cells. B cells differentiate into plasma cells that synthesize antibody. Activated macrophages participate in delayed-type hypersensitivity (type IV) reactions. Cytotoxic T cells also develop. Murine monoclonal antibodies are used to enumerate CD4$^-$ T lymphocytes by flow cytometry.

T$_H$0 cells are a subset of CD4$^-$ cells in both humans and mice based on cytokine production and effector functions. T$_H$0 cells synthesize multiple cytokines. They are responsible for effects intermediate between those of T$_H$1 and T$_H$2 cells, based on the cytokines synthesized and the responding cells. T$_H$0 cells may be precursors of T$_H$1 and T$_H$2 cells.

T$_H$1 cells are a subset of CD4$^-$ cells which synthesize interferon (IFN)-γ, IL-2 and tumor necrosis factor (TNF)-β. They are mainly responsible for cellular immunity against intracellular microorganisms and for delayed-type hypersensitivity reactions. They affect IgG2a antibody synthesis and antibody-dependent cell-mediated cytotoxicity. T$_H$1 cells activate host defense mediated by phagocytes. Intracellular microbial infections induce T$_H$1 cell development which facilitates elimination of the microorganisms by phagocytosis. T$_H$1 cells induce synthesis of antibody that activates complement and

serves as an opsonin that facilitates phagocytosis. The IFN-γ they produce enhances macrophage activation. The cytokines released by T$_H$1 cells activate NK cells, macrophages and CD8$^+$ T cells. Their main function is to induce phagocyte-mediated defense against infections, particularly by intracellular microorganisms.

T$_H$2 cells are a subset of CD4$^-$ cells which synthesize IL-4, IL-5, IL-6, IL-9, IL-10 and IL-13. They greatly facilitate IgE and IgG1 antibody responses, and mucosal immunity, by synthesis of mast cell and eosinophil growth and differentiation factors and facilitation of IgA synthesis. IL-4 facilitates IgE antibody synthesis. IL-5 is an eosinophil-activating substance. IL-10, IL-13 and IL-4 suppress cell-mediated immunity. T$_H$2 cells are principally responsible for host defense exclusive of phagocytes. They are crucial for the IgE and eosinophil response to helminthes, and for allergy attributable to activation of basophils and mast cells through IgE.

Cytotoxic T lymphocytes (CTLs) are a subset of antigen-specific effector T cells that have a principal role in protection and recovery from viral infection, mediate allograft rejection, participate in selected autoimmune diseases, participate in protection and recovery from selected bacterial and parasitic infections and are active in tumor immunity. They are CD8$^+$, class I major histocompatibility complex (MHC)-restricted, non-proliferating endstage effector cells. However, this classification also includes T cells that evoke one or several mechanisms to produce cytolysis, including perforin/granzyme, Fas ligand (FasL)/Fas and tumor necrosis factor (TNF)-α, synthesize various lymphokines by T$_H$1 and T$_H$2 lymphocytes and recognize foreign antigen in the context of either class I or class II MHC molecules.

Suppressor T cells (T$_S$ cells) constitute a T lymphocyte subpopulation that diminishes or suppresses antibody formation by B cells or downregulates the ability of T lymphocytes to mount a cellular immune response. T$_S$ cells may induce suppression that is specific for antigen, idiotype or non-specific. Some CD8$^+$ T lymphocytes diminish T helper CD4$^+$ lymphocyte responsiveness to both endogenous and exogenous antigens. This leads to suppression of the immune response. An overall immune response may be a consequence of the balance between helper T lymphocyte and suppressor T lymphocyte stimulation. Suppressor T cells are also significant in the establishment of immunologic tolerance, and are particularly active in response to unprocessed antigen. The inability to confirm the presence of receptor molecules on suppressor cells has cast a cloud over the suppressor cell; however, functional suppressor cell effects are indisputable. Some suppressor T lymphocytes are antigen specific and are important in the regulation of T helper cell function. Like cytotoxic T cells, T suppressor cells are MHC class I restricted. T cells may act as suppressors of various immune responses by forming inhibitory cytokines.

T cell receptor (TCR) is a T cell surface structure that comprises a disulfide-linked heterodimer of highly variable α and β chains expressed at the cell membrane as a complex with the invariant CD3 chains (Figure 18). Most T cells that bear this type of receptor are termed αβ T cells. A second receptor, the γδ TCR, is composed of variable γ and δ chains expressed with CD3 on a smaller subset of T lymphocytes that recognize different types of antigens. Both of these types of receptors are expressed with a disulfide-linked homodimer of ξ chains. The TCR is a receptor for antigen on CD4$^+$ and CD8$^+$ T lymphocytes that recognizes foreign peptide–self-MHC molecular complexes on the surface of antigen-presenting cells. In the predominant αβ TCR, the two disulfide-linked transmembrane α and β polypeptide chains each bear one N-terminal immunoglobulin (Ig)-like variable (V) domain, one Ig-like constant (C) domain, a hydrophobic transmembrane region and a short cytoplasmic region.

There are two types of **T cell antigen receptors**: TCR1, which appears first in ontogeny, and TCR2 (Figure 19). TCR2 is a heterodimer of two polypeptides (α and β); TCR1 consists of γ and δ polypeptides (Figure 19). Each of the two polypeptides constituting each receptor has a constant and a variable region (similar to immunoglobulin). Reminiscent of the diversity of antibody molecules, T cell antigen receptors can likewise identify a tremendous number of antigenic specificities (estimated to be able to recognize 10^{15} epitopes).

The TCR is a structure comprising a minimum of seven receptor subunits, whose production is encoded by six separate genes. Following transcription, these subunits are assembled precisely. Assimilation of the complete receptor complex is requisite for surface expression of TCR subunits. Numerous biochemical events are associated with activation of a cell through the TCR receptor. These events ultimately lead to receptor subunit phosphorylation.

T cells may be activated by the interaction of antigen, in the context of MHC, with the T cell receptor. This involves transmission of a signal to the interior through the CD3 protein to activate the cell.

αβ T cells are T lymphocytes that express αβ chain heterodimers on their surface. The vast majority of T cells are of the αβ variety. T lymphocytes that express an antigen receptor are composed of α and β polypeptide chains. This population, to which most T cells belong, includes all those that recognize peptide antigen presented by major histocompatibility complex (MHC) class I and class II molecules.

γδ T cells are early T lymphocytes that express γ and δ chains making up the T cell receptor of the cell surface. They constitute only 5% of the normal circulating T cells in healthy adults. γδ T cells 'home' to the lamina propria of the gut. Their function is not fully understood.

The **γδ T cell receptor** is a far less common receptor than the αβ TCR (Figure 19). It comprises γ and δ chains and occurs on the surface of early thymocytes and a small number of peripheral blood lymphocytes. The γδ TCR appears on double-negative CD4$^-$CD8$^-$ cells. Thus, the γδ heterodimer resembles its αβ counterpart in possessing both V and C regions, but has less diversity. TCR specificity and diversity are attributable to the multiplicity of germ line V gene segments subjected to somatic recombination in T cell ontogeny, leading to a complete TCR gene. Cells bearing the γδ receptor often manifest target cell killing that is not MHC restricted. Monoclonal antibodies to specific TCR V regions are being investigated for possible use in the future treatment of autoimmune diseases. γδ T cells are sometimes found associated with selected epithelial surfaces, especially in the gut. The TCR complex is made up of the antigen-binding chains associated at the cell level with

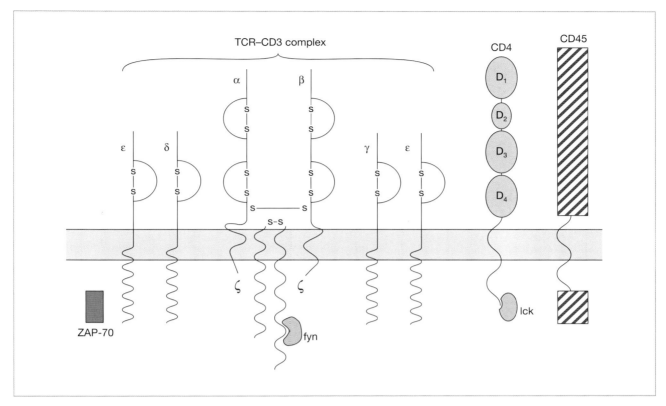

Figure 18   T cell receptor (TCR)–CD3 complex

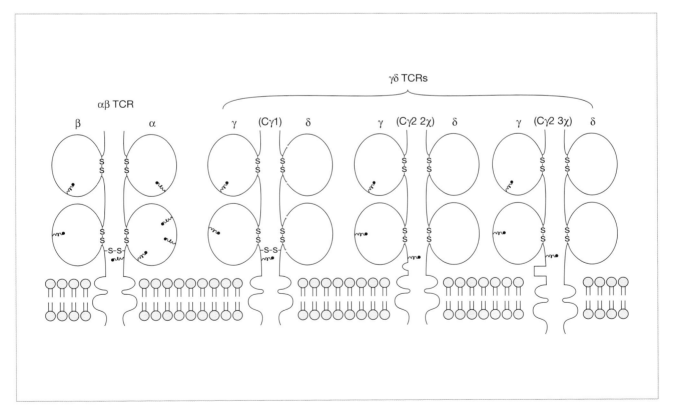

Figure 19   T cell receptor (TCR) showing αβ and γδ receptors

the signal transduction molecules CD3 together with zeta (ζ) and eta (η).

$\gamma\delta$ TCR-expressing cells might protect against microorganisms entering through the epithelium in the skin, lung, intestines, etc. $\gamma\delta$ TCR-bearing cells constitute a majority of T cells during thymic ontogeny and in the epidermis of the mouse. It is not known whether the epidermis/epithelium in the skin can function as a site for T cell education and maturation. $\gamma\delta$ TCR represents an evolutionary precursor of the $\alpha\beta$ TCR, as reflected by the relatively low percentages of cells expressing $\gamma\delta$ TCRs in adults and the fact that cells expressing the $\alpha\beta$ TCR carry out the principal immunologic functions. Diversity of the $\gamma\delta$ TCR and lymphokine synthesis by cells expressing the $\gamma\delta$ TCR attest to the significance of the cells in the immune system. Little is known concerning the types of antigen recognized by $\gamma\delta$ TCRs. They fail to recognize peptide complexes bound to polymorphic MHC molecules.

B lymphocyte B lymphocytes mature under the influence of the bursa of Fabricius in birds and in the bursa equivalent (bone marrow) in mammals. The bursa of Fabricius is an outpouching of the hindgut located near the cloaca in avian species that governs B cell ontogeny. This specific lymphoid organ is the site of migration and maturation of B lymphocytes (Figure 20). B cells occupy follicular areas in lymphoid tissues and account for 5–25% of all human blood lymphocytes that number 1000–2000 cells/mm^3. They constitute most of the bone marrow lymphocytes, one-third to one-half of the lymph node and spleen lymphocytes but less than 1% of those in the thymus. Non-activated B cells circulate through lymph nodes and spleen. They are concentrated in follicles and marginal zones around the follicles. Circulating B cells may interact and be activated by T cells at extrafollicular sites where the T cells are present in association with antigen-presenting dendritic cells. Activated B cells enter the follicles, proliferate and displace resting cells. They form germinal centers and differentiate into both plasma cells that form antibody and long-lived memory B cells. Those B cells synthesizing antibodies provide defense against microorganisms including bacteria and viruses. Surface and cytoplasmic markers reveal the stage of development and function of lymphocytes in the B cell lineage. Pre-B cells contain

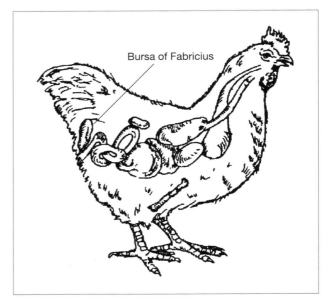

Figure 20 Bursa of Fabricius

cytoplasmic immunoglobulins, whereas mature B cells express surface immunoglobulin and complement receptors. B lymphocyte markers include CD9, CD19, CD20, CD24, Fc receptors, B1, BA-1, B4 and Ia.

A **B cell antigen receptor** (Figures 21 and 22) is an antibody expressed on antigen-reactive B cells that is similar to secreted antibody but is membrane-bound due to an extra domain at the Fc portion of the molecule. Upon antigen recognition by the membrane-bound immunoglobulin, non-covalently associated accessory molecules mediate transmembrane signaling to the B cell nucleus. The immunoglobulin and accessory molecule complex is similar in structure to the antigen receptor–CD3 complex of T lymphocytes. The cell surface membrane-bound immunoglobulin molecule serves as a receptor for antigen together with two associated signal-transducing Igα/Igβ molecules.

Plasma cells are antibody-producing cells. Immunoglobulins are present in their cytoplasm, and secretion of immunoglobulin by plasma cells has been directly demonstrated *in vitro*. Increased levels of immunoglobulins in some pathologic conditions are associated with increased numbers of plasma cells, and conversely, their number at antibody-producing sites increases following immunization. Plasma cells develop from B cells and are large spherical or ellipsoidal cells 10–20 μm in size. Mature plasma cells have

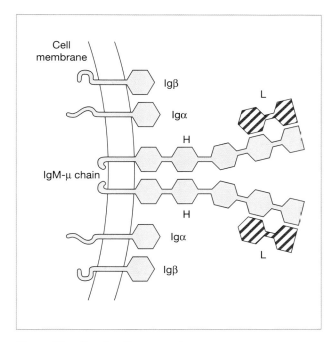

Figure 21   B cell antigen receptor

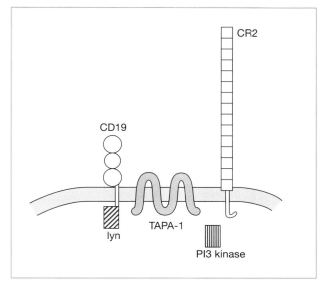

Figure 22   B cell coreceptor

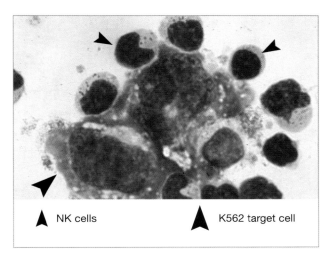

Figure 23   Natural killer (NK) cells

abundant cytoplasm, which stain deep blue with Wright's stain, and have an eccentrically located, round or oval nucleus, usually surrounded by a well-defined perinuclear clear zone. The nucleus contains coarse and clumped masses of chromatin, often arranged in a cartwheel fashion. The nuclei of normal, mature plasma cells have no nucleoli, but those of neoplastic plasma cells such as those seen in multiple myeloma have conspicuous nucleoli. The cytoplasm of normal plasma cells has conspicuous Golgi complex and rough endoplasmic reticulum, and frequently contains vacuoles. The nuclear to cytoplasmic ratio is 1 : 2. By electron microscopy, plasma cells show very abundant endoplasmic reticulum, indicating extensive and active protein synthesis. Plasma cells do not express surface immunoglobulin or complement receptors, which distinguishes them from B lymphocytes.

Natural killer (NK) cells (Figure 23) attack and destroy certain virus-infected cells. They constitute an important part of the natural immune system, do not require prior contact with antigen and are not major histocompatibility complex (MHC)-restricted by the MHC antigens. NK cells are lymphoid cells of the natural immune system that express cytotoxicity against various nucleated cells, including tumor cells and virus-infected cells. NK cells, killer (K) cells or antibody-dependent cell-mediated cytotoxicity

(ADCC) cells induce lysis through the action of antibody. Immunologic memory is not involved, as previous contact with antigen is not necessary for NK cell activity. The NK cell is approximately 15 μm in diameter and has a kidney-shaped nucleus with several, often three, large cytoplasmic granules. The cells are also called large granular lymphocytes (LGLs). In addition to the ability to kill selected tumor cells and some virus-infected cells, they also participate in ADCC by anchoring antibody to the cell surface through an Fcγ receptor. Thus, they are able to destroy antibody-coated nucleated cells. NK cells are believed to represent a significant part of the natural immune defense against spontaneously developing neoplastic cells and against infection by viruses. NK cell activity is measured by a ^{51}Cr-release assay employing the K562 erythroleukemia cell line as a target. NK cells secrete IFN-γ and fail to express antigen receptors such as immunoglobulin receptors or T cell receptors. Cell-surface stimulatory receptors and inhibitory receptors, which recognize self-MHC molecules, regulate their activation.

K (killer) cells, also called null cells, have lymphocyte-like morphology but functional characteristics different from those of B and T cells. They are involved in a particular form of immune response, the antibody-dependent cellular cytotoxicity (ADCC), killing target cells coated with IgG antibodies. A K cell is an Fc-bearing killer cell that has an effector function in mediating ADCC. An IgG antibody molecule binds through its Fc region to the K cell's Fc receptor. Following contact with a target cell bearing antigenic determinants on its surface for which the Fab regions of the antibody molecule attached to the K cell are specific, the lymphocyte-like K cell releases lymphokines that destroy the target. This represents a type of immune effector function in which cells and antibody participate. Besides K cells, other cells that mediate ADCC include NK cells, cytotoxic T cells, neutrophils and macrophages. A K cell is a large granular lymphocyte bearing Fc receptors on its surface for IgG, which makes it capable of mediating ADCC. Complement is not involved in the reaction. Antibody may attach through its Fab regions to target cell epitopes and link to the K cell through attachment of its Fc region to the K cell's Fc receptor, thereby facilitating cytolysis of the target by the K cell, or an IgG antibody may first link via its Fc region to the Fc receptor on the K cell surface and direct the K cell to its target. Cytolysis is induced by insertion of perforin polymer in the target cell membrane in a manner that resembles the insertion of C9 polymers in a cell membrane in complement-mediated lysis. Perforin is showered on the target cell membrane following release from the K cell.

Macrophages (Figure 25) are mononuclear phagocytic cells derived from monocytes in the blood that were produced from stem cells in the bone marrow. These cells have a powerful, although non-specific, role in immune defense. These intensely phagocytic

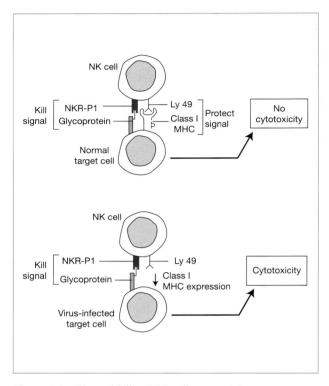

Figure 24   Natural killer (NK) cell cytotoxicity

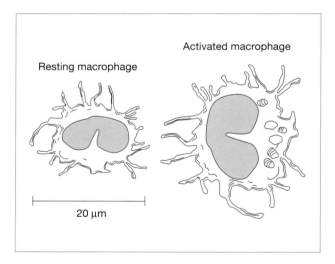

Figure 25   Schematic representation of a resting macrophage vs. an activated macrophage

cells contain lysosomes and exert microbicidal action against microbes that they ingest. They also have effective tumoricidal activity. They may take up and degrade both protein and polysaccharide antigens and present them to T lymphocytes in the context of major histocompatibility complex class II molecules. They interact with both T and B lymphocytes in immune reactions. They are frequently found in areas of epithelium, mesothelium and blood vessels. Macrophages have been referred to as adherent cells since they readily adhere to glass and plastic and may spread on these surfaces and manifest chemotaxis. They have receptors for Fc and C3b on their surfaces, stain positively for non-specific esterase and peroxidase, and are Ia antigen positive when acting as accessory cells that present antigen to CD4$^+$ lymphocytes in the generation of an immune response. Monocytes, which may differentiate into macrophages when they migrate into the tissues, make up 3–5% of leukocytes in the peripheral blood. Macrophages that are tissue bound may be found in the lung alveoli, as microglial cells in the central nervous system, as Kupffer cells in the liver, as Langerhans cells in the skin and as histiocytes in connective tissues, as well as macrophages in lymph nodes and peritoneum. Multiple substances are secreted by macrophages including complement components C1 through C5, factors B and D, properdin, C3b inactivators and β-1H. They also produce monokines such as interleukin-1, acid hydrolase, proteases, lipases and numerous other substances.

IFN-γ activates macrophages to increase their capacity to kill intracellular microorganisms. Macrophages are known by different names according to the tissue in which they are found, such as the microglia of the central nervous system, the Kupffer cells of the liver, alveolar macrophages of the lung and osteoclasts in the bone.

Monocytes are mononuclear phagocytic cells in the blood that are derived from promonocytes in the bone marrow. Following a relatively brief residence in the blood, they migrate into the tissues and are transformed into macrophages. They are less mature than macrophages, as suggested by fewer surface receptors, cytoplasmic organelles and enzymes than the latter. Monocytes are larger than polymorphonuclear leukocytes, are actively phagocytic and constitute 2–10% of the total white blood cell count in humans. The monocyte in the blood circulation is 15–25 μm in diameter. It has grayish-blue cytoplasm that contains lysosomes with enzymes such as acid phosphatase, arginase cachetepsin, collagenase, deoxyribonuclease, lipase, glucosidase and plasminogen activator. The cell has a reniform nucleus with delicate lace-like chromatin. The monocyte has surface receptors such as the Fc receptor for IgG and a receptor for CR3. It is

actively phagocytic and plays a significant role in antigen processing. Monocyte numbers are elevated in both benign and malignant conditions. Certain infections stimulate a reactive type of monocytosis, such as in tuberculosis, brucellosis, human immunodeficiency virus (HIV)-1 infection and malaria.

Dendritic cells are mononuclear phagocytic cells found in the skin as Langerhans cells, in the lymph nodes as interdigitating cells, in the paracortex as veiled cells in the marginal sinus of afferent lymphatics, and as mononuclear phagocytes in the spleen where they present antigen to T lymphocytes. Dendritic reticular cells may have non-specific esterase, Birbeck granules, endogenous peroxidase, possibly CD1, complement receptors CR1 and CR3, and Fc receptors. Dendritic cells (DC) are sentinels of the immune system. They originate from a bone marrow progenitor, travel through the blood and are seeded into non-lymphoid tissues. DC capture and process exogenous antigens for presentation as peptide–major histocompatibility complex (MHC) complexes at the cell surface and then migrate via the blood and afferent lymph to secondary lymph nodes. In the lymph nodes, they interact with T lymphocytes to facilitate activation of helper and killer T cells. DC have been named according to their appearance and distribution in the body. During the past decade, DC have been further characterized by lineage, by maturation stage, by functional and phenotype characteristics of these stages and by mechanisms involved in migration and function. DC are being considered as adjuvants in immunization protocols for antiviral or antitumor immunity. Immature DC are defined by cell surface markers that represent functional capacity. They express the chemokine receptors CCR-1, CCR-2, CCR-5, CCR-6 (only CD34$^+$ HPC-derived DC) and CXCR-1, commonly thought to allow DC to migrate in response to inflammatory chemokines expressed by inflamed tissues. Immature DC are phagocytic and have a high level of macropinocytosis, allowing them to process efficiently and present antigen on class I molecules. Expression of Fcγ (CD64) and the mannose receptors allow efficient capture of IgG immune complexes and antigens that expose mannose or fucose residues. The expression of E-cadherin allows DC to interact with tissue cells and remain in the tissues until activated. Following antigen processing, DC are remodeled. Fc and mannose receptors are downregulated, and there is a disappearance of acidic interacellular compartments, resulting in a loss of endocytic activity. During this maturation process, the level of MHC class II molecules and costimulatory molecules are unregulated, and there is a change in chemokine receptor expression. Maturing DC home to T cell areas of secondary lymph nodes, where they present antigen to naive T cells. *In vitro* culture of DC with CD40L, lipopolysaccharide (LPS) and TNF-α generates mature DC. These cells are very good stimulators of allogeneic T cell proliferation. The DC–T cell interaction is thought to be a two-way process. Evidence suggests that T cells interact with DC through CD40 ligation to enhance DC viability and their T cell stimulatory ability. Addition of CD40L induces DC to produce IL-12, which is known to support T$_{H1}$ responses. LPS stimulation generates a weaker *in vitro* immune response than the CD40L-stimulated DC.

The **mononuclear phagocyte system** consists of mononuclear cells with pronounced phagocytic ability that are distributed extensively in lymphoid and other organs. 'Mononuclear phagocyte system' should be used in place of the previously popular 'reticuloendothelial system' to describe this group of cells. Mononuclear phagocytes originate from stem cells in the bone marrow that first differentiate into monocytes that appear in the blood for approximately 24 h or more, with final differentiation into macrophages in the tissues. Macrophages usually occupy perivascular areas. Liver macrophages are termed Kupffer cells, whereas those in the lung are alveolar macrophages. The microglia represent macrophages of the central nervous system, whereas histiocytes represent macrophages of connective tissue. Tissue stem cells are monocytes that have wandered from the blood into the tissues and may differentiate into macrophages. Mononuclear phagocytes have a variety of surface receptors that enable them to bind carbohydrates or such protein molecules as C3 via complement receptor 1 and complement receptor 3; and IgG and IgE through Fcγ and Fcε receptors. The surface expression of MHC class II molecules enables both monocytes and macrophages to serve as antigen-presenting cells to CD4$^+$ T lymphocytes. Mononuclear phagocytes secrete a rich array of molecular substances with various functions. A few of these include: interleukin-

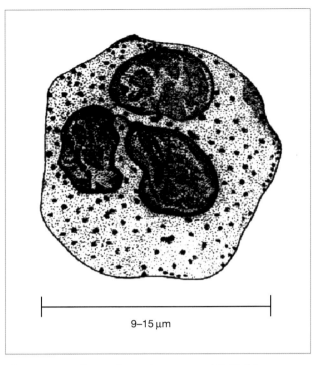

9–15 μm

Figure 26 Polymorphonuclear neutrophil (PMN)

1; tumor necrosis factor-α; interleukin-6; C2, C3, C4 and factor B complement proteins; prostaglandins; leukotrienes; and other substances.

Polymorphonuclear leukocytes (PMNs) (Figure 26) are white blood cells with lobulated nuclei that are often trilobed. These cells are of the myeloid cell lineage and in the mature form can be differentiated into neutrophils, eosinophils and basophils. This distinction is based on the staining characteristics of their cytoplasmic-specific or secondary granules. These cells, which measure approximately 13 μm in diameter, are active in acute inflammatory responses.

A **neutrophil leukocyte** is a peripheral blood polymorphonuclear leukocyte derived from the myeloid lineage. Neutrophils constitute 40–75% of the total white blood count numbering 2500–7500 cells/mm^3. They are phagocytic cells and have a multilobed nucleus and azurophilic and specific granules that appear lilac following staining with Wright's or Giemsa stain. They may be attracted to a local site by such chemotactic factors as C5a. They are the principal cells of acute inflammation and actively phagocytize invading microorganisms. Besides serving as the first line of cellular defense infection, they participate

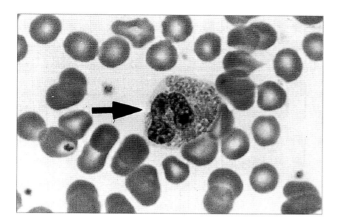

Figure 27 Eosinophil

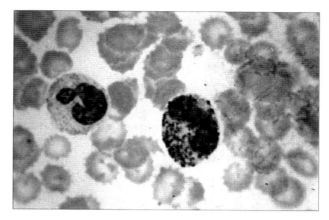

Figure 28 Neutrophil and basophil

in such reactions as the uptake of antigen–antibody complexes in the Arthus reaction.

A **neutrophil** expresses Fc receptors and can participate in antibody-dependent cell-mediated cytotoxicity. It has the capacity to phagocytize microorganisms and digest them enzymatically.

Eosinophils (Figure 27) are polymorphonuclear leukocytes identified as brilliant reddish-orange refractile granules in Wright- or Giemsa-stained preparations by staining of secondary granules in the leukocyte cytoplasm. Cationic peptides are released from these secondary granules when an eosinophil interacts with a target cell, and may lead to death of the target. Eosinophils make up 2–5% of the total white blood cells in man. After a brief residence in the circulation, eosinophils migrate into tissues by passing between the lining endothelial cells. It is believed that they do not return to the circulation. The distribution corresponds mainly to areas exposed to an external environment, such as skin, mucosa of the bronchi and gastrointestinal tract. Eosinophils are elevated during allergic reactions, especially type I immediate hypersensitivity responses, and are also elevated in individuals with parasitic infestations.

Basophils (Figure 28) are polymorphonuclear leukocytes of the myeloid lineage with distinctive basophilic secondary granules in the cytoplasm that frequently overlie the nucleus. These granules are storage depots for heparin, histamine, platelet-activating factor and other pharmacological mediators of immediate hypersensitivity. Degranulation of the cells with release of

these pharmacological mediators takes place following cross-linking by allergen or antigen of Fab regions of IgE receptor molecules bound through Fc receptors to the cell surface. They constitute less than 0.5% of peripheral blood leukocytes. Following cross-linking of surface-bound IgE molecules by specific allergen or antigen, granules are released by exocytosis. Substances liberated from the granules are pharmacological mediators of immediate (type I) anaphylactic hypersensitivity.

Mast cells are a normal component of the connective tissue that plays an important role in immediate (type I) hypersensitivity and inflammatory reactions by secreting a large variety of chemical mediators from storage sites in their granules upon stimulation. Their anatomical location at mucosal and cutaneous surfaces and about venules in deeper tissues is related to this role. They can be identified easily by their characteristic granules, which stain metachromatically. The size and shape of mast cells vary, i.e. 10–30 μm in diameter. In adventitia of large vessels, they are elongated; in loose connective tissue, they are round or oval; and the shape in fibrous connective tissue may be angular. On their surfaces, they have Fc receptors for IgE. Cross-linking by either antigen for which the IgE Fab regions are specific, or by anti-IgE or antireceptor antibody, leads to degranulation, with the release of pharmacological mediators of immediate hypersensitivity from their storage sites in the mast cell granules. Leukotrienes, prostaglandins and platelet-activating factor are also produced and released following Fcε receptor cross-linking. Mast cell granules are approximately 0.5 μm in diameter and are electron dense. They contain many biologically active compounds, of which the most important are heparin, histamine, serotonin and a variety of enzymes. Histamine is stored in the granule as a complex with heparin or serotonin. Mast cells also contain proteolytic enzymes such as plasmin and also hydroxylase, β-glucuronidase, phosphatase and a high uronidase inhibitor, to mention only the most important. Zinc, iron and calcium are also found. Some substances released from mast cells are not stored in a preformed state, but are synthesized following mast cell activation. These represent secondary mediators as opposed to the preformed primary mediators. Mast cell degranulation involves adenylate cyclase activation with rapid synthesis of cyclic adenosine monophosphate (AMP), protein kinase activation, phospholipid methylation and serine esterase activation. Mast cells of the gastrointestinal and respiratory tracts that contain chondroitin sulfate produce leukotriene C_4, whereas connective tissue mast cells that contain heparin produce prostaglandin D_2.

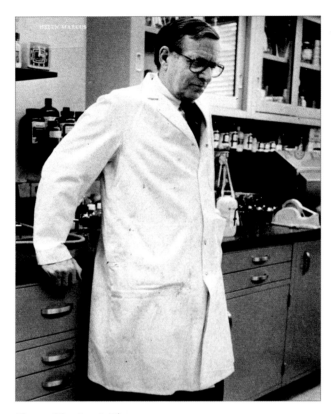

Figure 29   Lewis Thomas

TUMOR IMMUNITY

It has long been the dream of medical scientists to be able to resist cancer by immunological methods. William Coley, in 1891, observed that cancer patients who developed certain infections derived beneficial results. This led him to inject mixtures of bacterial toxins into cancer patients in an attempt to alter the pathogenesis of their malignant disease. His efforts met with success in 1893 when an inoperable tumor in a 16-year-old boy receiving bacterial toxin regressed and disappeared over several months of treatment. Coley applied his treatment to 250 other cancer victims whose survival ranged from 5 to 72 years. Perhaps because of the unavailability of sufficient immunological information to understand Coley's experiments at the time, their significance was not appreciated until years later. Shwartzman reported in his classic monograph on *The Phenomenon of Local Tissue Reactivity* in 1937 that the injection of one dose of endotoxin into a tumor site followed 24 h later by an intravenous injection of endotoxin resulted in a local Shwartzman reaction, leading to hemorrhage and necrosis in the tumor[23].

Studies on transplantable tumors in inbred strains of mice are discussed in Chapter 11 on 'Immunogenetics, immunologic tolerance, transfusion and transplantation'. In the 1950s, F. M. Burnet and Lewis Thomas (Figure 29) proposed a concept of immune surveillance to describe the interaction between tumor cells and the immune system[24,25]. They postulated that somatic mutations of cells with the potential to develop into malignant tumors are recognized as alien by antigenic determinants not present on normal cells, and are destroyed by immunocytes that police the bodily tissues to eliminate cells not recognized as self by seek-and-destroy tactics. They theorized that failure of the immune system to carry out this function could lead to proliferation of these aberrant cells into a tumor mass too great to be eliminated by immunological means. Indirect evidence offered in support of such a concept included the increased frequency of tumors in children with immunodeficiency of the T-cell system, tumors that appear in individuals on prolonged immunosuppressive therapy, as in transplant patients, and the increase in tumor incidence with advancing age.

One of the many paradoxes in cancer immunology is the phenomenon of immunological enhancement, in which antibodies favor the establishment of a tumor graft rather than hasten its rejection. Immunological enhancement was defined by Kaliss as the 'successful establishment of a tumor homograft and its progressive growth (usually to death of the host) as a consequence of the tumor's contact with specific antiserum in the host'[26]. This definition was later altered to the successful establishment or prolonged survival (conversely the delayed rejection) of an allogeneic graft. In 1932, Casey observed enhancement of Brown–Pearce sarcoma in rabbits[27]. He reported the presence of a principle termed XYZ factor in preserved preparations of Brown–Pearce sarcoma, which, upon injection into rabbits 2 weeks prior to transplantation of the tumor, resulted in an increased incidence of tumors, larger metastases and a briefer period of survival following transplantation. Snell and associates studied tumor enhancement using inbred strains of mice of known genetic constitution[28]. These investigators aimed at solving the mechanism and other aspects of immunological enhancement. Besides antibody, immune complexes comprising antigen and antibody were found to favor the establishment of a tumor by blocking or interfering with the immunological rejection mechanism. Carl and Ingegerd Hellström demonstrated immune complexes that acted as blocking factors in the serum of certain cancer patients[29]. They subsequently discovered unblocking factors capable of eliminating complexes that interfere with the immune system of the tumor-bearing host[30]. A renaissance of interest in Dr Coley's treatment occurred following the demonstration that tumor-bearing mice injected with bacillus Calmette–Guérin (BCG) attenuated tuberculosis vaccine showed regression of their tumors. After that, numerous clinical trials with BCG were carried out in selected tumor patients with considerable success. Malignant melanoma, breast cancer, mycosis fungoides and acute lymphoid leukemia are among tumors treated with some success by BCG immunotherapy[31]. Foley, in 1953, provided the first clear demonstration of specific antigenicity in a class of experimental tumors[32]. He found that ligation and atrophy of methylcholanthrene-induced sarcoma in mice of the C3H-He pure line were followed by immunity. In 1957, Prehn extended Foley's observation to provide conclusive evidence of an immune response to cancer-specific antigens of autochthonous tumors of putatively non-viral origin[33].

In 1965, Phil Gold described carcinoembryonic antigen (CEA) in the sera of patients with cancer of the colon[34]. At first there was great hope that the detection of this antigen in the blood sera of patients might aid in the diagnosis of cancer. Unfortunately, patients with other types of cancer as well as certain non-neoplastic diseases may experience derepression of α gene encoding its formation. It is still useful to monitor blood sera for the reappearance of CEA in patients who have undergone surgical excision of colonic cancer, to signal any recurrence or metastasis of the malignancy. Another cell-coded antigen that shows a more restricted association with one type of tumor than does CEA is α-fetoprotein observed in the sera of patients with hepatoma[35,36]. Regrettably, however, this is of little consequence for the patient in whom no effective therapy can be applied. Burkitt's lymphoma, a B-cell malignancy, which shows strong evidence of association with the Epstein–Barr virus, shows remission in some patients. This appears to have an immunologic basis.

Tumor antigens are cell surface proteins on tumor cells that can induce a cell-mediated and/or humoral immune response.

Tumor-associated antigens (Figure 30) are antigens designated as CA125, CA19-9 and CA195, among others, that may be linked to certain tumors such as lymphomas, carcinomas, sarcomas and melanomas, but the immune response to these tumor-associated antigens is not sufficient to mount a successful cellular or humoral immune response against the neoplasm. Three classes of tumor-associated antigens have been described. Class I antigens are very specific for a certain neoplasm and are absent from normal cells. Class II antigens are found on related neoplasms from separate individuals. Class III antigens are found on malignant as well as normal cells, but show increased expression in the neoplastic cells. Assays of clinical value will probably be developed for class II antigens, since they are associated with multiple neoplasms and are very infrequently found in normal individuals.

Prostate-specific antigen (PSA) is a marker in serum or tissue sections for adenocarcinoma of the prostate. PSA is a 34-kDa glycoprotein found exclusively in benign and malignant epithelium of the

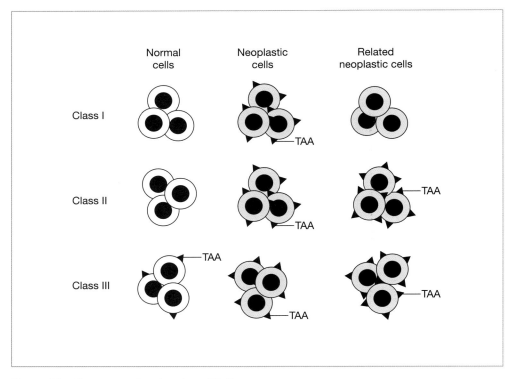

Figure 30 Tumor-associated antigen (TAA)

prostate. Men with PSA levels of 0–4.0 ng/ml, and a non-suspicious digital rectal examination, are generally not biopsied for prostate cancer. Men with PSA levels of 10.0 ng/ml and above typically undergo a prostate biopsy. About one-half of these men will be found to have prostate cancer. Certain kinds of PSA, known as bound PSA, link themselves to other proteins in the blood. Other kinds of PSA, known as free PSA, float by themselves. Prostate cancer is more likely to be present in men who have a low percentage of free PSA relative to the total amount of PSA. This finding is especially valuable in helping to differentiate between cancer and other benign conditions, thus eliminating unnecessary biopsies among men in that diagnostic gray zone who have total PSA levels between 4.0 and 10.0 ng/ml. The PSA molecule is smaller than prostatic acid phosphatase (PAP). In patients with prostate cancer, preoperative PSA serum levels are positively correlated with the disease. PSA is more stable and shows less diurnal variation than does PAP. PSA is increased in 95% of new cases for prostatic carcinoma compared with a 60% increase for PAP; PSA is increased in 97% of recurrent cases compared with a 66% increase of PAP. PAP may also be increased in selected cases of benign prostatic hypertrophy and

prostatitis, but these elevations are less than those associated with adenocarcinoma of the prostate. It is inappropriate to use either PSA or PAP alone as a screen for asymptomatic males. Transurethral resection (TUR), urethral instrumentation, prostatic needle biopsy, prostatic infarct or urinary retention may also result in increased PSA values. PSA is critical for the prediction of recurrent adenocarcinoma in post-surgical patients. PSA is also a useful immunocytochemical marker for primary and metastatic adenocarcinoma of the prostate.

Oncofetal antigens (Figure 31) are markers or epitopes present in fetal tissues during development but are not present, or found in minute quantities, in adult tissues. These cell-coded antigens may reappear in certain neoplasms of adults due to derepression of the gene responsible for their formation. Examples include carcinoembryonic antigen (CEA), which is found in the liver, intestine and pancreas of the fetus, but also in both malignant and benign gastrointestinal conditions. Yet it is still useful to detect recurrence of adenocarcinoma of the colon based upon demonstration of CEA in the patient's serum; α-fetoprotein (AFP) is demonstrable in approximately 70% of hepatocellular carcinomas.

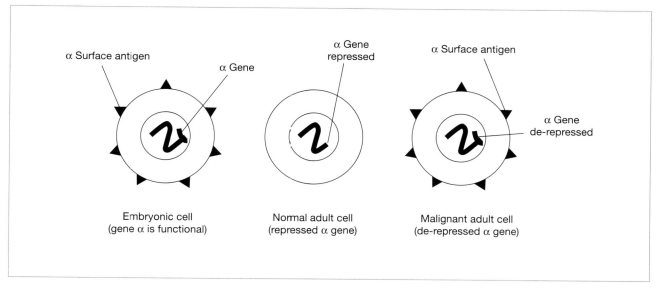

α Surface antigen

α Gene

α Gene repressed

α Surface antigen

α Gene de-repressed

Embryonic cell
(gene α is functional)

Normal adult cell
(repressed α gene)

Malignant adult cell
(de-repressed α gene)

Figure 31   Oncofetal antigen

A **fetal or oncofetal antigen** is expressed as a normal constituent of embryos and not in adult tissues. It is re-expressed in neoplasms of adult tissues, apparently as a result of derepression of the gene responsible for its formation.

Carcinoma-associated antigens are self antigens whose epitopes have been changed due to effects produced by certain tumors. Self antigens are transformed into a molecular structure for which the host is immunologically intolerant. Examples include the T antigen, which is an MN blood group precursor molecule exposed by the action of bacterial enzymes, and Tn antigen, which is a consequence of somatic mutation in hematopoietic stem cells caused by inhibition of galactose transfer to N-acetyl-D-galactosamine.

Embryonic antigens are protein or carbohydrate antigens synthesized during embryonic and fetal life that are either absent or formed in only minute quantities in normal adult subjects. Fetoproteins (AFP) and carcinoembryonic antigen (CEA) are fetal antigens that may be synthesized once again in large amounts in individuals with certain tumors. Their detection and level during the course of the disease and following surgery to remove a tumor, reducing the substance, may serve as a diagnostic and prognostic indicator of the disease process. Blood group antigens, such as the iI, which are reversed in their levels of expression in the fetus and in the adult, may show a re-emergence

of i antigen in adults in patients with thalassemia and hypoplastic anemia. Cold autoagglutinins specific for it may be found in infectious mononucleosis patients. Common acute lymphoblastic leukemia antigen (CALLA, CD10) is rarely found on peripheral blood cells of normal subjects, whereas CALLA cells coexpressing IgM and CD19 molecules may be found in fetal bone marrow and peripheral blood samples. CD10 may be expressed in children with common acute lymphoblastic leukemia.

The **melanoma antigen-1 gene (MAGE-1)** in humans was derived from a malignant melanoma cell line. It encodes for an epitope that is recognized by a cytotoxic T lymphocyte clone specific for melanoma. This clone was isolated from a patient bearing melanoma. **MAGE-1 protein** is found on one-half of all melanomas and one-quarter of all breast carcinomas, but is not expressed on the majority of normal tissues. Even though MAGE-1 has not been shown to induce tumor rejection, cytotoxic T lymphocytes in melanoma patients manifest specific memory for MAGE-1 protein.

Melanoma-associated antigens (MAAs) are antigens associated with the aggressive, malignant and metastatic tumors arising from melanocytes or melanocyte-associated nevus cells. Monoclonal antibodies have identified more than 40 separate MAAs. They are classified as MHC molecules, cation-binding proteins, growth factor receptors, gangliosides, high-molecular-weight extracellular matrix-binding molecules and nevomelanocyte differentiation antigens. Some of the antigens are expressed on normal cells, whereas others are expressed on tumor cells. Melanoma patient blood sera often contain anti-MAA antibodies, which are regrettably not protective. Monoclonal antibodies against MAAs aid studies on the biology of tumor progression, immunodiagnosis and immunotherapy trials.

Tumor cells may be subject to alterations in antigenic structure. **Antigenic transformation** refers to changes in a cell's antigenic profile as a consequence of antigenic gain, deletion, reversion or other process. **Antigenic gain** refers to non-distinctive normal tissue components that are added or increased without simultaneous deletion of other normal tissue constituents. **Antigenic deletion** describes antigenic determinants that have been lost or masked in the progeny of cells that usually contain them. Antigenic deletion may take place as a consequence of neoplastic transformation or mutation of parent cells resulting in the disappearance or repression of the parent cell genes. **Antigenic modulation** is the loss of epitopes or antigenic determinants from a cell surface following combination with an antibody. The antibodies either cause the epitope to disappear or become camouflaged by covering it. **Antigenic diversion** refers to the replacement of a cell's antigenic profile by the antigens of a different normal tissue cell. It is used in tumor immunology. **Antigenic reversion** is the change in antigenic profile characteristic of an adult cell to an antigenic mosaic that previously existed in the immature or fetal cell stage of the species. Antigenic reversion may accompany neoplastic transformation.

Tumor cells express **tumor-specific determinants or epitopes** present on tumor cells, but identifiable also in varying quantities and forms on normal cells. **Tumor-specific antigen (TSAs)** (Figure 32) are present on tumor cells, but not found on normal cells. Murine tumor-specific antigens can induce transplantation rejection in mice. **Tumor-specific transplantation antigens (TSTAs)** are epitopes that induce rejection of tumors transplanted among syngeneic (histocompatible) animals.

Tumor rejection antigen is an antigen that is detectable when transplanted tumor cells are rejected, also called tumor transplant antigen.

TATA is the abbreviation for tumor-associated transplantation antigen.

Designer lymphocytes are lymphocytes into which genes have been introduced to increase the cell's ability to lyse tumor cells. Tumor-infiltrating lymphocytes transfected with these types of genes have been used in experimental adoptive immunotherapy.

Cytotoxic T lymphocytes (CTLs) are specifically sensitized T lymphocytes that are usually CD8$^+$ and recognize antigens through the T cell receptor on cells of the host infected by viruses or that have become neoplastic. CD8$^+$ cell recognition of the target is in the context of MHC class I histocompatibility molecules. Following recognition and binding, death of the target cell occurs a few hours later. CTLs secrete lymphokines that attract other lymphocytes to the area and release serine proteases and perforins that produce ion channels in the membrane of the target, leading to cell lysis (Figure 32). Interleukin-2, produced by CD4$^+$ T cells, activates cytotoxic T cell precursors. Interferon-γ generated from CTLs activates macrophages. CTLs have a significant role in the rejection of allografts and in tumor immunity. A minor population of CD4$^+$ lymphocytes may also be cytotoxic, but they recognize target cell antigens in the context of MHC class II molecules.

Tumor-specific IgG antibodies may act in concert with immune system cells to produce antitumor effects. **Antibody-dependent cell-mediated cytotoxicity (ADCC)** (Figure 33) is a reaction in which T lymphocytes, natural killer (NK) cells, including large granular lymphocytes, neutrophils and macrophages may lyse tumor cells, infectious agents and allogeneic cells by combining, through their Fc receptors, with the Fc region of IgG antibodies, bound through their Fab regions to target cell surface antigens. Following linkage of Fc receptors with Fc regions, destruction of the target is accomplished through released cytokines. It represents an example of participation between antibody molecules and immune system cells to produce an effector function.

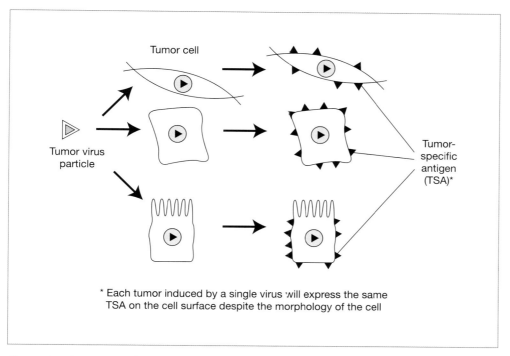

Figure 32   Tumor-specific antigens

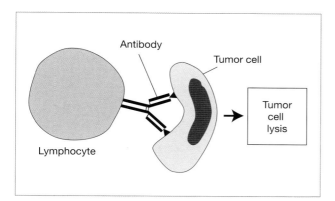

Figure 33   Antibody-dependent cell-mediated cytotoxicity (ADCC)

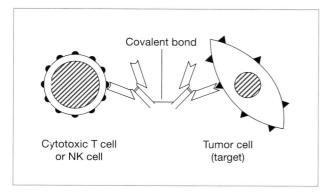

Figure 34   Heteroconjugate antibodies. NK, natural killer

Heteroconjugate antibodies (Figure 34) are antibodies against a tumor antigen coupled covalently to an antibody specific for a natural killer cell or cytotoxic T lymphocyte surface antigen. These antibodies facilitate binding of cytotoxic effector cells to tumor target cells. Antibodies against effector cell surface markers may also be coupled covalently with hormones that bind to receptors on tumor cells.

Immunosurveillance refers to the policing or monitoring function of immune system cells to recognize and destroy clones of transformed cells prior to their development into neoplasms, and to destroy tumors after they develop. Immunosurveillance is believed to be mediated by the cellular limb of the immune response. Indirect evidence in support of the concept includes:

(1) An increased incidence of tumors in aged individuals who have decreased immune competence;

(2) Increased tumor incidence in children with T-cell immunodeficiencies;

(3) The development of neoplasms (lymphomas) in a significant number of organ or bone marrow transplant recipients who have been deliberately immunosuppressed.

Immunoselection is the selective survival of cells due to their diminished cell surface antigenicity. This permits these cells to escape the injurious effects of either antibodies or immune lymphoid cells.

Immunological escape is a mechanism of escape in which tumors that are immunogenic continue to grow in immunocompetent syngeneic hosts in the presence of a modest *in vivo* antitumor immune response. Escape mechanisms may facilitate tumors in evading a fatal tumoricidal response and render them incapable of inducing such a response. Failure of tumor antigen presentation by MHC class I molecules, lack of costimulation and downregulation of tumor-destructive immune responses by tumor antigens, immune complexes and molecules such as transforming growth factor (TGF)-β and P15E are all believed to contribute to the inefficiency of tumor immunity.

Immunologic enhancement (tumor enhancement) describes the prolonged survival, conversely the delayed rejection, of a tumor allograft in a host as a consequence of contact with specific antibody. Antitumor antibodies may have a paradoxical effect. Instead of eradicating a neoplasm, they may facilitate its survival and progressive growth in the host. Both the peripheral and central mechanisms have been postulated. Coating of tumor cells with antibody was presumed, in the past, to interfere with the ability of specifically reactive lymphocytes to destroy them, but today a central effect in suppressing cell-mediated immunity, perhaps through suppressor T lymphocytes, is also possible. Enhancing antibodies are blocking antibodies that favor survival of tumor or normal tissue allografts.

Immunologic facilitation (facilitation immunologique) is the slightly prolonged survival of certain normal tissue allografts, e.g. skin, in mice conditioned with isoantiserum specific for the graft.

Immunotherapy employs immunologic mechanisms to combat disease. These include non-specific stimulation of the immune response with BCG immunotherapy in treating certain types of cancer, and the IL-2/lymphokine-activated killer (LAK) cell adoptive immunotherapy technique for treating selected tumors.

Biological response modifiers (BRMs) are a wide spectrum of molecules, such as cytokines, that alter the immune response. They include substances such as interleukins, interferons, hematopoietic colony-stimulating factors, tumor necrosis factor, B lymphocyte growth and differentiating factors, lymphotoxins and macrophage-activating and chemotactic factors, as well as macrophage inhibitory factor, eosinophils chemotactic factor, osteoclast-activating factor, etc. BRMs may modulate the immune system of the host to augment antirecombinant DNA technology and are available commercially. An example is α-interferon used in the therapy of hairy cell leukemia.

An **immunotoxin** (Figure 35) is produced by linking an antibody specific for target cell antigens with a cytotoxic substance such as the toxin ricin. Upon parenteral injection, its antibody portion directs the immunotoxin to the target and its toxic portion destroys target cells on contact. An immunotoxin may also be a monoclonal antibody or one of its fractions linked to a toxic molecule such as a radioisotope, a bacterial or plant toxin or a chemotherapeutic agent. The antibody portion is intended to direct the molecule to antigens on a target cell such as those of a malignant tumor, and the toxic portion of the molecule is for the purpose of destroying the target cell. Contemporary methods of recombinant DNA technology have permitted the preparation of specific hybrid molecules for use in immunotoxin therapy. Immunotoxins may have difficulty reaching the intended target tumor, may be quickly metabolized and may stimulate the development of anti-immunotoxin

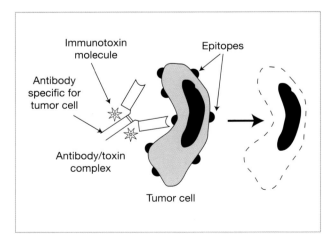

Figure 35   Immunotoxin

antibodies. Cross-linking proteins may likewise be unstable.

Among its uses is the purging of T cells from hematopoietic cell preparations used for bone marrow transplantation. It is a substance produced by the union of a monoclonal antibody or one of its fractions to a toxic molecule such as a radioisotope, a bacterial or plant toxin, or a chemotherapeutic agent. The antibody portion is intended to direct the molecule to antigens on a target cell, such as those of a malignant tumor, and the toxic portion of the molecule is for the purpose of destroying the target cell. Contemporary methods of recombinant DNA technology have permitted the preparation of specific hybrid molecules for use in immunotoxin therapy. Immunotoxins may have difficulty reaching the intended target tumor, may be quickly metabolized and may stimulate the development of anti-immunotoxin antibodies. Cross-linking proteins may likewise be unstable. Immunotoxins have potential for antitumor therapy and as immunosuppressive agents.

Magic bullet is a term coined by Paul Ehrlich in 1900 to describe what he considered to be the affinity of a drug for a particular target. He developed '606' (Salvarsan), an arsenical preparation, to treat syphilis. In immunology, it describes a substance that could be directed to a target by a specific antibody and injure the target once it arrives. Monoclonal antibodies have been linked to toxins such as diphtheria toxin or ricin, as well as to cytokines, for use as magic bullets.

Adoptive immunotherapy is the experimental treatment of terminal cancer patients with metastatic tumors unresponsive to other modes of therapy by the inoculation of lymphokine-activated killer (LAK) cells or tumor-infiltrating lymphocytes (TIL) together with interleukin (IL)-2. This mode of therapy has shown some success in approximately one-tenth of treated individuals with melanoma or renal cell carcinoma.

Lymphokine-activated killer (LAK) cells are lymphoid cells derived from normal or tumor patients which, when cultured in medium with recombinant interleukin (IL)-2, become capable of lysing natural killer (NK)-resistant tumor cells as revealed by ^{51}Cr-release cytotoxicity assays. These cells are also referred to as lymphokine-activated killer cells. Most LAK activity is derived from NK cells. The large granular

lymphocytes (LGLs) contain all LAK precursor activity and all active NK cells. In accord with the phenotype of precursor cells, LAK effector cells are also granular lymphocytes expressing markers associated with human NK cells. The asialo $Gm_1{}^+$ population, known to be expressed by murine NK cells, contains most LAK precursor activity. Essentially all LAK activity resides in the LGL population in the rat. LAK cell and IL-2 immunotherapy has been employed in human cancer patients with a variety of histological tumor types when conventional therapy has been unsuccessful. Approximately one-quarter of LAK- and IL-2-treated patients manifested significant responses, and some individuals experienced complete remission. Serious side-effects include fluid retention and pulmonary edema attributable to the administered IL-2.

Tumor immunity Numerous experimentally induced tumors in mice express numerous specific transplantation antigens which can induce an immune response that leads to the destruction of neoplastic cells *in vivo*. Lymphocytes play a critical role in the immunological destruction of many antigenic tumors. Both cell-mediated and antibody-mediated immune responses to human neoplasms have been identified and their targets characterized in an effort to develop clinically useful immunotherapy.

Tumor-infiltrating lymphocytes (TILs) are lymphocytes isolated from the tumor they are infiltrating. They are cultured with high concentrations of IL-2, leading to expansion of these activated T lymphocytes *in vitro*. TILs are very effective in destroying tumor cells and have proven much more effective than lymphokine-activating killer (LAK) cells in experimental models. TILs have 50–100 times the antitumor activity produced by LAK cells. TILs have been isolated and grown from multiple resected human tumors, including those from kidney, breast, colon and melanoma. In contrast to the non-B-non-T LAK cells, TILs nevertheless are generated from T lymphocytes and phenotypically resemble cytotoxic T lymphocytes. TILs from malignant melanoma exhibit specific cytolytic activity against cells of the tumor from which they were extracted, whereas LAK cells have a broad range of specificity. TILs appear unable to lyse cells of melanomas from patients other than those in whom the tumor originated. TILs may be tagged in order that they may be identified later.

REFERENCES

1. Coons AH, Creech HJ, Jones N, Berliner E. Demonstration of pneumococcal antigen in tissues by use of fluorescent antibody. *J Immunol* 1942;45:159

2. Landsteiner K, Chase MW. Experiments on transfer of cutaneous sensitivity to simple compounds. *Proc Soc Exp Biol Med* 1942;49:688–90

3. Virchow R, Ludwig K. *Die Cellularpathologic in ihrer Begrundung auf Physiologische und Pathologische Gewebelehre.* Berlin: Hirschwald, 1858

4. Murphy JB. *The Lymphocyte in Relation to Tissue Grafting, Malignant Disease and Tuberculous Infection, an Experimental Study.* Monographs of the Rockefeller Institute for Medical Research, No. 21. New York: Rockefeller Institute for Medical Research, 1926

5. Harris TN, Grimm E, Mertins E, Ehrich WE. Role of lymphocyte in antibody formation. *J Exp Med* 1945;981:73–83

6. Fagraeus A. Antibody production in relation to the development of plasma cells: *in vivo* and *in vitro* experiments. *Acta Med Scand* 1948;130(Suppl 1):3

7. Glick B, Chang TS, Jaap RG. The bursa of Fabricius and antibody formation production. *Poult Sci* 1956;35:224

8. Archer O, Pierce JC. Role of thymus in development of the immune response. *Fed Proc* 1961;20:26

9. Archer OK, Pierce JC, Papermaster BW, Good RA. Reduced antibody response in thymectomized rabbits. *Nature (London)* 1962;195:191–3

10. Miller JFAP. Immunological function of the thymus. *Lancet* 1961;2:748

11. Gowans JL. The recirculation of lymphocytes from blood to lymph in the rat. *J Physiol (London)* 1959;146:54–69

12. Harris TN, Hummeler K, Harris S. Electron microscope observations on antibody producing lymph node cells. *J Exp Med* 1966;123:161–72

13. Claman HN, Chaperon EA, Triplett RR. Thymus–marrow cell combinations. Synergism in antibody production. *Proc Soc Exp Biol Med* 1966;122:1167

14. Davies AJS, Leuchars E, Wellis V, *et al.* The failure of thymus-derived cells to produce antibody. *Transplantation* 1967;5:222; The thymus and the cellular basis of immunity. *Transpl Rev* 1969;1:43–91

15. Mitchison NA. Recognition of antibody by cells. *Prog Biophys* 1966;16:3–14

16. Gershon RK, Kondo K. Antigenic competition between heterologous erythrocytes. I. Thymic dependency. II. Effect of passive antibody administration. *J Immunol* 1971;106:1524–39

17. Jerne NK. Toward a network theory of the immune system. *Ann Immunol (Paris)* 1974;125c(1–2):373–89

18. Cantor H, Boyse EA. Functional subclasses of T lymphocytes bearing different Ly antigens. I. The generation of functionally distinct T-cell subclasses in a differentiative process independent of antigen. *J Exp Med* 1975;141:1376

19. Cantor H, Boyse EA. Functional subclasses of T lymphocytes bearing different Ly antigens. II. Cooperation between subclasses of Ly-cells in the generation of killer activity. *J Exper Med* 1975;141:1390

20. Köhler G, Milstein C. Continuous cultures of fused cells secreting antibody of predefined specificity. *Nature (London)* 1975;256:495–97

21. Potts M, Wheelar R. The quest for a magic bullet. *Medicine: Time*, August 11, 1980:75

22. Zinkernagel RM, Doherty PC. H-2 compatibility requirement for T-cell mediated lysis of target cells infected with lymphocytic choriomeningitis virus. *J Exp Med* 1975;141:1427

23. Shwartzman G. *The Phenomenon of Local Tissue Reactivity and its Immunological and Clinical Significance.* New York: Paul B. Hoeber, 1937

24. Burnet FM. Cancer – a biological approach. *Br Med J* 1957;779:841–7

25. Thomas L. Discussion. In Lawrence HS, ed. *Cellular and Humoral Aspects of the Hypertensive States.* London: Cassell, 1959:529–32

26. Kaliss N. Immunological enhancement of tumor homografts in mice. *Cancer Res* 1958;18:992

27. Casey AE. Experimental enhancement of malignancy in Brown Pearce rabbit tumor. *Proc Soc Exp Biol Med* 1932;29:816–18

28. Snell GD, Winn HJ, Stimpfling JH, *et al.* Depression by antibody of the immune response to homografts and its role in immunological enhancement. *J Exp Med* 1960;112:293

29. Hellstrom KE, Hellstrom I. Cellular immunity against tumor antigens. *Adv Cancer Res* 1969;12:167

30. Hellstrom I, Hellstrom KE. Colony inhibition studies on blocking and non-blocking serum effects on cellular immunity to Molony sarcomas. *Int J Cancer* 1970;5:195

31. Cruse JM, Lewis RE Jr. Immunotherapy of cancer. *EOS J Immunol Immunopharmacol* 1989;9:41–53

32. Foley EJ. Antigenic properties of methylcholanthrene-induced tumors in mice of the strain of origin. *Cancer Res* 1953;13:835

33. Prehn RT, Main JM. Immunity to methylcholanthrene-induced sarcomas. *J Natl Cancer Inst* 1957;18:796

34. Gold P, Freedman SO. Specific carcinoembryonic antigens in the human digestive system. *J Exp Med* 1965;122:467–81

35. Parmely MJ, Hsu HF. Rat alphafetoprotein: inhibitory activity on lymphocyte cultures. *Fed Proc* 1973;32:979

36. Murgita RA, Tomasi TB Jr. Suppression of the immune response by α-fetoprotein on the primary and secondary antibody response. *J Exp Med* 1975;141:269–86

CHAPTER 9

Autoimmunity

The historical development of autoimmunity has been presented in the past in widely scattered notes in the medical literature. In an attempt to assimilate an account of the metamorphosis of this fascinating chapter in the history of immunology, we present the following major advances in autoimmunity and their discoverers, who are no less fascinating than the subject itself. It should be pointed out that a comprehensive or exhaustive review of the literature of autoimmunity was not our intention. By contrast, we only outline the milestones in the development of autoimmunity, which has significance not only for selected disease mechanisms but also for many features of normal immune reactivity and immunoregulation.

In 1900, Ehrlich and Morgenroth[1] (Figure 1) found that the injection of self-antigens failed to elicit

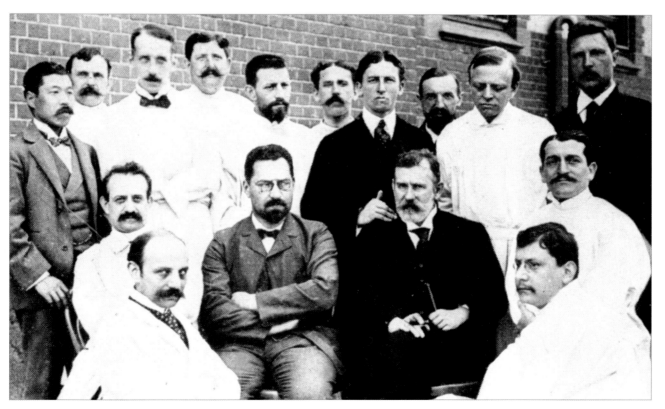

Figure 1   Professor Dr Paul Ehrlich and associates, Frankfurt-am-Main. Standing from left to right: Dr Shiga; Wunsch; Dr Noeggerath; Goeldner; unknown; Kaul; Dr Keyes; Kadereit; Dr Sticker; Dr Hans Sachs (mentor of Dr Ernest Witebsky). Seated: Dr Apolant; Dr Julius Morgenroth; Geheimrath Professor Dr Paul Ehrlich; Dr Max Neisser. Seated in front: Dr Embden, left; Dr Lippstein, right (with kind permission of Econ Verlag, Stuttgart)

an immune response in the autologous host. On discovering that goats immunized with their own erythrocytes failed to produce autoantibodies, Ehrlich formulated a concept of 'horror autotoxicus'[2] to explain the animal body's failure to mount an immune response against itself. Nevertheless, he recognized also that autoimmunity might occur as an aberration and lead to disease[2,3]. As Ehrlich and Morgenroth stated: 'In the explanation of many disease phenomena, it will in the future be necessary to consider the possible failure of the internal regulation, as well as the action of directly injurious exogenous or endogenous substances.' Apparently this latter report was overlooked in the confusion of the Great World War, and only the earlier concept of 'horror autotoxicus' prevailed in succeeding years, leading future generations of immunologists to be told incorrectly that Ehrlich had not appreciated the possibility that autoimmunity could constitute a part of the etiopathogenesis of selected disease states[2–4]. An investigator of rare genius and foresight, Ehrlich was already making contributions that still have relevance in cellular immunology and molecular genetics today, even before de Vries[5] rediscovered Mendel's basic principles of inheritance in 1901.

Subsequently, Donath and Landsteiner[6] showed that autoantibodies were responsible for paroxysmal cold hemaglobinuria in syphilis. Wassermann and colleagues[7] reported a diagnostic serologic test for syphilis based on autoantibodies. Meanwhile, many claims were made that one type of disease process or another had an autoimmune basis. These have been reviewed extensively[8–16]. For many years immunologists accepted Ehrlich's dictum that the animal body would not form harmful immunologic reactions against itself. Half a century later, Burnet[17,18] and Burnet and Fenner[19] expressed the concept as 'self-tolerance', and suggested the presence of a thymic censor which was supposed to prevent the appearance of forbidden clones.

Once early investigators began to use antigens from diverse sources, Metchnikoff[20] and other pathfinders in immunology[21] reported the development of cytotoxic antibodies in animals immunized with spermatozoa and tissue cells, thereby initiating the concept of autoallergy in which an animal mounts an autoimmune response against its own self-antigens. Early discoveries about eye diseases in which autoallergy was found to play a key role included phacoanaphylaxis, caused by inflammatory reactivity against protein antigens released from a traumatized lens capsule. Sympathetic ophthalmia was also found to occur as a result of autoallergic sensitization following trauma to one eye, leading to immunologic sensitization of the host against the uninjured companion eye[22–24].

Although the use of adjuvant substances to potentiate the immune response to antigens dates from the time of Pasteur, Freund and co-workers[25–30] established (1942) the efficiency of water-in-oil emulsions in potentiating the antibody response to a variety of antigens. The water-in-oil emulsion without added mycobacteria, known as 'incomplete' adjuvant, stimulated sensitivity of the immediate (immunoglobulin-mediated) variety, which was dependent upon antibody titers in the serum, in contrast to sensitivity of the delayed or tuberculin-type, which was mediated by sensitized lymphoid cells. It was soon found that the incorporation of various normal tissues into Freund's adjuvant, or similar adjuvant-like materials, could lead to the production of an autoimmune response in the animal body[26–28]. In 1951, Voisin and colleagues[31] produced aspermatogenesis experimentally by the injection of testicular tissue incorporated into Freund's adjuvant. It was postulated that the use of an adjuvant material such as Freund's adjuvant might cause stimulation of so-called 'forbidden clones', according to the clonal selection concept of acquired immunity, and that these 'forbidden clones', might augment an immune response against self-antigens leading to pathological sequelae. Witebsky[32] developed certain criteria later known as Witebsky's postulates that were patterned after Koch's postulates in bacteriology.

Ernest Witebsky (1901–69), German–American immunologist and bacteriologist who made significant contributions to transfusion medicine and to concepts of autoimmune diseases. He was a direct descendent of the Ehrlich school of immunology, having worked at Heidelberg with Hans Sachs, Ehrlich's principal assistant, in 1929. He went to Mt Sinai Hospital in New York in 1934 and became Professor at the University of Buffalo in 1936, where he remained until his death. A major portion of his work on autoimmunity was the demonstration with Noel R. Rose of experimental autoimmune thyroiditis.

According to these criteria, an autoimmune response should be considered the cause of a human disease if:

(1) It is regularly associated with that disease;

(2) Immunization of an experimental animal with antigen from the appropriate tissue causes the animal to make an immune response, i.e. form antibodies or develop a cell-mediated response;

(3) Associated with this response, the animal develops pathological changes that are basically similar to those of the human;

(4) The experimental disease can be transferred to non-immunized animals by serum or by lymphoid cells[32,33].

Of course, in human diseases, it is difficult to gather all of these criteria to establish a particular disease process as having an autoimmune etiology or pathogenesis. Witebsky's postulates reflect the thinking of that period concerning autoimmunity when a single cause was often believed to be responsible for an autoimmune disease. In comparison with Koch's postulates, where a single microorganism was proven to be the etiologic agent of an infectious disease, Witebsky's postulates were designed to follow the same pattern.

Many investigators suspected that viruses were especially significant etiologic agents of autoimmune diseases. Indeed, viruses do represent one of several factors important in the etiology and pathogenesis of autoimmunity. It was also widely held that disease resulted from qualitative abnormalities resulting in autoimmune disease. In recent years, several investigators have attempted to present a unifying concept of autoimmunity since the demonstration that autoimmune reactions may be physiologic as well as pathologic. Contemporary immunologic research has demonstrated clearly that self-reactivity is entirely normal. Indeed, normal immune function and immune regulation are dependent upon appropriate self–self interactions. It is now recognized that quantitative rather than qualitative abnormalities, including the relative quantities of autoantibody or immune complexes formed or the degree of stem cell proliferation, may lead to disease. Recent research demonstrates also that autoimmune diseases have a multifactorial etiology, where genetics, environmental and hormonal factors and defective immune regulation are now recognized to all act in concert to produce an autoimmune disease.

In contrast to the 'horror autotoxicus' concept of Ehrlich and Morgenroth[2,3] and Burnet's 'forbidden clone' explanation[17], Boyden[34], Grabar[35] and Kay and Makinodan[36] emphasized the physiologic regulatory functions of autoimmunity. In an attempt to explain how physiologic autoimmunity might be both physiologic and pathologic, and in an attempt to account for the various etiologic factors, Beutner and colleagues[37] presented a 'unified concept of autoimmunity'. They based this concept on the effects produced in vivo by autoantibodies or autoreactive T cells in the autologous host. Smith and Steinberg[38] described a new classification for autoimmune diseases, in the light of current information.

DEVELOPMENT OF IMMUNOBIOLOGY AND CELLULAR IMMUNOLOGY

Medawar[39] (1944–46) provided the first convincing proof that the rejection of grafts between individuals who are not related to one another, i.e. allografts or homografts, has an immunological basis. During the same period, Owen[40] described dizygotic cattle twins in which blood cells of one twin were tolerated immunologically by the other, i.e. they were chimeras.

Burnet and Fenner[19] at the Walter and Eliza Hall Institute (Figure 2) were beginning to take a view of antibody production different from that proposed by chemists adhering to the template theory of antibody production. The second edition of their classic monograph entitled The Production of Antibodies, published in 1949, contains an exposé of their developing concepts. Modifying their views through various explanations[19] that included a self-marker hypothesis to explain antibody production, Burnet[41] noted with interest that Jerne[42] had proposed a selective theory of antibody formation in 1955. Whereas Jerne[42] discussed various antibody populations, Burnet[41] and Talmage[43] independently emphasized replicating cells in a cell selection theory in 1957, leading to formulation of a new hypothesis which Burnet[17] termed the 'clonal selection theory of acquired immunity' in 1959. The template theory of antibody production which had been popular with the chemists for so many years could no longer explain these new biological revelations that included immunological tolerance, and it had never explained the secondary (or anamnestic) immune response. The *coup*

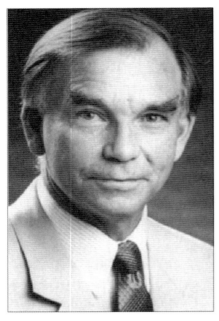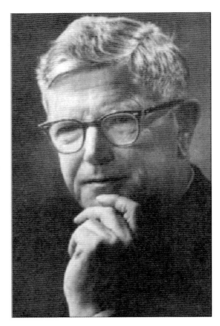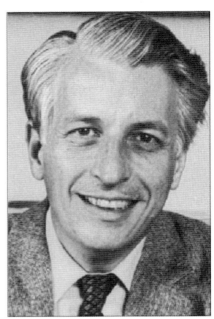

Figure 2 The Walter and Eliza Hall Institute Group. Left to right: Professor Ian Mackay; Sir Macfarlane Burnet; Sir Gustav Nossal

de grâce to this hypothesis was the observation that mature antibody-synthesizing cells contained no antigen. Burnet[17] proposed lymphoid cells genetically programmed to synthesize one type of antibody.

Antigen would have no effect on most lymphoid cells but would selectively stimulate those cells already synthesizing the corresponding antibody at a low rate. The cell surface antibody would serve as receptor for antigen and proliferate into a clone of cells producing antibody of that specificity. Burnet introduced the 'forbidden clone' concept to explain autoimmunity. Cells capable of forming antibody against a normal self-antibody were 'forbidden' and eliminated during embryonic life. Since that time various modifications of the clonal selection hypothesis have been offered.

The renaissance of cellular immunology developed following Burnet's description of the clonal selection theory of acquired immunity, which Nossal[44], Nossal and Pike[45] and Green and co-workers[46] proved to be correct.

In 1948, Fagraeus[47] established the role of the plasma cell in antibody formation. The fluorescent antibody technique[48,49] was a major breakthrough for identification of antigens in tissues and subsequently for demonstrating antibody synthesis by individual cells. While attempting to immunize chickens in which the bursa of Fabricius had been removed, Glick and colleagues[50] noted that antibody

production did not take place. This was the first evidence of bursa dependence of antibody formation. Good and associates[51] immediately realized the significance of this finding for immunodeficiencies of childhood. He and his associates in Minneapolis[51–53] and Miller[54] in England went on to show the role of the thymus in the immune response, and various investigators began to search for bursa equivalents in man and other animals. Thus, the immune system of many species was found to have distinct bursa-dependent, antibody-synthesizing and thymus-dependent, cell-mediated limbs. In 1959, Gowans[55] proved that lymphocytes actually recirculate. In 1966, Harris and co-workers[56] demonstrated clearly that lymphocytes could form antibodies. In 1966 and 1967, Claman and colleagues[57], Davies and colleagues[58] and Mitchison and associates[59] showed that T and B lymphocytes cooperate with one another in the production of an immune response. Various phenomena, such as the switch from forming one class of immunoglobulin to another by B cells, were demonstrated to be dependent upon a signal from T cells activating B cells to change from immunoglobulin IgM to IgG or IgA production. B cells stimulated by antigen in which no T cell signal was given continued to produce IgM antibody. Such antigens were referred to as thymus-independent antigens and others requiring T cell participation as thymus-dependent antigens.

Research focused next upon subpopulations of T lymphocytes. Mitchison and colleagues[59] described a subset of T lymphocytes demonstrating helper activity, i.e. helper T cells, whose hyperactivity is well recognized to lead to manifestations of autoimmunity. In 1971, Gershon and Kondo[60,61] described suppressor T cells that prevent development of autoimmune reactivity under normal circumstances. However, should their function become defective, autoimmunity may result. The concept of suppressor T cells has been brought into question because of the inability to characterize them by molecular biological analysis. However, the concept of immunosuppression, possibly through the action of cytokines, is unquestioned.

Subsequent studies concerned interactions among the various cell types of the immune system including interaction with antigen-presenting cells. Thus, elucidation of the T and B cell populations and subsets and their role in immunoregulation was requisite for improved understanding of autoimmune mechanisms. Especially critical to autoimmunity research was the discovery of the regulatory role of T cells in the immune response.

Benacerraf and colleagues[62], Benacerraf and McDevitt[63] and McDevitt and Chinitz[64] demonstrated the significant role played by gene products of the major histocompatibility complex in the specificity and regulation of T cell-dependent immune responses. For a review of genetic control of autoimmunity, the reader is referred to Rose and associates[65] and Vaughan[66].

In his network theory of immunity, Jerne[67] suggested that the formation of antibodies against idiotypic specificities on antibody molecules followed by the formation of anti-anti-idiotypic antibodies constituted a significant additional immunoregulatory process for proper functioning of the immune system. His postulates have been proven valid by numerous investigators. Tonegawa and colleagues[68] and Leder and associates[69] identified and cloned the genes that encode variable and constant regions of immunoglobulin molecules leading to increased understanding of the origin of diversity in antibody-combining sites.

In 1975, Köhler and Milstein[70] successfully fused splenic lymphocytes from mice forming antibody with tumor cells to produce what they called a 'hybridoma'. The spleen cells conferred the antibody-producing capacity while the tumor cells provided the capability for endless reproduction. Monoclonal antibodies are the valuable homogeneous products of hybridomas

with widespread application in diagnostic laboratory medicine. Human hybridomas formed by immortalization of lymphoid cells from patients with autoimmune disease, such as systemic lupus erythematosus (SLE), through fusion with a tumor cell line provide monoclonal antibodies that may be employed in the search for self-antigens eliciting autoimmune reactivity.

AUTOIMMUNE MANIFESTATIONS OF DISEASE

The historical development of autoimmunity associated with the etiopathogenesis of selected disease processes is presented in the following paragraphs.

Autoimmune hemolytic anemia

The association of autoantibodies with blood diseases dates from the observation by Donath and Landsteiner[6] that paroxysmal cold hemaglobinuria patients develop a hemolytic antibody in the serum that adsorbs to their red cells at relatively low temperatures, leading to lysis of the cells by complement upon warming to 37°C. Subsequently, Landsteiner[71] proposed that this antibody was a consequence of autoimmunization with altered tissue components, possibly assisted by the spirochete of syphilis.

Other early investigators such as Widal and colleagues[72] performed studies suggestive of a role for autohemagglutinins in acquired hemolytic icterus, and Chauffard and Vincent[73] and Chauffard[74] pointed to the action of hemolysins in the production of acute hemolytic anemia with hemoglobinuria. Dameshek and Schwartz[75] and Dameshek and colleagues[76] (Figure 3) described hemolytic antibodies in the blood sera of individuals with acute hemolytic anemia, pointing to the possibility that selected clinical hemolytic syndromes could be attributable to hemolysins in serum, rather than to intrinsically defective erythrocytes. They injected guinea-pigs with rabbit antibody against guinea-pig erythrocytes to produce experimental hemolytic syndromes, with associated spherocytosis, increased fragility of cells and reticulocytosis, closely resembling comparable human disorders.

Further investigation of immunologic aspects of human acquired hemolytic anemia was impeded by the lack of techniques for the detection of various types of

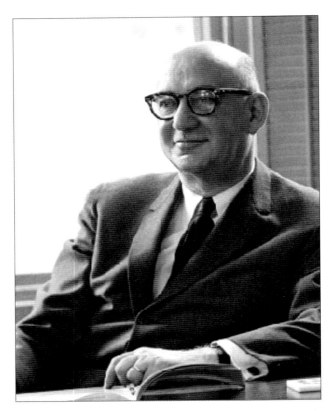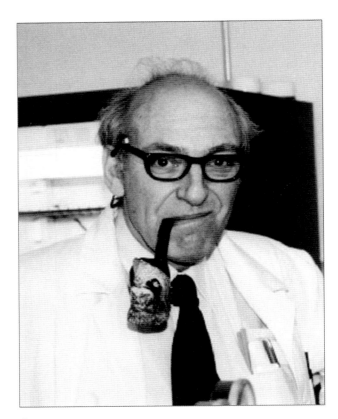

Figure 3   Dr William Dameshek (left); Dr H. Hugh Fudenberg (right)

antibodies against red cells, in particular those not demonstrable by agglutination *in vitro*. Coombs and colleagues'[77] introduction of the antiglobulin test for detection of red cells sensitized by incomplete rhesus isoantibodies represented the breakthrough needed for further progress. This technique was also found to be useful for detection of antibodies against red cells from selected idiopathic acquired hemolytic anemia cases[78,79]. Thus, this test came into widespread use for the detection of incomplete (i.e. non-agglutinating) autoantibodies against erythrocytes. Coombs[80] later credited Moreschi with development of a similar test after the turn of the century, even though this was unknown to Coombs and colleagues[80] when they developed the antiglobulin technique.

William Dameshek (1900–69), noted Russian–American hematologist who was among the first to understand autoimmune hemolytic anemias. He spent many years as editor-in-chief of the journal *Blood.*

Robin R. A. Coombs (1921–), British pathologist and immunologist who is best known for the Coombs'

test as a means for detecting immunoglobulin on the surface of a patient's red blood cells. The test was developed in the 1940s to demonstrate autoantibodies on the surface of red blood cells that failed to cause agglutination of the cells. It is a test for autoimmune hemolytic anemia. He has also contributed much to serology, immunohematology and immunopathology. *The Serology of Conglutination and Its Relation to Disease,* 1961; *Clinical Aspects of Immunology* (with Gell), 1963.

Morton and Pickles[81] developed other serological tests that included enzyme-treatment of erythrocytes to facilitate their agglutination by incomplete antibody. Other investigators[78,82,83] described techniques to elute and recover antibody bound to red blood cell surfaces, thus permitting the study of their autoantibody specificity. Antibodies in the circulation and on the surface of erythrocytes were found to shorten red cell survival. Mollison[84] showed that transfused normal ^{51}Cr-labeled red cells, as well as the patient's own erythrocytes, exhibited a remarkably briefer life span than the normal value of 110 days.

Dacie[79] suggested the serious nature of autoimmune acquired hemolytic anemia, pointing to the high mortality rate (>40%) in the warm antibody type, and emphasized the role of circulating autoantibodies against erythrocytes in the pathogenesis of the disease.

After Coombs and colleagues[77] introduced the antiglobulin test in 1945, autoantibodies were generally accepted to be etiologic factors in acquired hemolytic anemia. There was widespread introduction of the terms 'autoimmune' and 'autoallergic' into the medical literature. Subsequently, other blood diseases were shown to be associated with autoantibodies, e.g. antiplatelet antibodies in idiopathic thrombocytopenic purpura (ITP). Certain types of neutropenia, red cell aplasia and aplastic anemia have been linked also to autoantibodies and autoallergic cytotoxic reactions.

Ackroyd[85] performed most of the basic work on drug-induced blood dyscrasias associated with autoimmunity. For example, the drug sedormid elicits antibodies reactive not only with the drug but also with platelets, erythrocytes and even leukocytes bearing drug molecules, metabolites or even drug–antidrug complexes.

Immune complexes and tissue injury

Following the development of horse antitoxin for specific therapy in the treatment for both diphtheria and tetanus early in this century, clinicians noted an adverse reaction to large doses of antitoxin which they termed 'serum sickness'. In a series of elegant studies based upon this early model, Dixon and colleagues[86] developed an experimental model for serum sickness in the 1950s to demonstrate the basic principles of mechanisms of immunopathologic injury mediated by immune complexes. As antigen, they utilized iodinated bovine serum albumin and injected it into rabbits. They followed the elimination of the antigen in three phases, one of which was immune elimination, and studied the development of experimentally induced pathological lesions in the vessels, kidneys and joints of the animals, correlating this with the immune complex content of the blood serum. Cochrane[87] studied the role of polymorphonuclear leukocytes in nephrotoxic nephritis. Dixon and Wilson carried out fundamental investigations on the mechanism of immune complex-mediated injury in glomerulonephritis. As a result of studies by these and other investigators, immune complex disorders have been demonstrated to be dynamic processes implicated in the pathogenesis of a host of immunological diseases, including SLE and rheumatoid arthritis. In addition to their studies of immune complexes, Dixon and colleagues[86] continued to examine immunoregulatory dysfunction of immune system cells in SLE.

In an effort to unify the diverse descriptions of hypersensitivity phenomena, the British immunologists, Coombs and Gell[88] (Figure 4), developed a simplified classification of immunopathological phenomena that includes: type I, anaphylaxis; type II, cytotoxicity; type III, immune complex disease; type IV, delayed-type hypersensitivity. Immune complex disorders of the serum sickness variety belong in the type III hypersensitivity of the Coombs and Gell classification.

Systemic lupus erythematosus

First recognized as a distinct cutaneous disease in the early 1800s, SLE was described by Kaposi[89] as a multisystem disease. In 1895, Osler[90] called the disease 'erythema multiforme exudativum' pointing to its visceral complications. The first immunological abnormality observed in SLE was a false-positive serological test for syphilis. Pathologic lesions in the blood vessels and connective tissues of SLE cases were reported in the 1920s and 1930s. Gross[91], studying autopsy materials from SLE cases, discovered 'hematoxylin-stained bodies'. In 1935, G. Baehr and associates reported the 'wire-loop' appearance of affected glomeruli in lupus. Klemperer[92] emphasized the fibrinoid changes in lupus, but these were found also in other diseases of unknown pathogenesis. Thus, 'fibrinoid necrosis' was widely used as a descriptive term concerning SLE and related disorders. Klemperer coined the term 'collagen disease' to include rheumatic fever, rheumatoid arthritis, subacute and chronic glomerulonephritis, SLE, dermatomyositis and scleroderma. It was his intention to point out the common pathogenic features of these conditions and to use the term 'collagen disease' as a topographic rather than an etiopathogenetic description. Unfortunately, 'collagen disease' came into widespread use by clinicians with incorrect connotations.

The serologic breakthrough came with the development of autoantibody tests, beginning with the lupus erythematosus (LE) cell test by Hargreaves and colleagues[93] in 1948. Although positive in only 50–70% of SLE patients and not specific for SLE, since it was also positive in some other connective tissue diseases such as rheumatoid arthritis, this test permitted the identification of previously occult mild cases and

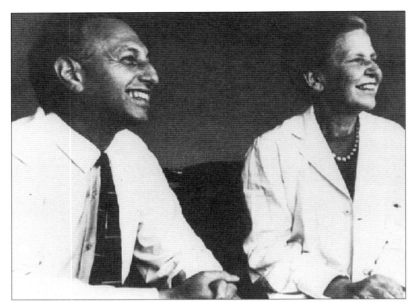
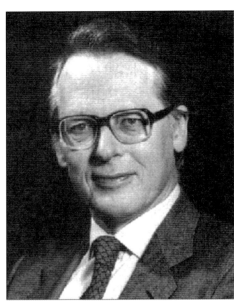

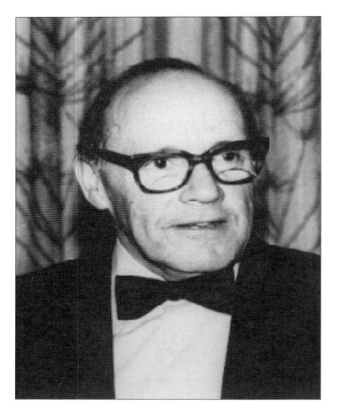

Figure 4 The British Autoimmunity Group. Top, left to right: Professor Ivan Roitt; Professor Deborah Doniach; Professor J. Irvine. Bottom: Professor R. R. A. Coombs

introduced the concept of autoantibodies in SLE. Miescher[94] (Figure 5) described antinuclear antibodies, thus establishing SLE as an immunological disease. Other prominent investigators of molecular aspects of autoimmune diseases, including SLE, are also shown in

Figure 5, i.e. Talal, Theofilopoulos and Steinberg. Anti-DNA antibodies were described by several investigators. Other autoantibody tests developed subsequently included the fluorescent antinuclear antibody test (FANA)[95], which became the most common single laboratory finding in SLE, since it is positive in 95–98% of SLE cases.

By 1957, several independent teams of investigators, including the United States group of W. C. Robbins and associates described antibodies against DNA (Figure 6). Following introduction of the Farr[96] ammonium sulfate technique to increase the sensitivity of the test for native (double-stranded) DNA antibodies in 1968, this method gained widespread clinical acceptance as a laboratory feature of SLE. Tan and Kunkel[97] described the anti-Sm antibody which was found to be virtually diagnostic for SLE even though it was present in only 28–32% of SLE patients.

Later investigations centered around the disordered suppressor T cell function in SLE (Figure 7). Miller and Schwartz[98] reported abnormal suppressor cell activity in 11 of 15 SLE patients as well as in 13 of 50 healthy first-degree relatives, including 12 females. Thus, observations in humans, as well as in experimental animal models of this disease, suggested that the immunologic defect in SLE was influenced by genetics. Hormones were believed also to have a significant role in the expression of immunologic parameters in SLE. Thus, the pathogenesis of SLE was recognized to be influenced by genetic, hormonal and infective mechanisms.

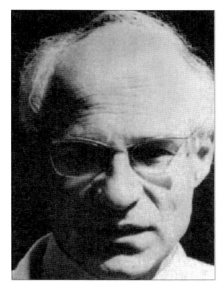
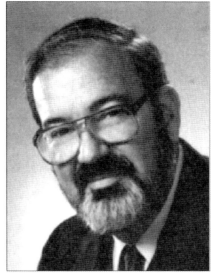
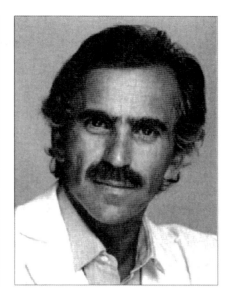

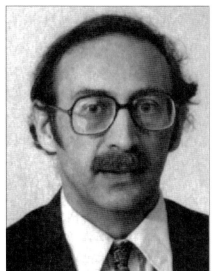

Figure 5 Top, left to right: Professor Peter Miescher; Professor Norman Talal; Argyrios N. Theofilopoulos, MD. Bottom: Alfred D. Steinberg, MD

Rheumatoid arthritis and rheumatoid factor

Meyer[99] observed coincidentally that selected human sera were able to agglutinate sheep red cells sensitized with rabbit amboceptor during the performance of routine complement fixation tests for syphilis. Waaler[100] and Rose and associates[101] reinvestigated the finding to determine whether it had relevance for rheumatoid arthritis, even though the original patient had suffered from chronic bronchitis. Limited agglutinating activity was present in most of the sera Waaler studied, yet this activity was accentuated in certain rheumatoid sera. Subsequent studies failed to demonstrate that rheumatoid factors in the sera of rheumatoid arthritis patients were qualitatively any different from those in the sera of patients with other diseases, or even of normal subjects.

Noel Richard Rose (1927–), American immunologist and authority on autoimmune disease, who first discovered, with Witebsky, experimental autoimmune thyroiditis (Figure 8). Dr Noel Rose's discovery in the mid-1950s that rabbits could be immunized to their own thyroid protein overturned the established dogma of 'horror autotoxicus' and showed unequivocally that autoimmunity could be the cause of disease. With Witebsky, he also demonstrated that patients with chronic thyroiditis develop similar antibodies to their own thyroid antigen, implicating autoimmunity as the cause of this human disease. The initial experiments were followed by others that elucidated the pathogenesis of autoimmune disease in animals and humans. In the 1970s, he described, for the first time, the critical role of genetics in conferring susceptibility to autoimmune disease and showed that the major histocompatibility complex includes the major susceptibility gene. In the 1980s, he showed how virus infections can serve as the trigger for autoimmune disease of the heart. These discoveries open the way to improved treatments and new prevention strategies for this group of diseases. Rose's pioneering investigations initiated the modern era of research on autoimmune disease.

Dr Rose has served as Professor of Microbiology at SUNY, Buffalo, Professor and Chair of Immunology and Microbiology at Wayne State University, Detroit and as Professor and Chair of Immunology and

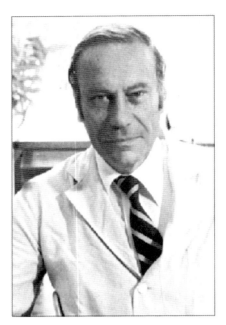
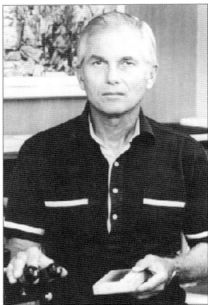
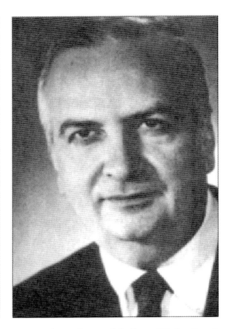

Figure 6 Left to right: H. G. Kunkel, MD, Rockefeller University; Frank J. Dixon, MD, Research Institute of Scripps Clinic; Baruj Benacerraf, MD, Harvard Medical School

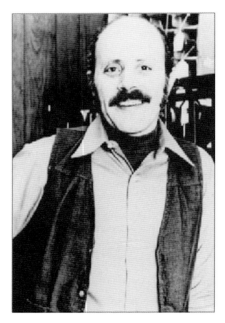
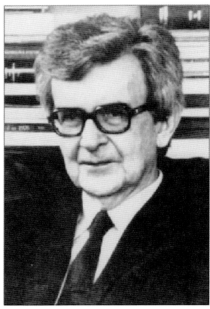
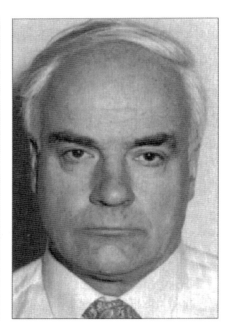

Figure 7 Representatives of contributors to immunoregulation. Left to right: Richard Gershon, MD: suppressor T cells; Niels K. Jerne, MD: natural selection theory of antibody formation, and network theory of immunoregulation; N. A. Mitchison, MD: helper T cells

Infectious Diseases at The Johns Hopkins University. The author of more than 600 articles and editor of numerous books and leading journals in the field, he is presently Director of The Johns Hopkins Center for Autoimmune Disease Research and the WHO/PAHO Collaborating Center for Autoimmune Disorders.

Dean[102] demonstrated that a thermostable globulin from normal guinea pig serum could agglutinate red cells sensitized with dilute antiserum. This was attributable to a euglobulin unrelated to complement. He emphasized the significance of antigen access for this globulin to produce maximal agglutination or

IgM rheumatoid factors were found not to be species-restrictive, indicating the sharing of active sites on the Fc fragment of human IgG with corresponding structures on immunoglobulin molecules of many other mammalian species. Milgrom and Witebsky[107] immunized rabbits with aggregated autologous globulin and discovered that the rabbits produced antibodies with greater reactivity for human globulin than for rabbit globulin.

Many of the studies on immunoglobulins, including rheumatoid factors, were conducted by Kunkel and co-workers[9,108] at the Rockefeller University. Among these individuals were Franklin and co-workers[103–105], Fudenberg and co-workers[109–111], Edelman and colleagues[112] and a host of others. For further historical notes on rheumatoid factor, consult Waller[113].

Henry George Kunkel (1916–83), American physician and immunologist. The primary focus of his work was immunoglobulins. He characterized myeloma proteins as immunoglobulins and rheumatoid factor as an autoantibody. He also discovered IgA and idiotypy and contributed to immunoglobulin structure and genetics. Kunkel received the Lasker Award and the Gairdner Award. A graduate of Johns Hopkins Medical School, he served as Professor of Medicine at the Rockefeller Institute for Medical Research.

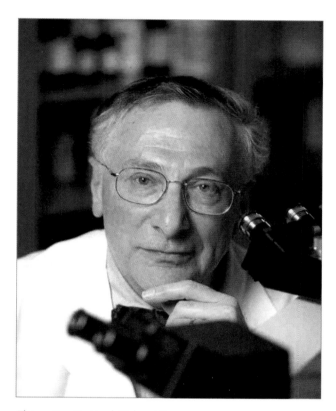

Figure 8   Dr Noel Richard Rose

precipitation. This agglutinating globulin had the peculiar ability to enhance the action of an extremely dilute antibacterial serum. Agglutinating 'activating factor' was later called 'rheumatoid factor', reflecting its association with rheumatoid arthritis.

Subsequent studies demonstrated that sera from rheumatoid arthritis patients could agglutinate not only certain streptococci but other bacteria as well. Attempts to correlate reactivity against bacteria with the progress of the disease led to inconclusive and contradictory results.

The demonstration that rheumatoid factor reacted best with denatured gammaglobulin led to the concept that it might be an autoantibody. Franklin[103] and Franklin and co-workers[104,105] found both 19S rheumatoid factor and 7S gammaglobulin as a 22S complex when the sera of rheumatoid arthritis patients were studied by ultracentrifugation. Epstein and colleagues[106] showed the ability of rheumatoid factor and gammaglobulin to give a positive precipitin reaction. The demonstration that autologous IgG was able to block the interaction of rheumatoid factor and globulin coating-sensitized cells further substantiated the concept of rheumatoid factor as an autoantibody.

It was difficult to accept that human IgG served as the antigen for stimulation of rheumatoid factor synthesis. Early investigators, such as Cecil and colleagues[114], attempted to show that microorganisms had stimulated formation of these factors. With the demonstration that IgG molecules possessed Gm groups capable of stimulating anti-immunoglobulin antibodies, it became more plausible to consider IgM rheumatoid factor as an antibody against native IgG, which was weakly antigenic in the autologous host. There still remained the difficulty of explaining antibodies against IgG in the serum of normal individuals, as well as those with a variety of diseases other than rheumatoid arthritis. The Fc region of denatured IgG molecules was found to be the primary antigen reactive with rheumatoid factor. Rheumatoid factors are natural humoral antibodies whose levels are markedly increased by the etiologic agent or agents of rheumatoid arthritis and, occasionally, the agents of other disease states. Despite a multitude of studies, the role of rheumatoid factor in the pathogenesis of rheumatoid arthritis remains an enigma.

Further studies of rheumatoid arthritis revealed that antigen–antibody complexes became entrapped on the synovial surface and in fibrocartilage followed by activation of various biological amplification mechanisms, including complement, kinins, clotting, fibrinolysis and phagocytosis. Lymphocytes and plasma cells in the subsynovium were found to produce rheumatoid factor and IgG molecules that were secreted into the joint space, perhaps perpetuating inflammation. The discovery of rheumatoid arthritis in agammaglobulinemic children and the fact that rheumatoid factor did not produce ill effects following infusion into healthy volunteers discouraged a pathogenic role for rheumatoid factor in rheumatoid arthritis. Nevertheless, immune complexes containing IgG rheumatoid factor and cryoglobulins were implicated in the pathogenesis of rheumatoid vasculitis. Regrettably, investigation of immune complexes was not able to account for joint inflammation or vasculitis. Abnormal cellular immune phenomena in rheumatoid arthritis were found to include anergy, depressed lymphoblastogenesis, depressed mixed leukocyte culture reactivity and diminished antibody-dependent cell-mediated cytotoxicity of synovial fluid lymphocytes. Possible explanations for the uncontrolled synthesis of rheumatoid factor antibodies against native IgG have included chronic antigenic stimulation, enhanced T helper cell function or diminished T suppressor function.

Sjögren's syndrome

This disorder was described as a triad of keratoconjunctivitis sicca, xerostomia and rheumatoid arthritis[115]. In one manifestation the sicca component predominates, whereas in the other the sicca occurs in conjunction with either rheumatoid arthritis or another disorder. Sjögren's syndrome has been associated with the presence of specific antibodies and T lymphocyte sensitization against salivary duct antigens. Patients were hypergammaglobulinemic and demonstrated serum antinuclear factor and antibody reactive by the autoimmune complement fixation test. Anderson and colleagues[116] showed precipitating antibodies reactive with organ extracts in the sera of 10 of 29 patients with Sjögren's syndrome. The presence of antinuclear antibodies and a positive test for rheumatoid factor suggested a resemblance of Sjögren's

syndrome to both SLE and rheumatoid arthritis. As evidenced by lymphoid infiltrate of the salivary glands, patients with Sjögren's syndrome were shown to manifest many different kinds of lymphoproliferation, most as benign lymphoid infiltrate of the salivary and lacrimal glands, but also sometimes as lymphocytic infiltrate of the lungs, kidneys and other organs. Occasional patients developed lymphoproliferation leading to lymphoma or Waldenström's macroglobulinemia.

Autoimmune thyroiditis

Oswald[117] described the globulin that R. Hutchison extracted from the thyroid as 'thyroglobulin'. Subsequently, Hektoen and Shulhof[118] and Hektoen and colleagues[119] demonstrated that thyroglobulin antibodies were not species-restricted. Rabbit antibodies specific for horse, dog and human thyroglobulin all cross-reacted with bovine thyroglobulin. Rabbit antiporcine thyroglobulin cross-reacted with horse, beef, monkey, human, rat and sheep, as well as swine thyroglobulin. In 1958, Witebsky and colleagues[120] (Figure 9) confirmed Hektoen's observation using purified thyroglobulin. An antibody against thyroid cross-reacted with thyroid extracts of selected but not all species tested. Thus, thyroglobulin was proved to be organ-specific, yet less broadly cross-reactive than in the case of the lens proteins[121] or the brain[122]. Although Lerman[123] could not elicit antibody against rabbit thyroid by the injection of rabbit thyroglobulin, he did observe that rabbit antibody against human thyroglobulin would precipitate rabbit thyroglobulin.

Rose and Witebsky[124–126] challenged rabbits with rabbit thyroid extract incorporated into Freund's adjuvant. Upon finding that an antibody reactive with rabbit thyroid extract was produced, they proceeded to ascertain whether an autoantibody had been formed. Thyroidectomized or hemithyroidectomized rabbits were inoculated with autologous thyroid extracts incorporated into Freund's complete adjuvant. Antibodies were produced not only against their own thyroid glands but against those of other rabbits and thyroids of other species. Histopathological examination revealed reduced colloid and infiltration by lymphoid, phagocytic and eosinophilic cells, further substantiating the autoimmune nature of rabbit antirabbit thyroid antibody[127–130].

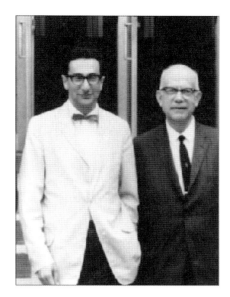
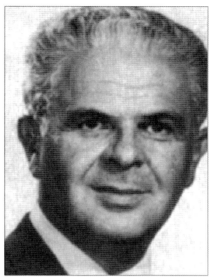
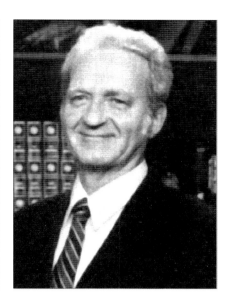

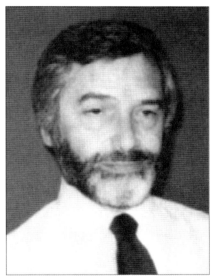

Figure 9 The Buffalo Immunology Group. Top from left to right: Professor Noel Rose; Professor Ernest Witebsky; Professor Felix Milgrom; Professor Ernst Beutner. Bottom: Professor Sidney Shulman

Following the demonstration by Witebsky and colleagues[32] that ammonium sulfate fractionated rabbit thyroglobulin incorporated into Freund's complete adjuvant could elicit antibodies in the autologous host that were reactive with rabbit thyroid extract, Beutner and associates[131] showed by immunofluorescence that antibodies against rabbit thyroid would stain rabbit thyroid gland colloid containing thyroglobulin. Reactivity was shown to be thyroid specific.

Although first considered to be anatomically isolated in the follicles of the thyroid gland, and not in contact with immunocompetent cells under normal conditions, relatively low levels of circulating thyroglobulin were subsequently demonstrated. T cells were found to be tolerant of low doses of thyroglobulin in the circulation, whereas B cells remained immunocompetent. In the absence of a signal from the T cell, B cells fail to mount an autoimmune response against thyroglobulin.

Roitt and colleagues[132] observed a positive precipitation reaction following interaction between serum of Hashimoto's thyroiditis patients and human thyroglobulin *in vitro*. This represented the first proof that humans with thyroid disease contained circulating antibodies reactive with thyroglobulin. For further historical details of autoimmune thyroiditis, refer to Rabin[127].

Insulin-dependent (type 1) diabetes mellitus

Inflammatory lesions termed 'insulitis' in the pancreatic islets of diabetics at onset suggested that autoimmunity might have a central role in the pathogenesis of type 1 or insulin-dependent diabetes mellitus (IDDM)[133,134]. The immunologic attack appeared to be directed specifically against insulin-producing β cells, even though at least three other cell types were present in the pancreatic islets. Glucagon-containing α cells, somatostatin-containing δ cells and pancreatic polypeptide-containing (PP) cells increased in relative proportion to the markedly reduced mass of β cells[135]. Immunologic phenomena discovered in association with IDDM included evidence of cell-mediated immunity[136–138], killer cell activity[136] and circulating antibody[139,140], reactive with the pancreatic islets. Considering the significance of the major histocompatibility complex in immunoregulation, it was interesting to note that certain human leukocyte antigen (HLA) types, especially HLA-DR3 and -DR4, were found to be closely associated with IDDM. Thus, the presence of predisposing conditions associated with these alleles pointed to a significant role for autoimmunity in this disease. Therefore, it became clear that suppression of the immune response might represent a potential mode of therapy in IDDM.

Antibodies specific against pancreatic islet cells were found in the circulation of insulin-dependent diabetics. Either environmental factors or loss of immunoregulatory control were credited with initiating autoimmunity against insulin-producing β cells. Several types of antibodies against both cytoplasmic and surface antigenic determinants of pancreatic islet cells have been linked to the onset of IDDM. Islet cell surface antibodies attracted special interest owing to their preferential β cytotoxicity[140].

Historically, observations relating to cell-mediated autoimmune phenomena in the pathogenesis of diabetes preceded the recognition of humoral autoimmunity in this disease. Two-thirds of patients with short-duration juvenile-onset diabetes mellitus exhibited striking mononuclear cellular infiltrate, principally lymphocytes, in and around the islets of Langerhans at autopsy[141,142]. In addition, many patients with type I diabetes mellitus had associated autoimmune disorders[143,144].

Nerup and associates[138] described inhibition of leukocyte migration in response to an extract of porcine insulin in diabetics by comparison with controls. Delayed-type hypersensitivity was demonstrated by intracutaneous injection of the insulin extract. Liver or kidney extracts and porcine insulin had no effect on lymphocyte migration. Migration inhibition had no association with a history of insulin therapy[145]. Studies by Huang and Maclaren[136] demonstrated that cell-mediated cytotoxicity could participate in the pathogenesis of type I diabetes. To establish the role of cell-mediated immunity in type I diabetes, Buschard and colleagues[146] reported passive transfer of diabetes from humans to nude mice by injection of peripheral mononuclear cells derived from newly diagnosed patients with insulin-dependent diabetes. A valuable

asset for experimental studies of type I diabetes was recognition of the spontaneously diabetic BB rat. Studies of the disease in this species have revealed the genetic basis for transmission of the syndrome, the insulin-dependent feature of physiologic abnormalities and the role of immune phenomena in pathogenesis. It is anticipated that future studies will reveal effector cells leading to β cell destruction and the antigenic targets against which the immune attack is directed.

Other autoimmune endocrinopathies: autoimmunity of adrenal and gonads, parathyroid and pituitary

This is reviewed by Doniach and colleagues[147]. Following the successful introduction of antibiotic therapy for tuberculosis, most Addison's disease cases were found to be due to autoimmune destruction of the adrenal cortex. Approximately 60% of Addisonian patients demonstrated antibodies reactive with adrenocortical cells in all three layers. An incidence of 88% adrenal antibodies in HLA-A1, B5, DR3 haplotype patients demonstrated the influence of genetic predisposition in development of this disease. Antibodies against steroid cells were shown to be cross-reactive with steroid-secreting cells in both the placenta and gonads.

Milgrom and Witebsky[148] and Witebsky and Milgrom[149] differentiated clearly between antigens of the adrenal medulla and cortex in their investigations of experimental immune adrenalitis (for further details, refer to references 8, 148 and 149).

Blizzard and colleagues[150] first studied idiopathic hypoparathyroidism immunologically and found positive immunofluorescence on parathyroid substrates with 38% of patient sera and with 6% of controls. Parathyroid gland atrophy and clinical associations placed this disease with the organ-specific autoimmune diseases. Antibodies against pituitary prolactin cells were first shown in polyendocrine disease. Subsequently, antibodies against some other types of pituicytes were discovered.

Pernicious anemia and autoimmunity

Pernicious anemia together with its associated gastric atrophy were described between 1850 and 1870, and the therapeutic effect of liver and the extrinsic and intrinsic factor concept were developed between 1920 and 1930.

Next came the identification of vitamin B_{12} as extrinsic factor and its structural analysis (1948–55).

The recognition of pernicious anemia as an autoimmune disease (1962–65) was based upon the identification of autoantibodies against gastric parietal cells and intrinsic factor, and the association between gastric antibodies and defective absorption of vitamin B_{12}. Other supportive evidence was the association of this disease with other autoimmune disorders, as well as the ability of prednisolone to facilitate regeneration of gastric mucosal atrophy.

In the 1950s, continued use of hog intrinsic factor to treat pernicious anemia reduced its effectiveness with time. In 1958, Taylor and Morton[151] found that rabbits injected with intrinsic factor developed anti-intrinsic factor activity, and Schwartz[152] demonstrated development of an inhibitor of hog intrinsic factor activity in the serum of patients treated with this factor. Further interest in gastric autoimmunity stemmed from Tudhope and Wilson's report[153] that there was a different incidence of pernicious anemia in patients with thyroid disease compared with the general population. As Mackay and Whittingham[154] pointed out, this linkage and the possibility that spontaneous hypothyroidism might be a consequence of autoimmune thyroiditis fueled speculation of an association between autoimmune reactivity against gastric cells and pernicious anemia.

Irvine and colleagues[155] found positive complement fixation reactions using sera from pernicious anemia patients and gastric mucosa as antigen. He also demonstrated serological cross-reactivity between individuals with pernicious anemia and patients with Hashimoto's thyroiditis, employing gastric and thyroid tissue antigens. Immunofluorescence was employed subsequently to demonstrate that the reactive antigen in pernicious anemia was that associated with parietal cells.

Subsequent studies were directed toward antibodies against intrinsic factor reactive *in vitro*. Two different antibodies were shown to react with separate reactive sites on the molecule and were referred to as blocking and binding antibodies[156]. Whereas parietal cell antibody was shown by immunofluorescence in 90–95% of pernicious anemia cases, only 50–55% of subjects showed antibody against intrinsic factor. It was then suggested that antibody against intrinsic factor in gastric juice rather than in serum might be a reliable indicator of gastric autoimmune reactivity.

Mackay and Burnet[137] set up criteria for the diagnosis of autoimmune diseases that included:

(1)   Hypergammaglobulinemia;

(2)   Serum antibodies;

(3)   Lymphoid infiltration of the affected tissue;

(4)   Responsiveness of the disease to corticosteroids;

(5)   Association of the disease with clinical and serological features of other autoimmune diseases in that patient and/or blood relatives.

Pernicious anemia fulfilled several of these, i.e. antibody against both parietal cells and intrinsic factor, lymphoid infiltration of the stomach, regeneration of atrophic gastric mucosa in response to prednisolone therapy and the demonstration of clinical and serological overlap between pernicious anemia and Hashimoto's thyroiditis–thyrotoxicosis–myxedema complex of diseases.

The central question in autoimmunity has always been whether autoantibodies are the cause or result of a given disease process. In the case of pernicious anemia, a positive correlation was demonstrated between the presence of gastric antibodies and impaired vitamin B_{12} absorption. For further details concerning the history of pernicious anemia, the reader is referred to the review article by Mackay and Whittingham[154].

Autoimmunity and the liver

Autoimmunity has been implicated in liver disease since 1908 when Fiessinger[157] cited by Paronetto and Popper[158] concluded from his serologic and experimental study that autoantibodies against liver could be induced following hepatic injury.

The demonstration of an autoimmune component in chronic active hepatitis was shown in Melbourne in 1955 when Joske and King[159] demonstrated that two 'active chronic viral hepatitis' patients had positive LE cell tests. Mackay and co-workers[160] reported five more cases, including predominantly females with hypergammaglobulinemia. Observing that some manifestations, such as arthralgia, suggestive of SLE were present, they termed the condition 'lupoid hepatitis', which they believed to be the result of autoimmunization. Complement fixation assays of the serum of patients with lupoid hepatitis, primary biliary cirrhosis (PBC) and SLE revealed reactivity with saline extracts of human tissues, especially liver and kidney[161]. Further support for autoimmunity was provided by the use of immunofluorescence after 1960 to show positive antinuclear antibody in many patients with chronic active hepatitis whose LE cell tests were negative[162].

Johnson and associates[163] reported smooth muscle antibodies in chronic active hepatitis patients. Antibody titers appeared to be positively correlated with disease activity. These antibodies were also found in PBC as well as in selected other conditions, such as the low titers found in acute viral hepatitis.

Walker and colleagues[164] described antimitochondrial antibodies in PBC patients. Subsequently, these antibodies were found also in some chronic active hepatitis patients. The fluorescent antibody technique was found to be useful for detection of both smooth muscle and mitochondrial antibodies. Other antibodies found in liver disease included antinuclear and antiliver antibodies. Antinuclear and antismooth muscle antibodies were characteristically seen in chronic active hepatitis patients. Other identifiable antibodies were those against mitochondria, microsomes, cardiolipin, thyrogastric antigens, gammaglobulins and erythrocytes. Immune complexes did not appear to contribute significantly to hepatocellular damage in chronic active hepatitis. By contrast, so-called antiliver antibodies demonstrated much variation from one case to another and little correlation with severity, progression or even presence of disease.

Since studies of humoral antibodies failed to explain pathogenetic mechanisms responsible for development of selected liver diseases, efforts were made to show a role for cell-mediated immunity, which was suggested by the histologic appearance of lymphocytes, histiocytes and large pyroninophylic cells in liver sections from patients with certain hepatic diseases. *In vitro* studies included lymphocyte stimulation by plant mitogens or hepatic tissue antigens. Soborg and Bendixen[165] showed cell-mediated immunity by use of the leukocyte migration inhibition technique. Most of 34 untreated chronic active hepatitis patients showed positive *in vitro* correlates of cell-mediated immunity. Another study by Miller and colleagues[166] showed cell-mediated immunity, as revealed by the lymphocyte migration inhibition technique, in 11 of 16 cases of chronic active hepatitis and seven of 12 cases of PBC. Bacon and co-workers[167] found evidence of cell-mediated immune reactivity using whole liver cell extracts as antigens in 24 of 32 patients with either chronic active hepatitis or PBC.

Autoimmune neurologic disorders

Tissue injury produced by immune reactions was first described as a cause of disease in the nervous system[168]. Occasional individuals who received the Pasteur vaccine for rabies virus, following its introduction in 1885, developed neurological signs and symptoms attributable to acute inflammation in the central nervous system (CNS). This was induced by an immune response against the nervous tissue in which the virus was cultured during attenuation. In 1933 and 1935, Rivers and colleagues[169] and Rivers and Swentker[170] reported development of acute disseminated encephalomyelitis in monkeys that had received repeated inoculations of CNS tissue extracts or emulsions. They observed a close similarity between this experimental disease and the encephalomyelitis found in occasional subjects following rabies vaccination. They suggested that the myelin injury might be attributable to an immune response to CNS antigens. Subsequently, Kabat and colleagues[171–173] and Morgan[174] reported independently that incorporation of either homologous or heterologous CNS tissue into Freund's complete adjuvant could induce experimental allergic encephalomyelitis (EAE) in monkeys.

Waksman and Adams[175] pointed out that most histological studies of EAE had been made on animals with advanced disease rendering unsuitable interpretation of the interrelationships among cells present in the lesions. To remedy this problem, they administered antigen by a technique known to provide clinical evidence of EAE in rabbits and guinea pigs 9–10 days following a single injection. The animals were killed at daily intervals beginning on the fifth day, which permitted the investigators to show that lymphocytes and small mononuclear cells were the first to infiltrate the area, apparently having been derived from circulating blood by emigration from adjacent vessels.

They observed that many of the cells remained close to the vessel where they originated, either in meninges or in Virchow–Robin spaces. Yet many others migrated into the adjacent parenchyma and increased in number by mitosis. The infiltrating cells then underwent progressive metamorphosis into typical histiocytes, which Waksman and Adams[175] suggested were directly responsible for demyelination in areas of infiltration. Thus, specific injury to the nervous system tissue was shown to be mediated by cells, an observation which was supported indirectly by failure to correlate the presence of circulating antibody with development of CNS lesions.

Later studies demonstrated that the primary antigen was myelin basic protein (MBP), and pointed to the close resemblance between EAE and multiple sclerosis, the principal demyelinating disease of humans.

Myasthenia gravis

Although myasthenia gravis (MG) was probably first described by Willis[176] in 1685, and approximately seven cases had been reported by the turn of the century, it was not until 1901 that Laquer and Weigert[177] reported association of a thymic tumor with MG. Subsequently, thymectomy was found to improve the clinical status of some myasthenic patients with thymic tumor, even though it would be more than a half century before Good and associates[51] and Miller[54] described the cardinal role of the thymus in the immune response. Recent research has focused on whether the physiological defect could be presynaptic, with diminished quantities of acetylcholine, or postsynaptic, with acetylcholine receptor defects. This was resolved by Fambrough and associates[178], who demonstrated conclusively that the number of functional acetylcholine receptors is diminished in MG. Ito and colleagues[179] demonstrated that this decrease in acetylcholine receptors could account for the physiological changes in the disease. Patrick and Lindstrom[180] immunized rabbits with acetylcholine receptors purified from the electric organ of the electric eel, to develop an experimental model of MG that closely resembles the human disease. Serum from immunized animals was capable of transferring the disease passively to previously untreated recipients. Such antibodies have since been demonstrated in MG patients whose condition has been improved by plasma exchange[181] or thoracic duct drainage[182].

Autoimmune reactions of the skin

Increased understanding of bullous diseases, including pemphigus, began with Civatte's description of acantholysis and with Lever's delineation of pemphigus from pemphigoid syndromes. Beutner and Jordan[183] found that serum from patients with pemphigus vulgaris contained an antibody reactive with intercellular substances of stratified squamous epithelium. Eight of 13 patients' sera produced what has become known as a classic 'chicken wire' reaction pattern when examined by indirect immunofluorescence microscopy. Normal skin adjacent to a blister of one pemphigus patient exhibited gammaglobulin in the intercellular space. Subsequent studies by these authors and others confirmed deposition of an IgG antibody in involved as well as in uninvolved areas of skin. Chorzelski and colleagues[184] described antibodies in 23 of 35 patients with active pemphigus. They showed that antibody titers decreased as some patients responded to therapy. By contrast, exacerbations of the disease were noted in conjunction with the rising titer. The authors emphasized the significance of performing serial serologic tests in patient treatment. A subsequent report by Jordan and co-workers[185] pointed to the diagnostic significance of direct immunofluorescence microscopy of skin biopsy specimens.

Beutner and colleagues[186] were able to identify the reactive principle in the serum of pemphigus patients as well as autoantibodies because in two patients the serum reacted with the patient's own normal skin. The antibodies also demonstrated tissue specificity by fixing only to squamous epithelium whether from skin, oral mucosa, esophagus, anus, vagina or cornea[184].

CONCLUSION

We have presented only an outline of representative major developments in the fascinating saga of autoimmunity, which have been brought about not only by immunologists but also largely through the efforts of endocrinologists.

General features of autoimmunity Failure or interruption of the mechanisms that maintain self-tolerance in B cells, T cells or both can lead to autoimmunity. Genetic susceptibility and environmental triggers, such as infections, are also principal contributory factors. Autoimmune diseases, which may be either systemic or organ-specific, are mediated by several effector mechanisms of tissue injury.

Determinant spreading is an amplification mechanism in inflammatory autoimmune disease in which the initial T lymphocyte response diversifies through induction of T cells against additional autoantigenic determinants. The response to the original epitope is followed by intramolecular spreading, activation of

Table 1 Chronology of events in the development of autoimmunity

Date	Events
1900	Ehrlich and Morgenroth[3] study blood of six goats, finding that there are clumping reactions between certain ones, not published until 1901, the 'horror autotoxicus' theory
1904	Donath–Landsteiner: antibody[6]
1910	Elschnig[22]: sympathetic ophthalmia described
1912	von Wassermann et al.[7]: syphilis autoantibodies
1922	Verhoff and Lemoine[24] established phacoanaphylaxis, hypersensitivity to lens protein
1933–35	Rivers and co-workers[169,170]: experimental acute disseminated encephalomyelitis in monkeys
1938	Dameshek and co-workers[75,76]: autoimmune hemolytic anemia
1942–46	Freund[29]: Freund's complete adjuvant which enhances antibody response to antigen and directs response to development of delayed hypersensitivity
1944	Medawar[39]: the mechanism of tissue transplant rejection is immunological
1945	Coombs et al.[77] develop the antiglobulin test for incomplete Rh antibody
1945	Owen[40]: bovine twins which share feral circulation are chimeras
1951	Voisin et al.[31]: autoimmune aspermatogenesis
1953	Billingham, Brent, Medawar: 'actively acquired tolerance' of foreign cells, proof for Burnet and Fenner's[19] theory of antibody production
1947–49	Kabat et al.[171,172]: autoimmunity to brain tissue encephalomyelitis
1948	Hargreaves et al.[93]: lupus erythematosus (LE) cells described
1955	Jerne[42]: natural selection theory of immunity
1956	Glick et al.[50]: B cells from bursa
1956	Witebsky and Rose[129]: autoimmune thyroiditis
1956	Roitt et al.[132]: autoantibodies in Hashimoto's thyroiditis
1957	Burnet[41] and Talmage[43] propose independently 'cell selection theories'
1957	Waldenström, Kunkel, Franklin, Fudenberg, Edelman: macroglobulins with antibody activity, cold agglutinins, rheumatoid factor
1959	Burnet's[17] clonal selection theory of antibody production
1960	Burnet, Medawar: Nobel Prize for work on acquired immunological tolerance
1960s–70s	Benacerraf and co-workers[62,63]: immune response genes
1961–62	Miller[54], Good et al.[51]: thymus dependence of immune responses
1966–67	Claman et al.[57], Davies et al.[58], Mitchison: T–B cell cooperation
1970	Mitchison, Rajewsky and Taylor[59] describe helper T cells
1970	Gershon and Kondo[60]: suppressor T cell
1973	Fambrough et al.[178], Patrick and Lindstrom[180]: role of decrease of acetylcholine receptors in myasthenia gravis
1974	Jerne[67]: network theory of immune regulation; Nobel Prize, 1984
1975	Cantor and Boyse: T cell subclasses distinguished by their Ly antigens, cell cooperation in the cell-mediated lympholysis (CML) reaction
1975	Köhler and Milstein[70]: monoclonal antibodies from hybridomas; Nobel Prize, 1984
1980	Dausset et al., Benacerraf and Snell: Nobel Prize for immunogenetics research, major histocompatibility complex

Continued...

Table 1 Continued...

Date	Events
1980	Kaplan, Olsson: human hybridomas
1981	Gershon et al.[187]: described contrasuppressor T cells
1982–84	monoclonal antibodies from hybridomas formed from lymphocytes of patients with autoimmune diseases: employed in search for specificity of antigens eliciting autoimmune reactions, e.g. Schwartz and Miller's studies of human hybridomas formed from lymphoid cells of systemic lupus erythematosus (SLE) patients
1986	Mossman et al. T_H1 and T_H2 CD4$^+$ T cells

Examples of significant further advances in autoimmunity in the past two decades include the following[188,189]:

– animal models of autoimmune diseases

– MHC genetics–disease associations

– non-MHC gene associations

– improved understanding of peripheral and central tolerance in autoimmunity

– central versus peripheral deletion

– improved knowledge of clonal deletion and clonal anergy in autoimmunity

– negative selection

– central deletion in the thymus or bone marrow protects against devastating autoimmune phenomena

– physiologic autoimmunity

– the receptor-binding properties of normal T cells and B cells includes the capacity to accommodate epitopes on autoantigens

– improved understanding of regulatory T cells in autoimmunity

– cytokine participation in the pathogenesis of autoimmune diseases

– regulatory and pathogenic cytokines and cytokine networks

– antibodies to multiple epitopes on a single subcellular organelle being involved in a single auto-immune disease

– antigen as the driver of autoimmunity

– advances in therapy of autoimmune diseases

T lymphocytes for other cryptic or subdominant self-determinants of the same antigen during chronic and progressive disease; intermolecular spreading involves epitopes on other unrelated self-antigens. A multideterminant protein antigen has dominant, subdominant and cryptic T cell epitopes. The dominant epitopes are the ones most efficiently processed and presented from native antigen. By contrast, cryptic determinants are inefficiently processed and/or presented. Only by immunization with a peptide that often requires no additional processing can a response to a cryptic determinant be mounted. Subdominant determinants fall between these two types.

Autoimmune diseases have a strong genetic predisposition. Most are polygenic. The inheritance of numerous genetic polymorphisms contributes to disease susceptibility of the autoimmune-associated genes, with those of the major histocompatibility complex (MHC), especially class II MHC genes, exerting the greatest influence. Several genes have been identified in knockout mice and patients that affect the maintenance of tolerance to self-antigens. Viral and bacterial infections may facilitate the development and exacerbation of autoimmunity. Besides susceptibility genes and infections, additional factors related to the development of autimmunity include anatomic alterations in tissues, including inflammation, ischemic injury or trauma, that may lead to the release of sequestered self-antigens not normally in contact with immune system cells. Hormones have a role in some human and experimental autoimmune diseases.

In summary, a failure of self-tolerance may lead to autoimmunity. Infectious, or other environmental stimuli may initiate autoimmunity in genetically susceptible hosts. Most autoimmune diseases are influenced by multiple genes, and many susceptibility genes facilitate development of disease. MHC genes are the major contributors, with other genes influencing the selection of self-reactive lymphocytes and the development of self-tolerance. Mechanisms whereby infections facilitate autoimmunity include enhanced expression of co-stimulators in tissues and cross-reactions between microbial antigens and self-antigens. Contemporary therapy of autoimmune diseases is aimed at keeping the injurious effects of autoimmune reactivity to a minimum. Future treatment will be designed to inhibit specific lymphocyte responsiveness against self-antigens and to induce tolerance in these cells.

Autoimmunity is an immune reactivity involving either antibody-mediated (humoral) or cell-mediated limbs of the immune response against the body's own (self) constituents, i.e. autoantigens. When autoantibodies or autoreactive T lymphocytes interact with self-epitopes, tissue injury may occur, e.g. in rheumatic fever the autoimmune reactivity against heart muscle sacrolemmal membranes occurs as a result of cross-reactivity with antibodies against streptococcal antigens (molecular mimicry). Thus, the immune response can be a two-edged sword, producing both beneficial (protective) effects while also leading to severe injury to host tissues. Reactions of this deleterious nature are referred to as hypersensitivity reactions that are subgrouped into four types.

Abrogation of tolerance to self-antigens often leads to autoimmunity. This may result from altered regulation of lymphocytes reactive with self or in aberrations in self-antigen presentation. Many factors participate in the generation of autoimmunity. Autoimmune reactants may be a consequence, and not a cause, of a disease process. Autoimmune diseases may be organ specific, such as autoimmune thyroiditis, or systemic, such as systemic lupus erythematosus. Different hypersensitivity mechanisms, classified from I to IV, may represent mechanisms by which autoimmune diseases are produced. Thus, antibodies or T cells may be the effector mechanisms mediating tissue injury in autoimmunity. CD4+ helper T cells control the immune response to protein antigens. Therefore, defects in this cell population may lead to high-affinity autoantibody production specific for self-antigens. MHC molecules, which are often linked genetically to the production of autoimmune disease, present peptide antigens to T lymphocytes. Various immunologic alterations may lead to autoimmunity. Experimental evidence supports the concept that autoimmunity may result from a failure of peripheral T lymphocyte tolerance, but little is known about whether or not loss of peripheral B cell tolerance is a contributory factor in autoimmunity. Processes that activate antigen presenting cells in tissues, thereby upregulating their expression of co-stimulators and leading to the formation of cytokines, may abrogate T lymphocyte anergy. The mouse model of human systemic lupus erythematosus involves *lpr/lpr* and *gld/gld* mice that succumb at 6 months of age to profound systemic autoimmune disease with nephritis and autoantibodies. The *lpr/lpr* is associated with a defect in the gene that encodes **Fas**, which determines the molecule that induces cell death. The *gld/gld* is attributable to a point mutation in the **Fas ligand**, which renders the molecule unable to signal. Thus, abnormalities in the Fas and Fas ligand prolong the survival of helper T cells specific for self-antigens since they fail to undergo activation-induced cell death. Thus, this deletion failure mechanism involves peripheral tolerance rather than central tolerance. A decrease of regulatory T cells which synthesize lymphokines that mediate immunosuppression and maintain self-tolerance might lead to autoimmunity, even though no such condition has yet been described.

Autoantigens are normal body constituents recognized by autoantibodies specific for them. T cell receptors may also identify autoantigen (self-antigen) when the immune reactivity has induced a cell-mediated T lymphocyte response.

An **autoantibody** recognizes and interacts with an antigen present as a natural component of the individual synthesizing the autoantibody (Figure 10). The

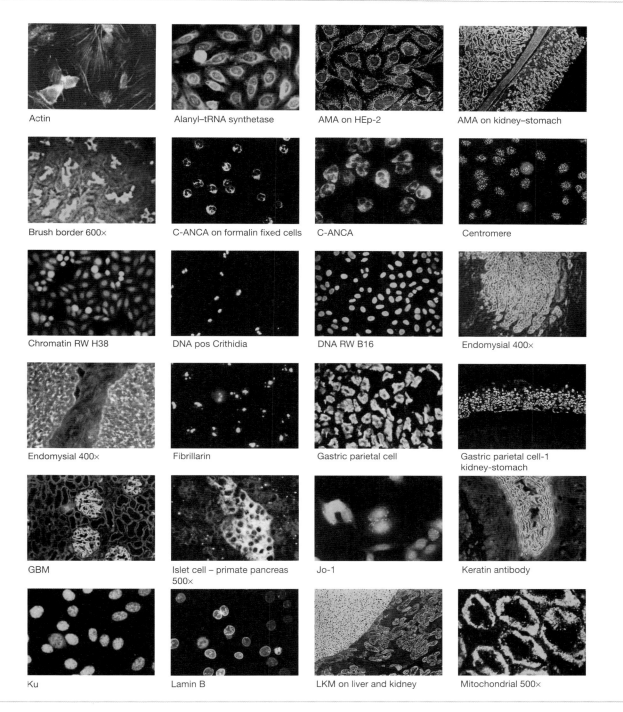

Figure 10 Examples of immunofluorescent stains of antibodies associated with various autoimmune diseases. *Continued overleaf*

ability of these autoantibodies to 'cross-react' with corresponding antigens from other members of the same species provides a method for *in vitro* detection of such autoantibodies. **Autoallergy** is a tissue injury or disease induced by immune reactivity against self-antigens.

Horror autotoxicus (historical) is the term coined by Paul Ehrlich *(circa* 1900) to account for an individual's failure to produce autoantibodies against his own self-constituents, even though they are excellent antigens or immunogens in other species. This lack of immune reactivity against self was believed to

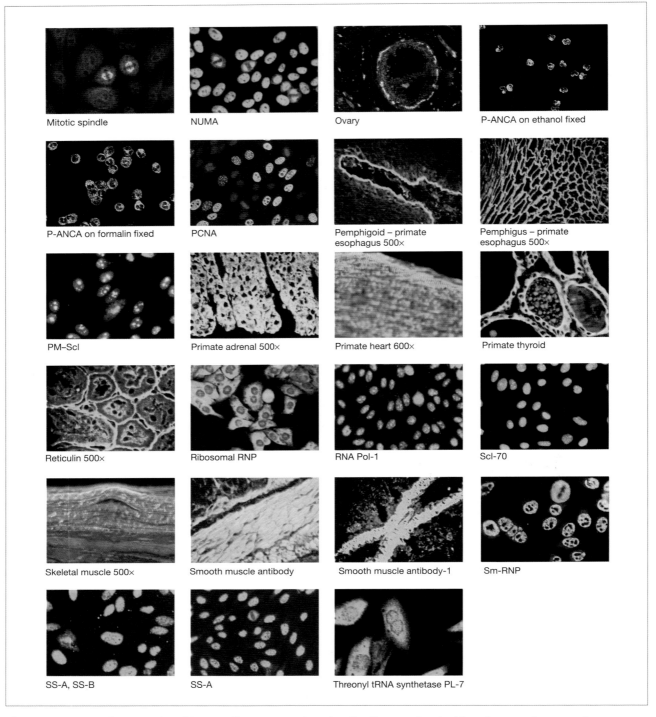

Mitotic spindle

NUMA

Ovary

P-ANCA on ethanol fixed

P-ANCA on formalin fixed

PCNA

Pemphigoid – primate esophagus 500×

Pemphigus – primate esophagus 500×

PM–Scl

Primate adrenal 500×

Primate heart 600×

Primate thyroid

Reticulin 500×

Ribosomal RNP

RNA Pol-1

Scl-70

Skeletal muscle 500×

Smooth muscle antibody

Smooth muscle antibody-1

Sm-RNP

SS-A, SS-B

SS-A

Threonyl tRNA synthetase PL-7

Figure 10 *Continued*   Examples of immunofluorescent stains of antibodies associated with various autoimmune diseases

protect against autoimmune disease. This lack of self-reactivity was postulated to be a fear of poisoning or destroying one's self. Abrogation of horror autotoxicus leads to autoimmune disease. Horror autotoxicus was later (1959) referred to as self-tolerance by F. M. Burnet.

Autoallergy is tissue injury or disease induced by immune reactivity against self-antigens.

Autosensitization is the development of reactivity against one's own antigens, i.e. autoantigens, that occurs in autoimmunity or in autoimmune disease.

Witebsky's criteria According to criteria suggested by Ernest Witebsky, an autoimmune response should be considered as the cause of a human disease if:

(1) It is regularly associated with that disease;

(2) Immunization of an experimental animal with the antigen from the appropriate tissue causes it to make an immune response (form antibodies or develop allergy);

(3) Associated with this response the animal develops pathological changes that are basically similar to those of the human;

(4) The experimental disease can be transferred to a non-immunized animal by serum or by lymphoid cells.

Altered self refers to the concept that the linkage of non-self peptide to MHC yields a peptide–MHC structure different from any found in normal cells of the individual.

An **autoimmune response** is an antibody or T cell immune response to self-antigens.

Autoreactive T lymphocytes in selected diseases may represent a failure of normal regulation, or, autoreactive T cells present in a normal healthy individual may be a necessary aspect of the immune system. Autoreactive T cells develop from mature antigen-dependent precursor cells that have changed physiologically in a manner that restores their thymic selected ability to respond to self. Any mechanism that returns T cells to a resting state would halt autoreactive expansion until stimulation is induced once again by a specific foreign antigen. Chronic stimulation in the presence of continuous expression of high levels of MHC class II molecules together with abnormal immune regulation can lead to severe and persistent inflammation.

Cytokine autoantibodies are autoantibodies that may inhibit cytokine functions and lead to cytokine deficiency. Autoimmune disease may occur and the action of the cytokine may be inhibited. By contrast, these autoantibodies may serve as cytokine-specific carriers in the circulation. For example, insulin autoantibodies may prolong the release of active insulin to the tissues leading to hypoglycemia in non-diabetics and a significant decrease in the exogenous insulin requirement in diabetic patients. Acquired immune deficiency syndrome (AIDS) patients may develop autoantibodies against interleukin-2 (IL-2), and antibodies against tumor necrosis factor-α (TNF-α) have been used successfully to treat rheumatoid arthritis. Both normal and inflammatory disease patients may develop autoantibodies against IL-1α. Cytokine activity is enhanced even in the presence of cytokine autoantibodies *in vivo* by a mechanism that delays rapid catabolism of cytokines from the circulation. The clinical relevance of cytokine autoantibodies *in vivo* remains to be determined. However, these autoantibodies portend a poor prognosis in any disease. Methods for cytokine autoantibody detection include bioassays, immunometric assays and blotting techniques.

Some mechanisms in **drug-induced autoimmunity** are similar to those induced by viruses. Autoantibodies may appear as a result of the helper determinant effect. With some drugs such as hydantoin, the mechanism resembles that of the Epstein–Barr virus (EBV). The generalized lymphoid hyperplasia also involves clones specific for autoantigens. A third form is that seen with α-methyldopa. This drug induces the production of specific antibodies. The drug attaches to cells *in vivo* without changing the surface antigenic makeup. The antibodies, which often have anti-e (Rh series) specificity, combine with the drug on cells, fix complement and induce a bystander type of complement-mediated lysis. Another form of drug-induced autoimmunity is seen with nitrofurantoin, in which the autoimmunity involves cell-mediated phenomena without evidence of autoantibodies.

Natural autoantibodies are polyreactive antibodies of low affinity that are synthesized by CD5$^+$ B cells that constitute 10–25% of circulating B lymphocytes in normal individuals, 27–52% in those with rheumatoid arthritis and less than 25% in systemic lupus erythematosus patients. Natural autoantibodies may appear in first-degree relatives of autoimmune disease patients as well as in older individuals. They may be predictive of disease in healthy subjects. They are often present in patients with bacterial, viral or parasitic infections and may have a protective effect. In contrast to natural antibodies, autoantibodies may increase in disease and may lead to tissue injury. The blood group isohemagglutins are also termed natural antibodies, even though they are believed to be of heterogenetic immune origin as a consequence of stimulation by microbial antigens.

Pathologic autoantibodies are autoantibodies generated against self antigens that induce cell and tissue injury following interaction with the cells bearing epitopes for which they are specific. Many autoantibodies are physiologic, representing an epiphenomenon during autoimmune stimulation, whereas others contribute to the pathogenesis of tissue injury. Autoantibodies that lead to red blood cell destruction in autoimmune hemolytic anemia represent pathogenic autoantibodies, whereas rheumatoid factors such as IgM anti-IgG autoantibodies have no proven pathogenic role in rheumatoid arthritis.

Sequestered antigen is anatomically isolated and not in contact with the immunocompetent T and B lymphoid cells of the immune system. Examples include myelin basic protein, sperm antigens and lens protein antigens. When a sequestered antigen such as myelin basic protein is released by one or several mechanisms including viral inflammation, it can activate both immunocompetent T and B cells. An example of the sequestered antigen release mechanism of autoimmunity is found in experimental and postinfectious encephalomyelitis. Cell-mediated injury represents the principal mechanism in experimental and postviral encephalitis. In vasectomized males, antisperm antibodies are known to develop when sperm antigens become exposed to immunocompetent lymphoid cells. Likewise, lens protein of the eye that enters the circulation as a consequence of either crushing injury to an eye or exposure of lens protein to immunocompetent cells inadvertently through surgical manipulation may lead to an antilens protein immune response. Autoimmunity induced by sequestered antigens is relatively infrequent, and is a relatively rare cause of autoimmune disease.

Sex hormones and immunity Females have been recognized as more susceptible to certain autoimmune diseases than males, which immediately led to suspicion that sex hormones might play a role. The exact mechanisms through which sex steroids interact with the immune system remain to be determined, but it is known that these hormones have a direct effect on immune system cells or indirectly through cells that control growth and development of the immune system or through organs that are ultimately destroyed by autoimmune reactions. Female mice synthesize more antibody in response to certain antigens than do males, but humans injected with vaccines show essentially identical antibody responses regardless of sex. Murine cell-mediated responses to selected antigens were stronger in females than in males. Sex steroids have a profound effect on the thymus. Androgen or estrogen administration to experimental animals led to thymic involution, whereas castration led to thymic enlargement. The thymus is markedly involuted during pregnancy, and achieves its normal size and shape following parturition. Sex steroids have numerous targets that include the bone marrow and thymus where the precursors of immunity originate and differentiate. Further studies have investigated how sex hormones control cytokine genes. Thus, sex steroid hormones affect the development and function of various immune system cells.

In an **autoimmune disease**, pathogenic consequences, including tissue injury, may be produced by autoantibodies or autoreactive T lymphocytes interacting with self epitopes, i.e. autoantigens. The mere presence of autoantibodies or autoreactive T lymphocytes does not prove that there is any cause and effect relationship between these components and a patient's disease. To show that autoimmune phenomena are involved in the etiology and pathogenesis of human disease, Witebsky suggested that certain criteria be fulfilled (see Witebsky's criteria). In addition to autoimmune reactivity against self constituents, tissue injury in the presence of immunocompetent cells corresponding to the tissue distribution of the autoantigen, duplication of the disease features in experimental animals injected with the appropriate autoantigen and passive transfer with either autoantibody or autoreactive T lymphocytes to normal animals offer evidence in support of an autoimmune pathogenesis of a disease. Individual autoimmune diseases are discussed under their own headings, such as systemic lupus erythematosus, autoimmune thyroiditis, etc. Autoimmune diseases may be either **organ specific**, such as thyroiditis and diabetes, or **systemic**, such as systemic lupus erythematosus.

Autoimmune disease animal models Studies of human autoimmune disease have always been confronted with the question of whether immune phenomena, including the production of autoantibodies, represent the cause or a consequence of the disease. The use of animal models has helped to answer many of these questions. By using the rat, mouse, guinea-pig, rabbit, monkey, chicken or dog, among other species, many of these questions have been answered. A broad spectrum of human autoimmune diseases has been clarified through the use of animal models that differ in detail but have nevertheless provided insight into pathogenic mechanisms, converging pathways and disturbances of normal regulatory function related to the development of autoimmunity.

REFERENCES

1. Ehrlich P, Morgenroth J. Über Hämolysine. 3. Mitteilung. *Berl Klin Wschr* 1900;37:453

2. Ehrlich P, Morgenroth J. Über Hämolysine. 3. Mitteilung. *Berl Klin Wschr*, 1901. In Himmelweit. ed. *Collected Papers of Paul Ehrlich*. Oxford: Pergamon Press, 1957;2:205

3. Ehrlich P, Morgenroth J. Über Hämolysine 3. Mitteilung. *Berl Klin Wschr*, 1901. (In Himmelweit, ed, *Collected Papers of Paul Ehrlich*. Oxford: Pergamon Press, 1957;2:246

4. Adams DD. Autoimmune mechanisms. In Davies AJD, ed. *Autoimmune Endocrine Disease*. New York: Wiley & Sons, 1982:1–39

5. Vries H. de: *Die Mutationstheorie. Versuche und Beobachtungen über die Entstehung von Arten im Pflanzenreich*. Leipzig: Veit, 1901–3

6. Donath J, Landsteiner K. Über paroxysmale Hämoglobinurie. *Münch Med Wschr* 1904;51:1590–3

7. von Wassermann A, Neisser A, Bruck C. Eine serclodiagnostische Reaktion bei Syphilis. *DT Med Wschr* 1906;32:745

8. Glynn LE, Holborow EJ. *Autoimmunity and Disease*. London: Clowes & Sons, 1965

9. Kunkel HG, Tan EM. Autoantibodies and disease. *Adv Immunol* 1964;4:351

10. Lachmann PJ. Auto-allergy. In Gell PGH, Coombs RRA, Lachmann PJ, eds. *Clinical Aspects of Immunology*. Oxford: Blackwell, 1975

11. Mackay IR, Masel M, Burnet FM. Thymic abnormality in systemic lupus erythematosus. *Australas Ann Med* 1964;13:5

12. Miescher PA, Dayer JM. Autoimmune hemolytic anemias. In Miescher PA, Müller-Eberhard HJ, eds. *Textbook of Immunopathology*, 2nd edn. New York: Grune & Stratton, 1976:649–61

13. Spry CJ. Autoallergic diseases. In Hobard MJ, McConnell I, eds. *The Immune System*. Oxford: Blackwell, 1975:287

14. Talal N, Fye K, Moutsopoulos H. Autoimmunity. In: Fundenberg HH, Stites DP, Caldwell JL, *et al.*, eds. *Basic and Clinical Immunology*. Los Altos: Lange, 1976:151

15. Vaughan JH. Autoallergic diseases: concepts and general considerations. In Samter M, Talmage DW, Rose NR, eds. *Immunological Diseases*. Boston: Little, Brown, 1972:87

16. Witebsky E. The question of self-recognition by the host and problems of autoantibodies and their specificity. *Cancer Res* 1961;21:1216

17. Burnet FM. *The Clonal Selection Theory of Acquired Immunity*. Nashville: Vanderbilt University Press, 1959

18. Burnet FM. Autoimmune disease as a breakdown in immunological homeostasis. In *Cellular Immunology*. Cambridge: Cambridge University Press, 1970:255

19. Burnet FM, Fenner F. *The Production of Antibodies*, 2nd edn. London: Macmillan, 1949

20. Mechnikov II. *Immunity in Infective Diseases* (transl from the French by Binnie FG). London: Cambridge University Press, 1907:101–4

21. Metalnikoff S. Etudes sur la Spermatoxine. *Ann Inst Pasteur (Paris)* 1900;14:577

22. Elschnig A. Die antigene Wirkung des Augenpigmentes. *Graefes Arch Ophthal* 1910;76:509

23. Silverstein AM. History of immunology. In Paul WE, ed. *Fundamental Immunology*. New York: Raven Press, 1984

24. Verhaff FH, Memoine AN. Endophthalmitis phacoanaphylactica. *Trans Int Cong Ophthalmol (Washington)* 1922;1:234

25. Freund J. The effect of paraffin oil and mycobacteria on antibody formation and sensitization. *Am J Clin Pathol* 1951;21:645

26. Freund J, Lipton MM, Thompson GE. Aspermatogenesis in the guinea pig induced by a single injection of homologous testicular material, paraffin oil, and killed mycobacteria. *Bull NY Acad Med* 1953;24:739

27. Freund J, Lipton MM, Thompson GE. Aspermatogenesis in the guinea pig induced by testicular tissue and adjuvants. *J Exp Med* 1953;97:711

28. Freund J, Lipton MM, Thompson GE. Impairment of spermatogenesis in the rat after cutaneous injection of testicular suspension with complete adjuvants. *Proc Soc Exp Biol Med* 1954;87:408

29. Freund J, McDermott K. Sensitization to horse serum by means of adjuvants. *Proc Soc Exp Biol Med* 1942;49:548–53

30. Freund J, Thompson KJ, Somer HE, Pisani TM. Antibody formation and sensitization with the aid of adjuvants. *J Immunol* 1948;60:383

31. Voisin G, Delaunay A, Barber M. Lésions testiculaires provoquées chez le cobaye par injection d'extraits de testicules homologues. *C R Hebd Séanc Acad Sci (Paris)* 1951;232:1264–6

32. Witebsky E, Rose NR, Terplan K, *et al.* Chronic thyroiditis and autoimmunization. *J Am Med Assoc* 1957;164:1439–47

33. Witebsky E. Historical roots of present concepts of immunopathology. In Grabar P, Miescher PA, eds. *Immunopathology. 1st Int Symp.* Basel: Schwabe, 1959:9–10

34. Boyden S. Pathology. Autoimmunity and inflammation. *Nature (London)* 1964;201:200

35. Grabar P. Hypothesis. Autoantibodies and immunologic theories: an analytical review. *Clin Immunol Immunopathol* 1975;4:453–66

36. Kay MMB, Makinodan T. Immunobiology of aging: evaluation of current status. *Clin Immunol Immunopathol* 1976;6:394

37. Beutner EH, Chorzelski TP, Binder WL. Nature of autoimmunity: pathologic versus physiologic responses and a unifying concept. In Beutner EH, Chorzelski TP, Bean, eds. *Immunopathology of the Skin.* New York: Wiley & Sons, 1979:147–80

38. Smith HR, Steinberg AD. Autoimmunity – a perspective. *Annu Rev Immunol* 1983;1:175–210

39. Medawar PB. The behavior and fate of skin autografts and skin homografts in rabbits. *J Anat* 1944;78:176–99

40. Owen RD. Immunogenetic consequences of vascular anastomoses between bovine twins. *Science* 1945;102:400–1

41. Burnet FM. A modification of Jerne's theory of antibody production using the concept of clonal selection. *Aust J Sci* 1957;20:67

42. Jerne NK. The natural-selection theory of antibody formation. *Proc Natl Acad Sci USA* 1955;41:849–57

43. Talmage DW. Allergy and immunology. *Annu Rev Med* 1957;8:239

44. Nossal GBJ. *Antigens, Lymphoid Cells and the Immune Response.* New York: Academic Press, 1971

45. Nossal GJV, Pike BL. Clonal anergy: persistence in tolerant mice of antigen-binding B lymphocytes incapable of responding to antigen or mitogen. *Proc Natl Acad Sci USA* 1980;77:1602

46. Green I, Vassali P, Nussenzweig V, Benacerraf B. Specificity of the antibodies produced by single cells following immunization with antigens bearing two types of antigenic determinants. *J Exp Med* 1967;125:511

47. Fagraeus A. Antibody production in relation to the development of plasma cells: *in vivo* and *in vitro* experiments. *Acta Med Scand* 1948;130(Suppl):3

48. Coons AH, *et al.* The demonstration of pneumococcal antigen in tissues by the use of fluorescent antibody. *J Immunol* 1942;45:159–80

49. Coons AH, Kaplan MH. Localization of antigen in tissue cells. *J Exp Med* 1950;91:1

50. Glick B, Chang TS, Jaap RG. The bursa of Fabricius and antibody formation production. *Poult Sci* 1956;35:224

51. Good RA, Dalmasso AO, Martinez C, *et al.* The role of the thymus in development of immunologic capacity of rabbits and mice. *J Exp Med* 1962;116:773–96

52. Archer O, Pierce JC. Role of thymus in development of the immune response. *Fed Proc* 1961;20:26

53. Archer OK, Pierce JC, Papermaster BW, Good RA. Reduced antibody response in thymectomized rabbits. *Nature (London)* 1962;195:191–3

54. Miller JFAP. Immunological function of the thymus. *Lancet* 1961;2:748–9

55. Gowans JL. The recirculation of lymphocytes from blood to lymph in the rat. *J Physiol (London)* 1959;146:54–69

56. Harris TN, Hummeler K, Harris S. Electron microscope observations on antibody producing lymph node cells. *J Exp Med* 1966;123:161–72

57. Claman HN, Chaperon EA, Triplett RR. Thymus–marrow cell combinations. Synergism in antibody production. *Proc Soc Exp Biol Med* 1966;122:1167

58. Davies AJS, *et al.* The failure of thymus-derived cells to produce antibody. *Transplantation* 1967;5:222

59. Mitchison NA, Rajewsky K, Taylor RB. Cooperation of antigenic determinants of cells in the induction of antibodies. In Sterzl J, Riha I, eds. *Developmental Aspects of Antibody Formation and Structure.* Prague: Academia, 1970;2:547–61

60. Gershon RK, Kondo K. Cell interactions in the induction of tolerance: the role of thymic lymphocytes. *Immunology* 1970;18:723–37

61. Gershon RK, Kondo K. Antigenic competition between heterologous erythrocytes. I. Thymic dependency. II. Effect of passive antibody administration. *J Immunol* 1971;106:1524–39

62. Benacerraf B, *et al.* Immune response genes of the major histocompatibility complex. *Immunol Rev* 1978;38:70–119

63. Benacerraf B, McDevitt HO. Histocompatibility-linked immune response genes. *Science* 1972;175:273–9

64. McDevitt HO, Chinitz A. Genetic control of the antibody response: relationship between immune response and histocompatibility (H-2) type. *Science* 1969;163:1207–8

65. Rose NR, Bigazzi PE, Warner NL. *Genetic Control of Autoimmune Disease.* New York: Elsevier/North-Holland, 1978

66. Vaughan JH. Autoimmune and histocompatibility (HLA)-associated diseases: general considerations. In Samter M, ed. *Immunological Diseases*, 3rd edn. Boston: Little, Brown, 1978;2:1029–37

67. Jerne NK. Towards a network theory of the immune system. *Ann Immunol (Paris)* 1974;125C:373

68. Tonegawa S, *et al*. Organization of immunoglobulin genes. *Cold Spring Harbor Symp Quant Biol* 1977;42:921–31

69. Leder P, *et al*. The cloning of mouse globulin and surrounding gene sequences in bacteriophage lambda. *Cold Spring Harbor Symp Quant Biol* 1977;42:915–20

70. Köhler G, Milstein C. Continuous cultures of fused cells secreting antibody of predefined specificity. *Nature (London)* 1975;256:495–7

71. Landsteiner K. *The Specificity of Serological Reactions*. New York: Dover Press, 1962:102

72. Widal F, Abrami P, Burle M. Les ictères d'origine hémolytique. *Arch Mal Cœur* 1908;1:193–231

73. Chauffard MA, Vincent C. Hémoglobinurie hémolysinique avec ictère polycholique aigu. *Sem Méd (Paris)* 1909;29:601

74. Chauffard MA. Pathogène de l'ictère congénital de l'adulte. *Sem Méd (Paris)* 1907;27:25–9

75. Dameshek W, Schwartz SO. Presence of hemolysins in acute hemolytic anemia, preliminary note. *N Engl J Med* 1938;218:75–80

76. Dameshek W, Schwartz SO, Gross S. Haemolysins as the cause of clinical and experimental haemolytic anaemias. With particular reference to the nature of spherocytosis and increased fragility. *Am J Med Sci* 1938;196:769

77. Coombs RRA, Mourant AE, Race RR. A new test for the detection of weak and 'incomplete' Rh agglutinins. *Br J Exp Pathol* 1945;6:255–66

78. Dacie JV. *Practical Haematology*, 2nd edn. London, Churchill, 1956:124

79. Dacie JV. *The Haemolytic Anaemias, Congenital and Acquired. II. The Autoimmune Anaemias*. London: Churchill, 1962

80. Coombs RRA. History and evaluation of the antiglobulin reaction and its application in clinical and experimental medicine. *Am J Clin Pathol* 1970;53:131–5

81. Morton JA, Pickles MM. Use of trypsin in detection of incomplete antiRh antibodies. *Nature (London)* 1947;159:779

82. Kidd P. Elution of an incomplete type of antibody from the erythrocytes in acquired haemolytic anaemia. *J Clin Pathol* 1949;2:103

83. Wiener W. Eluting red cell antibodies; a method and its application. *Br J Haematol* 1957;3:276

84. Mollison PL. *Blood Transfusion in Clinical Medicine*, 2nd edn. Oxford: Blackwell, 1956

85. Ackroyd JF. The cause of thrombocytopenia in sedormid purpura. *Clin Sci* 1949;8:269

86. Dixon RJ, Vasquez JJ, Weigle WO, Cochrane CG. Pathogenesis of serum sickness. *Arch Pathol* 1958;65:18

87. Cochrane CG. A role of polymorphonuclear leukocytes in nephrotoxic nephritis. *J Exp Med* 1965;122:99–116

88. Coombs RRA, Gell PGH. Classification of allergic reactions responsible for clinical hypersensitivity and disease. In Gell PGH, Coombs RRA, eds. *Clinical Aspects of Immunology*. Oxford: Blackwell, 1975:761

89. Kaposi MK. Neue Beiträge zur Kenntnis des Lupus erythematosus. *Arch Derm Syph* 1872;4:36–78

90. Osler W. On the visceral complications of erythema exudativum multiforme. *Am J Med Sci* 1895;110:629

91. Gross L. The heart in atypical verrucous endocarditis (Libman–Sacks). In *Contributions to the medical sciences in honor of Dr Emanual Libman by his pupils, friends and colleagues*, New York: International Press, 1932;2:527–50

92. Klemperer P. Concept of collagen disease. *Am J Pathol* 1950;26:505–19

93. Hargreaves MD, Richmond H, Morton R. Presentation of two bone marrow elements; 'tart' cell and 'L.E. cell'. *Proc Staff Meet Mayo Clin* 1948;23:25–8

94. Miescher P. Immune-nucléo-phagocytose expérimentale et phénomène L.E. *Exp Med Surg* 1953;11:173–9; Nucléophagocytose et phénomène L.E. *Schweiz Med Wschr* 1953;83:1042–3

95. Friou GJ. Clinical application of lupus serum–nucleoprotein reaction using fluorescent antibody technique. *J Clin Invest* 1957;36:890

96. Farr RS. A quantitative immunochemical measure of the primary interaction between I*BSA and antibody. *J Infect Dis* 1958;103:239–62

97. Tan EM, Kunkel HG. Characteristics of a soluble nuclear antigen precipitating with sera of patients with systemic lupus erythematosus. *J Immunol* 1966;96:464–71

98. Miller KB, Schwartz RS. Familial abnormalities of suppressor cell function in systemic lupus erythematosus. *N Engl J Med* 1979;301:803–2

99. Meyer K. Über Hämagglutininvermehrung und hämagglutinationsfördernde Wirkung bei menschlichen Seren. *Z Immun Forsch* 1922;34:229

100. Waaler E. On the occurrence of a factor in human serum activating the specific agglutination of sheep blood corpuscles. *Acta Pathol Microbiol Scand* 1940;17:172

101. Rose HM, Ragan C, Pearce F, Lipman MD. Differential agglutination of normal and sensitized sheep erythrocytes by sera of patients with rheumatoid arthritis. *Proc Soc Exp Biol Med* 1948;68:1

102. Dean HR. On the factors concerned in agglutination. *Proc R Soc* 1912;98:416

103. Franklin EC. The interaction of rheumatoid factor and γ-globulins. *Minerva Med* 1961;2:804

104. Franklin EC, Holman HR, Muller-Eberhard HJ, Kunkel HG. An unusual protein component of high molecular weight in the serum of certain patients with rheumatoid arthritis. *J Exp Med* 1957;103:425

105. Franklin EC, Kunkel HG, Muller-Eberhard HJ, Holman HR. Relation of high molecular weight proteins to the

serological reactions in rheumatoid arthritis. *Ann Rheum Dis* 1957;16:315

106. Epstein W, Johnson A, Ragan C. Observations on a precipitin reaction between serum of patients with rheumatoid arthritis and a preparation (Cohn fraction II) of human gamma globulin. *Proc Soc Exp Biol Med* 1956;91:235

107. Milgrom F, Witebsky E. Rabbit antibodies against γ-globulins resembling the rheumatoid factor. *Fed Proc* 1960;19:197

108. Kunkel HG, Ward JR. Clinical and laboratory findings in seven patients with rheumatoid arthritis with large amounts of high molecular weight rheumatoid factor complex. *Arthritis Rheum* 1959;2:95

109. Fudenberg HH, Franklin FC. Rheumatoid factors and the etiology of rheumatoid arthritis. *Ann NY Acad Sci* 1965;124:884

110. Fudenberg H, Kunkel HG. Specificity of the reaction between rheumatoid factor and γ-globulin. *J Exp Med* 1961;114:257

111. Fudenberg HH, Stiehm ER, Franklin EC, *et al*. Antigenicity of hereditary human γ-globulin (Gm) factors – biological and biochemical aspects. *Cold Spring Harbor Symp Quant Biol* 1964;29:463

112. Edelman GM, Kunkel HG, Franklin EC. Interaction of the rheumatoid factor with antigen-antibody complexes and aggregated γ-globulin. *J Exp Med* 1958;108:105

113. Waller M. Present status of the theumatoid factor. *CRC Crit Rev Clin Lab Sci* 1971;2:173–209

114. Cecil RL, Hicholls EF, Stainsby WJ. Rheumatoid arthritis. *Am J Med Sci* 1931;191:12

115. Sjögren H. A new conception of keratoconjunctivitis sicca (transl by Hamilton JB). Sydney: Australasian Medical Publishing, 1943

116. Anderson JR, Gray KG, Beck JS, Kinnear WF. Precipitating auto-antibodies in Sjögren's disease. *Lancet* 1961;2:456

117. Oswald A. Die Eiweisskörper der Schilddrüsen. *Hoppe-Seyler's Z Physiol Chem* 1899;27:14

118. Hektoen L, Schulhof K. The preciptin reaction of thyroglobulin. *Proc Natl Acad Sci USA* 1925;11:481

119. Hektoen L, Fox H, Schulhof K. Specificness in the precipitin reaction of thyroglobulin. *J Infect Dis* 1927;40:641

120. Witebsky E, Rose NR, Shulman S. The autoantibody nature of the thyroiditis antibody and the role of thyroglobulin in the reaction. *Lancet* 1958;1:808–9

121. Uhlenhuth P. *Zur Lehre von der Unterscheidung verschiedener Eiweissenarten mit Hilfe spezifischer Sera.* Jena: Fischer, 1903.

122. Witebsky E, Steinfeld J. Untersuchungen über spezifische Antigenfunktionen von Organen. *Z ImmunForsch* 1928;58:3–4

123. Lerman J. Endocrine action of thyroid antibodies. *Endocrinology* 1942;31:558

124. Witebsky E, Rose NR. Studies on organ specificity. IV. Production of rabbit thyroid antibodies in the rabbit. *J Immunol* 1956;76:408–16

125. Rose NR, Witebsky E. Studies on organ specificity. V. Changes in thyroid glands of rabbits following active immunization with rabbit thyroid extracts. *J Immunol* 1956;76:417–27

126. Rose NR, Witebsky E. Experimental autoimmune thyroiditis. In Miescher PA, Müller-Eberhard HJ, eds. *Textbook of Immunopathology.* New York: Grune & Stratton, 1968:150–63

127. Rabin BS. Autoimmune thyroiditis: historical aspects and laboratory diagnosis. *Va Med* 1970;97:37–42

128. Witebsky E. Experimental evidence for the role of autoimmunization in chronic thyroiditis. *Proc R Soc Med* 1957;50:955–8

129. Witebsky E, Rose NR. Studies on organ specificity. IV. Production of rabbit thyroid antibodies in the rabbit. *J Immunol* 1956;76:408–16

130. Witebsky E, Rose NR, Paine JR, Egan RW. Thyroid-specific autoantibodies. *Ann NY Acad Sci* 1957;69:660–77

131. Beutner EH, Witebsky E, Rose NR, Gerbasi JR. Localization of thyroid and spinal cord autoantibodies by the fluorescent antibody technique. *Proc Soc Exp Biol Med* 1958;97:712

132. Campbell PN, Doniach D, Hudson RV, Roitt IM. Autoantibodies in Hashimoto's disease (lymphadenoid goitre) preliminary communication. *Lancet* 1956;271:820–1

133. Gepts W. Morphological pathology of the islets of Langerhans in juvenile diabetes. In *Etiology and Pathogenesis of Insulin-Dependent Diabetes Mellitus.* New York: Raven Press, 1981:1–12

134. Gepts W, Le Compte PM. The pancreatic islets in diabetes. *Am J Med* 1981;70:105–15

135. Orci L, *et al*. Hypertrophy and hyperplasia of somatostatin-containing D cells in diabetes. *Proc Natl Acad Sci USA* 1973;73:1338–42

136. Huang SW, Maclaren NK. Insulin-dependent diabetes: a disease of autoaggression. *Science* 1976;192:64–6

137. Mackay IR, Burnet FM. *Autoimmune Diseases: Pathogenesis, Chemistry and Therapy.* Springfield, Thomas: 1963

138. Nerup J, Anderson OO, Bendixen G, *et al*. Antipancreatic cellular hypersensitivity in diabetes mellitus. *Diabetes* 1971;20:424–7

139. Bottazzo GF, Florin-Christensen A, Doniach D. Islet-cell antibodies in diabetes mellitus with autoimmune polyendocrine deficiencies. *Lancet* 1974;2:1279–82

140. Lernmark A, *et al*. Islet-cell-surface antibodies in juvenile diabetes mellitus. *N Engl J Med* 1978;299:375–80

141. Gepts W. Pathologic anatomy of the pancreas in juveinile diabetes mellitus. *Diabetes* 1965;14:619–33

142. LeCompte PM. 'Insulitis' in early juvenile diabetes. *Arch Pathol* 1958;66:450–7

143. Eisenbarth G, Jackson R. Immunogenetics of polyglandular failure and related disease. In Farid, ed. *HLA in Endocrine and Metabolic Disorders*. New York: Academic Press, 1981:

144. Eisenbarth GS, Wilson PW, Ward F, *et al*. The polyglandular failure syndrome: disease inheritance, HLA type, and immune function. *Ann Intern Med* 1978;91:528–33

145. MacCuish AC, *et al*. Cell-mediated immunity to human pancreas in diabetes mellitus. *Diabetes* 1975;23:693–7

146. Buschard K, Madsbad S, Rygaard J. Passive transfer of diabetes mellitus from man to mouse. *Lancet* 1978;1:908–10

147. Doniach D, Bottazzo, GF, Drexhage HA. The autoimmune endocrinopathies. In Lachmann PJ, Peters, eds. *Clinical Aspects of Immunology*, 4th edn. Oxford: Blackwell, 1982:903–37

148. Milgrom F, Witebsky E. Immunologic studies on adrenal glands. I. Immunization with adrenals of foreign species. *Immunology* 1962;5:46

149. Witebsky E, Milgrom F. Immunological studies on adrenal glands. II. Immunization with adrenals of the same species. *Immunology* 1962;5:67

150. Blizzard RM, Chee D, David W. The incidence of parathyroid and other antibodies in the sera of patients with idiopathic adrenal insufficiency (Addison's disease). *Clin Exp Immunol* 1966;2:19

151. Taylor KB, Morton JA. An antibody to Castle's intrinsic factor. *Lancet* 1958;1:29

152. Schwartz M. Intrinsic factor antibody in serum from patients with pernicious anaemia. *Lancet* 1960;2:1263

153. Tudhope GR, Wilson GM. Anaemia in hypothyroidism. *Q J Med* 1960;29:513

154. Mackay IR, Whittingham S. The saga of pernicious anemia. *NZ Med J* 1968;67:391–6

155. Irvine WJ, Davies SH, Delamore IW, Williams AW. Immunological relationship between pernicious anaemia and thyroid disease. *Br Med J* 1962;2:454

156. Roitt IM, Doniach D, Shapland C. Intrinsic-factor antibodies. *Lancet* 1964;2:469

157. Fiessinger N. Histogenèse des processus de cirrhose hépatique. Lésion parenchymateuse et cirrhose. In Maloine, ed. *Etude Histologique Expérimentale et Pathologique*. Paris: Thesis, 1908.

158. Paronetto F, Popper H. Hetero-, iso-, and autoimmune phenomena in the liver. In Miescher PA, Müller-Eberhard HJ, eds. *Textbook of Immunopathology*, 2nd edn. New York: Grune & Stratton, 1976:789–817

159. Joske RA, King WE. The L.E. cell phenomenon in active chronic viral hepatitis. *Lancet* 1955;2:477

160. Mackay IR, Taft LI, Cowling DC. Lupoid hepatitis. *Lancet* 1956;2:1323

161. Mackay IR, Larkin L. The significance of the presence in human serum of complement-fixing antibodies to human tissue antigens. *Australas Ann Med* 1958;7:251

162. Holborow EJ, Asherman GL, Johnson GD, *et al*. Antinuclear factor and other antibodies in blood and liver diseases. *Br Med J* 1963;1:656

163. Johnson SD, Holborow EJ, Glynn IE. Antibody to smooth muscle in patients with liver disease. *Lancet* 1965;2:878

164. Walker JG, Doniach D, Roitt IM, Sherlock S. Serological tests in diagnosis of primary biliary cirrhosis. *Lancet* 1965;1:827

165. Soborg M, Bendixen G. Human leucocyte migration as a parameter of hypersensitivity. *Acta Med Scand* 1967;191:247

166. Miller J, *et al*. Cell-mediated immunity to a human liver-specific antigen in patients with active chronic hepatitis with primary biliary cirrhosis. *Lancet* 1972;2:296

167. Bacon PA, Berry H, Brown R. Cell-mediated immune reactivity in liver disease. *Gut* 1972;13:427

168. Paterson, PY. Autoimmune neurological disease: experimental animal systems and implications for multiple sclerosis. In Talal N, ed. *Autoimmunity*. New York: Academic Press, 1977:643–92

169. Rivers TM, Sprunt DH, Berry GP. Observations on attempt to produce acute disseminated encephalomyelitis in monkeys. *J Exp Med* 1933;58:39–53

170. Rivers TM, Schwentker FF. Encephalomyelitis accompanied by myelin destruction experimentally produced in monkeys. *J Exp Med* 1935;61:689

171. Kabat EA, Wolf A, Bezer AE. Rapid production of acute disseminated encephalomyelitis in rhesus monkey by injection of heterologous and homologous brain tissue with adjuvants. *J Exp Med* 1947;85:117–30

172. Kabat EA, Wolf A, Bezer AE. Studies on acute disseminated encephalomyelitis produced experimentally in rhesus monkeys; disseminated encephalomyelitis produced in monkey with their own brain tissue. *J Exp Med* 1949;89:395–8

173. Kabat EA, Wolf A, Bezer AE, Murray JP. Studies on acute disseminated encephalomyelitis produced experimentally in Rhesus monkeys. VI. Changes in cerebrospinal fluid proteins. *J Exp Med* 1951;93:615–33

174. Morgan IM. Allergic encephalomyelitis in monkeys in response to injection of normal monkey nervous tissue. *J Exp Med* 1947;85:131–40

175. Waksman BH, Adams RD. A histologic study of the early lesion in experimental allergic encephalomyelitis in the guinea pig and rabbit. *Am J Pathol* 1962;41:135

176. Willis T. *The London Practice of Physick*. London: Basset & Crooke, 1685

177. Laquer L, Weigert C. Beiträge zur Lehre von der Erb'schen Krankheit. 2. Pathologisch-anatomischer Beiträge zur Erb'schen Krankheit (myasthenia gravis). *Neurol Zentbl* 1901;20:594–601

178. Fambrough DM, Drachman DB, Sathamurti S. Neuromuscular junction in myasthenia gravis; decreased acetylcholine receptors. *Science* 1973;182:293–5

179. Ito Y, *et al*. Acetylcholine receptors and end-plate electro-physiology in myasthenia gravis. *Brain* 1978;10:345–68

180. Patrick J, Lindstrom J. Autoimmune response to acetyl-choline receptor. *Science* 1973;180:871–2

181. Pinching AJ, Peters DK, Newsom DJ. Remission of myasthenia gravis following plasma exchange. *Lancet* 1976;2:1373–5

182. Bertstrom K, *et al*. The effect of thoracic duct lymph drainage in myasthenia gravis. *Eur Neurol* 1973;9:157–67

183. Beutner EH, Jordon RE. Demonstration of skin antibodies in sera of pemphigus vulgaris patients by indirect immunofluorescent staining. *Proc Soc Exp Biol Med* 1964;117:505–10

184. Chorzelski TP, Von Weiss JF, Lever WF. Clinical significance of autoantibodies in pemphigus. *Arch Derm* 1966;93:570–6

185. Jordan RE, Triftshauser CT, Schroeter AL. Direct immunofluorescent studies of pemphigus and bullous pemphigoid. *Arch Dermatol* 1971;103:486–91

186. Beutner EH, Lever WF, Witebsky E, *et al*. Autoantibodies in pemphigus vulgaris: response to an intercellular substance of epidermis. *J Am Med Assoc* 1965;192:682–8

187. Gershon RK, *et al*. Contrasuppression, a novel immunoregulatory activity. *J Exp Med* 1981;153:1533–46

188. Lahita RG, ed. *Textbook of the Autoimmune Diseases*. Philadelphia, PA: Lippincott Williams and Wilkins, 2000

189. Rose NR, Mackay IR, eds. *The Autoimmune Diseases*, 3rd edn. San Diego, CA: Academic Press, 1998

CHAPTER 10

Immunohematology

Immunohematology is the study of blood group antigens and antibodies and their interactions in health and disease. Both the cellular elements and serum constituents of the blood have distinct profiles of antigens. There are multiple systems of blood cell groups, all of which may stimulate antibodies and interact with them. These may be associated with erythrocytes, leukocytes or platelets.

Another dream in early times was the possibility of performing blood transfusions (Figure 1). A well-documented early attempt was the effort to rejuvenate Pope Innocent VIII in 1492 with the blood of three young men, which ended disastrously for all four. Several Italians in the early part of the 1600s claimed that they had performed transfusions. Harvey's work on the circulation of the blood paved the way for a better

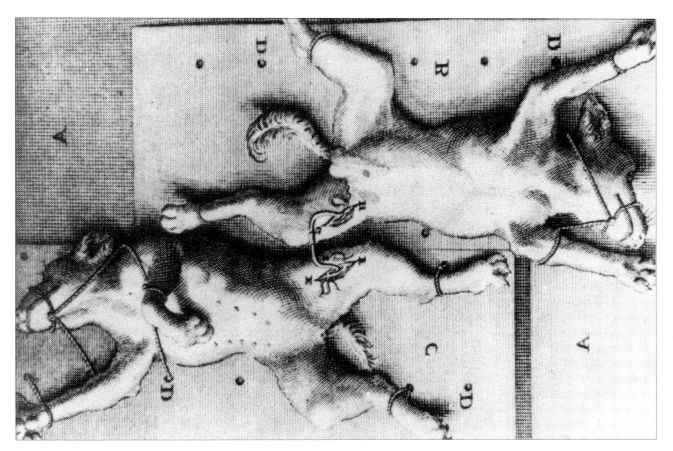

Figure 1 Early blood transfusions in dogs

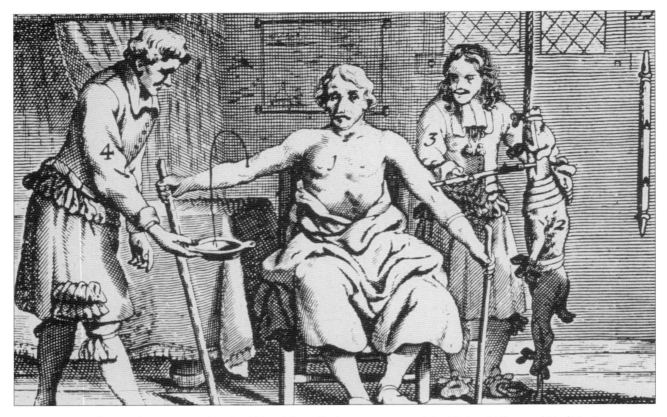

Figure 2   Transfusion of a patient with animal blood (from Scultatus, courtesy of the National Library of Medicine)

understanding of the flow of blood in the body. Robert Boyle published a proposal in the *Philosophical Transactions* in 1667 for Richard Lower to experiment with transferring blood from one living animal to another, at Gresham College (Figures 2 and 3). In the same year at Montpellier, in southern France, a professor of philosophy, Jean Denis, began a series of transfusions of animal blood into humans. The amounts of blood given were small and he was probably not able to introduce enough blood to produce death, although he reported predictable adverse effects. In November, Richard Lower claimed to have transfused 9 oz of lamb's blood into a young man, reported by Samuel Pepys. In December, Denis again attempted to give calf blood to a manic depressive patient, without fatal results; indeed, observers thought him much improved. A third transfusion was planned and the man died in mysterious circumstances. Denis accused the man's wife of poisoning him and was himself accused of causing the death but was acquitted. However, further experiments with transfusion came to an end for 150 years.

In 1800, Paul Scheel made an extensive study of the literature of attempted transfusions. His work was reviewed by James Blundell, an English obstetrician who tried animal experiments from sheep to dogs, which invariably failed. He revived a moribund obstetric patient with a transfusion of human blood in 1818, opening a new era (Figure 4). There continued to be great difficulties in the way of achieving human transfusion, for example with coagulation. Landsteiner's elucidation of the blood groups in 1901 (Figures 5–8) and the advent of sodium citrate as an anticoagulant in World War I finally made the matching of bloods comprehensible, and transfusions could become a medical possibility[1,2].

An article in the *Berliner klinische Wochenschrift* in 1900 by Ehrlich and Morgenroth, which described blood groups in goats based on antigens of their red cells[3], led Karl Landsteiner, a Viennese pathologist (Figure 5), successfully to identify the human ABO blood groups[4] (Figure 6). He took samples of his own blood, and from his colleagues Sturli and Ardhein, Dr Pletschnig and his assistant Zaritsch. The small tables Landsteiner used to illustrate his reasoning bear the names of these colleagues[5] (Figure 7). In 1902, Sturli and Alfred von Descastello, under Landsteiner's

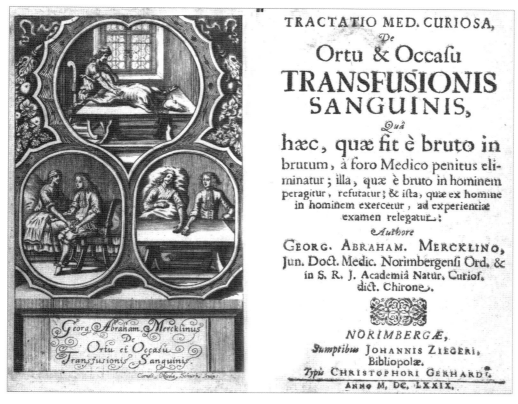

Figure 3   Engraved title page from G. A. Merklin, *Tractatio Med: Curioso de Ortu et Sanguinis*, 1679. This is one of the best early pictures of blood transfusion (from the Cruse Collection, Middleton Library, University of Wisconsin)

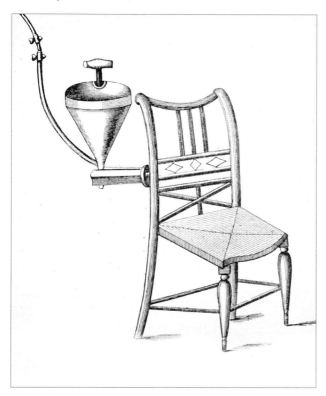

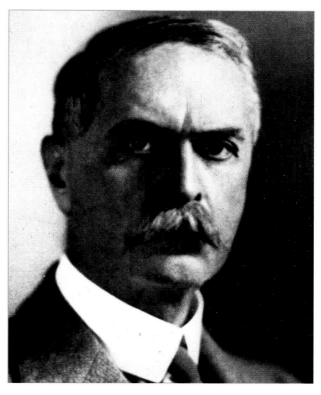

Figure 4   Transfusion chair developed by James Blundell, father of modern blood transfusion therapy

Figure 5   Karl Landsteiner, discoverer of the ABO human blood groups and Nobel Laureate in Medicine, 1930

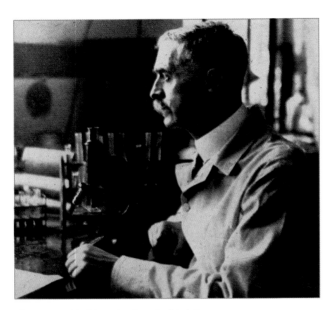

Figure 6 Karl Landsteiner in his laboratory

Tabelle I, betreffend das Blut sechs anscheinend gesunder Männer.

Sera	Dr. St.	Dr. Plecn.	Dr.Sturl.	Dr.Erdh.	Zar.	Landst.
Dr. St.	—	+	+	+	+	—
Dr. Plecn.	—	—	+	+	—	—
Dr. Sturl.	—	+	—	—	+	—
Dr. Erdh.	—	+	—	—	+	—
Zar.	—	—	+	+	+	—
Landst.	—	+	+	+	+	—

Blutkörperchen von:

Tabelle II, betreffend das Blut von sechs anscheinend gesunden Puerperae.

Sera	Seil.	Linsm.	Lust.	Mittelb.	Tomsch.	Graupf.
Seil.	—	—	+	—	—	+
Linsm.	+	—	+	+	+	+
Lust.	—	—	+	+	+	+
Mittelb.	—	—	+	—	+	+
Tomsch.	—	—	+	—	—	+
Graupn.	+	—	—	+	+	+

Blutkörperchen von:

Figure 7 Table illustrating ABO blood groups (*Wien Klin Wschr* 1901;14:1123–34)

Landsteiner, Zur Kenntnis der antifermentativen etc. Wirkungen des Blutserums. 357

Nachdruck verboten.

Zur Kenntnis der antifermentativen, lytischen und agglutinierenden Wirkungen des Blutserums und der Lymphe.

[Aus dem pathol.-anat. Univ.-Institute des Prof. Weichselbaum in Wien.]

Von Dr. **Karl Landsteiner** in Wien.

I. Zur Serumdiagnostik der Fermente.

Durch die Arbeiten von Fermi[1]), Pernossi[1]), Hammarsten, Hahn[2]), Röden[3]), Hildebrandt[4]) und Morgenroth[5]) wurde festgestellt, daß dem Blutserum die Fähigkeit zukomme, die Wirkung mancher Fermente aufzuheben. Fermi und Hahn führten ihre Untersuchungen an verdauenden Fermenten aus, Röden und Morgenroth am Labenzym.

Die Hoffnung, dieses eigentümliche Verhalten des Serums zur Untersuchung der Fermente benutzen zu können, ist leicht begreiflich, und es hat Morgenroth[6]) Versuche in Aussicht gestellt, die mit Hilfe der Einwirkung von Serum beweisen, daß im Lab verschiedene wirksame Gruppen vorhanden sind. In anderer Weise versuchte v. Dungern[7]) die antifermentativen Serumwirkungen zu verwerten, indem er Tiere mit verschiedenen Mikrobien immunisierte und zeigte, daß das resultierende Serum spezifisch gegen die Fermente der eingeführten Bakterien wirke. Es handelt sich in diesen Versuchen also um eine Art von Serodiagnostik von Bakterien auf dem Umwege über ihre Fermente. Wie es scheint, ist eine praktische Verwertung dieses Verhaltens bis jetzt nicht erzielt worden.

Versuche, die ich anstellte, gingen darauf aus, das Serum als Hilfsmittel zur Unterscheidung solcher tierischen Fermente zu benutzen, die auf anderem Wege keine Differenzen erkennen lassen. Ich wählte das tryptische Ferment als Objekt der Untersuchung. Dabei ging ich von der Vermutung aus, daß die gleich benannten Fermente verschiedener Tierspecies ebenso jeder Art eigentümlich sein könnten wie die wirksamen Serumstoffe, die Hämoglobine und gewisse andere Bestandteile der roten Blutkörperchen und tierischen Zellen überhaupt.

Die Erkenntnis der gesetzmäßigen Besonderheit sehr ähnlicher, zunächst nicht unterscheidbarer Stoffe bei den verschiedenen Species gelang bisher zum Teil durch chemische Untersuchung, namentlich durch die Serumreaktionen, andererseits führten physiologische und morphologische Ueberlegungen zu ähnlichen Schlüssen. So hat erst vor kurzem Rabl[8]) auf Grund der Erfahrungen bei Transplantationsversuchen und seiner Untersuchungen über den Bau der Linse des Auges auf die Konstanz der Unterschiede homologer Strukturen bei den verschiedenen Tierspecies hingewiesen.

1) Zeitschr. f. Hyg. Bd. XVIII. u. a. a. O.
2) Berl. klin. Wochenschr. 1897. p. 499.
3) Cit. nach Hahn.
4) Virch. Arch. Bd. CXXXI.
5) Centralbl. f. Bakt. etc. Bd. XXVI. No. 11, 12.
6) l. c.
7) Ref. Münch med. Wochenschr. 1898. p. 1040.
8) 71. Versamml. deutscher Naturforscher.

Figure 8 Title page of Landsteiner's article describing the human blood groups

Blood type	Red blood cell surface antigen	Antibody in serum
A	A antigen	Anti-B
B	B antigen	Anti-A
AB	AB antigens	No antibody
O	No A or B antigens	Both anti-A and anti-B

Figure 9 ABO blood group antigens and antibodies

direction (Figures 6–13), designated one more group[6], which was actually not named 'AB' until 10 years later when von Dungern and Hirszfeld (Figure 14), studying the genetic inheritance of blood types, designated the fourth type and gave Landsteiner's 'C' group the designation O[7]. It was for this discovery, rather than his elegant studies on immunochemical specificity, that he won the Nobel Prize in Medicine 30 years later. After 5 years of training in chemistry under the tutelage of Emil Fischer, Eugen von Bamberger and Arthur Hantzsch, and the beginning of his work on the specificity of serological reactions using chemically modified antigens, Dr Landsteiner served in Max von Grüber's Institute for 2 years. After von Grüber's departure for Munich, he became an assistant to Anton Weichselbaum, also of the Vienna University Faculty of Medicine, in 1897. In 1908, he was appointed to the staff of the Imperial

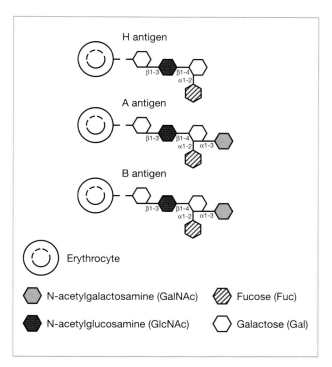

Figure 10 Chemical structure of A, B and H antigens of the ABO blood group system

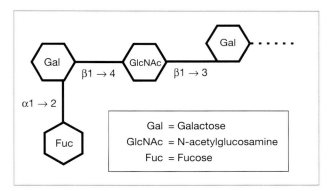

Figure 12 Chemical structure of H antigen, which is a specificity of the ABO blood group system

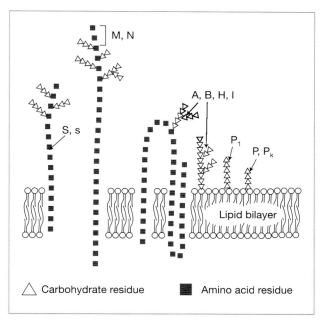

Figure 11 Schematic representation of membrane glycoproteins and glycosphingolipids that carry blood group antigens

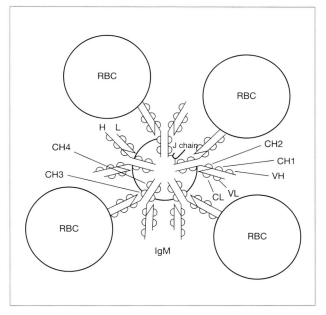

Figure 13 Schematic representation of the agglutination of human red blood cells (RBCs) by the natural isohemagglutinins, which are antibodies of the IgM class

Wilhelminen Hospital as head of the Department of Pathology. His years in Vienna were his most fruitful, with more than 170 papers. After a brief sojourn in Holland after World War I, he was invited to join the Rockefeller Institute for Medical Research by Simon Flexner in 1923. He continued there for the rest of his life, completing 346 papers during his enormously productive career[8]. Several of the investigators who trained under his direction, including Merrill W. Chase, gained scientific acclaim in their own right in subsequent years. Among those who worked with him in the field of immunohematology were Alexander Wiener

(Figure 15) and Philip Levine (Figures 16 and 17). Distinguished investigators who worked with Dr Landsteiner in other fields of immunology are mentioned in other sections of this book. Landsteiner and Levine discovered the M and N blood group antigens by injecting human erythrocytes into rabbits. The

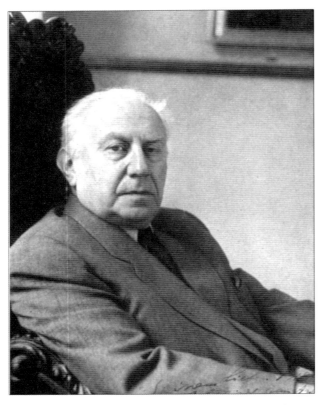

Figure 14 Dr Ludwik Hirszfeld, who with Emil von Dungern studied the genetics of blood groups

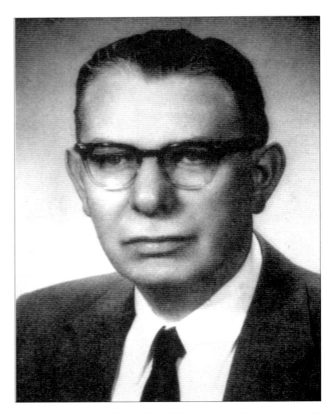

Figure 15 Dr Alexander Wiener, co-discoverer with Landsteiner of the Rh blood group system

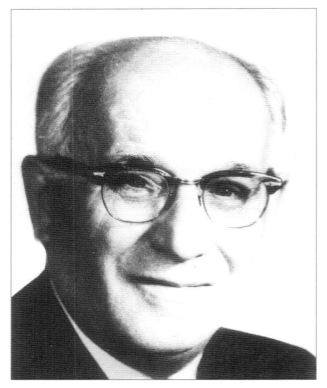

Figure 16 Dr Philip Levine, colleague of Landsteiner and co-discoverer of the MNS blood group system

antisera which they raised were able to divide human blood into three groups, M, N and MN, based on the antigenic content. They showed that these antigens were under the genetic control of codominant alleles[9,10]. Landsteiner and Wiener described the rhesus (Rh) factor in 1940[11,12] (Figures 18–20). At first thought to be a simple system involving a single antigen, it was shown to be genetically, immunologically and clinically complex. In studies on M-like factors on the erythrocytes of rhesus monkeys, antisera raised by injecting rabbits with rhesus red cells cross-reacted with human erythrocytes containing M antigen. It was subsequently demonstrated that the red cells of about 85% of the human population reacted with antisera against rhesus red cells (Figures 21–23). Thus, those individuals who shared an antigen with the rhesus monkey red cells were termed Rh_o positive and those who did not were termed Rh_o negative. It was subsequently demonstrated that multiple pregnancies with Rh (D) positive fetuses in Rh negative mothers leads to stimulation of maternal anti-D antibodies of the IgG class which cross the placenta and cause lysis of fetal red cells. Ronald Finn (Figure 24), studying Kleihauer's slides stained for fetal

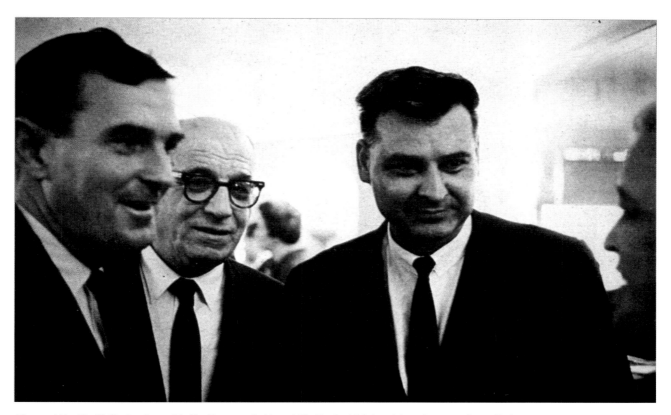

Figure 17   Dr Philip Levine with Dr Gorman (left) and Dr Freda (right) at his retirement from Ortho

hemoglobin, suggested that freeing a mother's blood of fetal cells would prevent Rh sensitization, thereby preventing erythroblastosis fetalis in subsequent pregnancies. Subsequently, anti-D antibody was used for this purpose. Unless the mother is treated with antibody against the D antigen after parturition, hemolytic disease of the newborn (erythroblastosis fetalis) may result in subsequent births. Race and Sanger (Figure 25) offered an alternative genetic concept of the Rh blood groups with a three allele theory rather than a single locus with a large series of alleles proposed by Wiener. Race and Sanger developed a system of nomenclature, i.e. CDE/cde, different from that of Wiener. Besides those mentioned above, other red blood cell antigens discovered in the intervening years included Kell, Diego, P, Duffy, the I blood group system and soluble antigens such as the Lewis and Lutheran antigens that are in the secretions and are adsorbed to the red cell surface[2]. Although most red cell groups are inherited as autosomal characteristics, the Xg^a blood group system is sex linked. Historically, new red blood cell antigens were discovered as a result of transfusion incompatibility reactions that could not be explained on the basis of existing or known antigens. Until the late 1950s

Haplotype	Fisher–Race	Wiener	Frequency (%)	
			Whites	African-American
R^1	CDe	Rh_1	42	17
r	cde	rh	37	26
R^2	cDE	Rh_2	14	11
R^0	cDe	Rh_0	4	44
r'	Cde	rh'	2	2
r''	cdE	rh''	1	<1
R^z	CDE	Rh_z	very rare	very rare
R^y	CdE	rh^y	very rare	very rare

Figure 18   Principal Rh genes and their frequencies of occurrence among Whites and African-Americans

immunohematology concerned itself almost exclusively with the immunology of the red cell. Since that time, however, tissue-typing techniques have demonstrated that human leukocyte antigens (HLA) in humans are present on leukocytes[13–15] but are absent on erythrocytes. Since most blood group studies employed red cells, this might explain the delay in their discovery. Since these are significant for organ and bone marrow transplantation, improvements in techniques for tissue typing using patient and donor lymphocytes progressed at a rapid pace. Pioneers in this field of human histocompatibility testing included Bernard Amos, a student

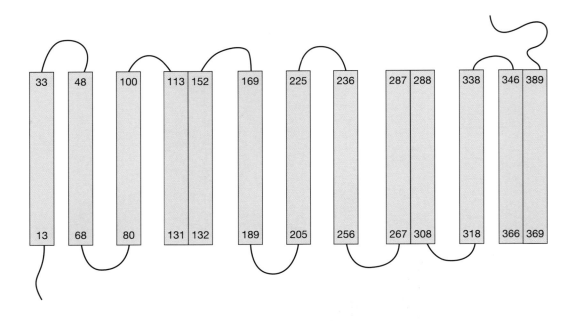

Figure 19   Schematic representation of the suggested molecular structure of the Rh polypeptide

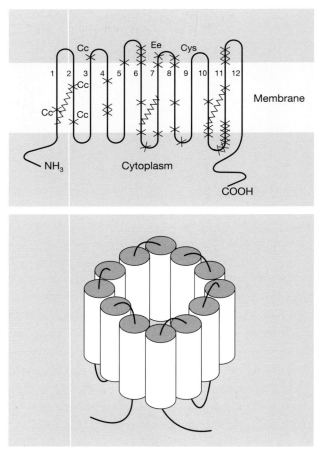

Figure 20   Schematic representation of Cc, Ee and D polypeptide topology within the erythrocyte membrane

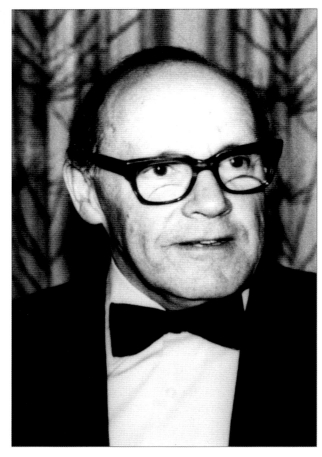

Figure 21   Dr R. R. A. Coombs, after whom the Coombs' antiglobulin test is named

of Peter Gorer, Kissmeyer-Nielsen, Van Rood, Ceppelini, Fritz Bach, Paul Terasaki and a host of others. Genes for the major histocompatibility complex (MHC) in man were localized to the short arm of chromosome 6. These include HLA-A, HLA-B, HLA-C, HLA-D and HLA-DR. The transplantation of bone marrow and solid organ grafts such as the kidney is facilitated by HLA typing.

Carlo Alberto Moreschi (1876–1921) (Figure 26) graduated as Doctor of Medicine at Pavia in 1900. He was assistant to Pfeiffer, Ehrlich and Ascoli and in 1920 was named Ordinarius in clinical medicine at Sassari and Messina Universities. He pursued studies on anaphylaxis, bacteriolysis and complement fixation reactions. Starting from the specific inhibition reaction perfected by Landsteiner and colleagues (1902) to study haptens, Moreschi reported in 1907 a new method to identify serological antibodies, which drew praise from Landsteiner in 1909. Coombs, Mourant and Race, in the 1940s, developed the anti-human globulin (Coombs) test based on the same principle as Moreschi's earlier report.

Karl Landsteiner (1868–1943), discoverer of the ABO and other blood group systems including MN and the Rh factor; developed artificial haptens to investigate antibody specificity, received the Nobel Prize in Medicine or Physiology in 1930 for discovery of the human blood groups.

Landsteiner was born in Vienna on June 14, 1868. The son of a journalist, he attended the University of Vienna from 1885 to 1891 when he graduated as MD. He maintained a strong interest in chemistry and took special instruction in organic chemistry under Emil Fischer and Eugen von Bamberger. In 1896, he became Assistant at the Institute of Hygiene directed by Max von Grüber where he was introduced to immunology and serology, which occupied his research interests for the remainder of his career. Two years later, he transferred to pathology. He coauthored nine papers with Donath, including a report on paroxysmal hemoglobinuria. Landsteiner was appointed Research Assistant at the Vienna Pathological Institute in 1898 where he remained until 1908 when he was appointed Chief of Pathology at the Royal Imperial Wilhelminen Hospital in Vienna and adjunct profes-

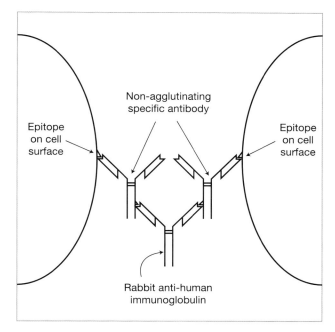

Figure 22 Schematic representation of the Coombs' antiglobulin test

sor in the Medical Faculty of the University of Vienna. Following World War I the newly formed Republic of Austria was chaotic, and experienced inflation and fuel and food shortages. Fleeing disruptive working conditions, Landsteiner left for The Hague in The Netherlands in 1919, where he accepted a position in the Catholic Hospital. He was lured to the Rockefeller Institute for Medical Research in New York City at the invitation of the Institute's Director, Dr Simon Flexner, in 1923, where he was made a Full Member and given a modest laboratory. He became an American citizen in 1929 and died in New York City on 26 June 1943.

Landsteiner discovered the human blood groups in 1900 when he found that the blood serum of some individuals could cause the agglutination of red cells from others. This led him to characterize red blood cells according to their antigens, leading subsequently to a description of the ABO blood groups. The development of citrates as anticoagulants in 1914 by Richard Lewisohn, together with Landsteiner's blood grouping, led to the widespread practice of blood transfusion. In 1927, Landsteiner and Phillip Levine discovered the additional blood group antigens M and N, which are not of significance in transfusion since human blood serum does not contain isoagglutinins (antibodies) against them, differentiating MN from the ABO groups.

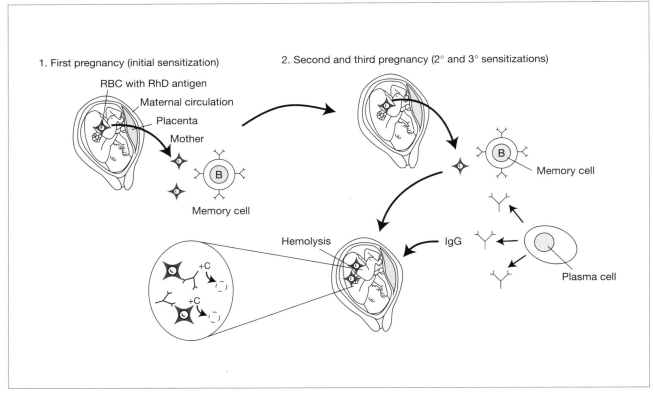

Figure 23   Representation of the mechanism of hemolytic disease of the newborn

In 1940, Landsteiner, Levine and Wiener discovered the Rh blood group system when they found that antibodies raised in rabbits and guinea pigs immunized with blood from a rhesus monkey were able to agglutinate the red blood cells of many humans, who were termed Rh positive, whereas those not possessing it were termed Rh negative. This factor was shown to be important in hemolytic disease of the newborn.

Landsteiner investigated poliomyelitis between 1908 and 1922. He discovered that a rhesus monkey became paralyzed following the injection of brain and spinal cord from a polio victim. After finding no bacteria in the monkey's nervous system, Landsteiner concluded that a virus must be the causative agent. He perfected a technique to diagnose poliomyelitis. Landsteiner discovered that an extract of ox hearts could replace the antigen derived from livers of babies with congenital syphilis, for use in the Wassermann test for syphilis.

With his excellent background in chemistry, medicine and pathology, Landsteiner continued his serology and immunology work at the Rockefeller Institute. He examined the effect of position on

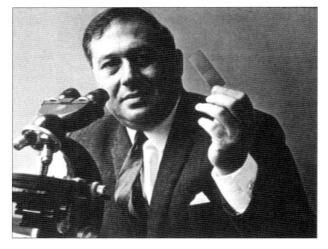

Figure 24   Dr Finn, analyzing Kleihauer's slides, realized that if the blood of the new mother that contained many dark fetal cells could be treated so that no fetal cells appeared, she would be spared Rh sensitization, and her next baby would not be ill

attached radicals. He discovered that immunochemical specificity was altered by the *ortho*, *meta* or *para* position on aromatic rings of stereoisomers. He found that position was more important than the nature of the radical.

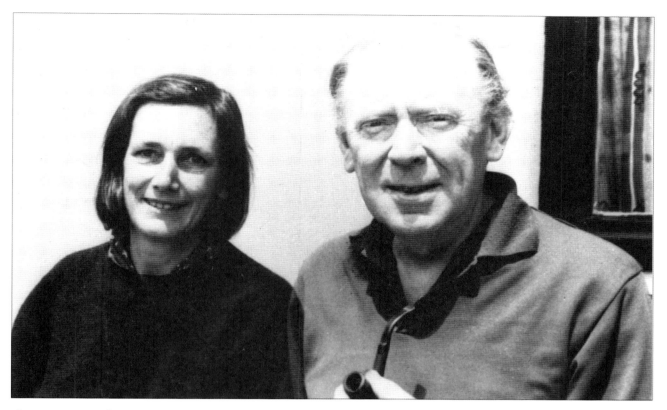

Figure 25 Drs Ruth Sanger and Robert Race, who developed the three allele theory and the C, D, E nomenclature for the Rh blood group system

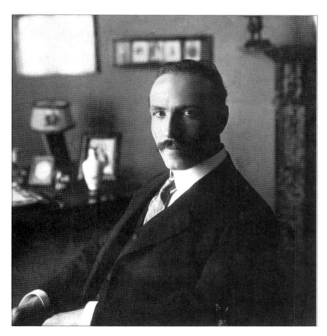

Figure 26 Dr Carlo Alberto Moreschi

Landsteiner further showed that partial antigens termed haptens were unable to elicit antibody formation, but could react with those formed in response to a complete antigen comprising a hapten bound to a carrier molecule. He demonstrated carrier-specific and hapten-specific antibodies. His extensive investigations on immunochemical specificity were first summarized in his book entitled *Die Specifizitat der serologischen Reactionen* published in 1933. The English translation was published in 1936, and a revised edition appeared following his death in 1945 entitled *The Specificity of Serological Reactions*. He found that haptens could combine with pre-existing antibodies to produce allergic desensitization. Landsteiner's work laid a foundation for much of modern immunology, including the construction of synthetic vaccines as a representative application of his research.

Philip Levine (1900–87), Russian–American immunohematologist. With Landsteiner, he conducted pioneering research on blood group antigens, including discovery of the MNP system. His work contributed much to transfusion medicine and transplantation immunobiology.

The **ABO blood group system** was the first described of the human blood groups based upon carbohydrate alloantigens present on red cell membranes. Anti-A or anti-B isoagglutinins (alloantibodies) are present only in the blood sera of individuals not possessing that specificity, i.e. anti-A is found in the serum of group B individuals and anti-B is found in the serum of group A individuals. This serves as the basis for grouping humans into phenotypes designated A, B, AB and O. Type AB subjects possess neither anti-A nor anti-B antibodies, whereas group O persons have both anti-A and anti-B antibodies in their serum. Blood group methodology to determine the ABO blood type makes use of the agglutination reaction. The ABO system remains the most important in the transfusion of blood and is also critical in organ transplantation. Epitopes of the ABO system are found on oligosaccharide terminal sugars. The genes designated as A/B, Se, H and Le govern the formation of these epitopes and of the Lewis (Le) antigens (Figure 10). The two precursor substances type I and type II differ only in that the terminal galactose is joined to the penultimate N-acetylglucosamine in the β 1–3 linkage in type I chains, but in the β 1–4 linkage in type II chains.

Landsteiner's rule (historical)   Landsteiner (1900) discovered that human red blood cells could be separated into four groups based on their antigenic characteristics. These were designated as blood groups O, A, B and AB. He found naturally occurring isohemagglutinins in the sera of individuals specific for the (ABO) blood group antigen which they did not possess (i.e. anti-A and anti-B isohemagglutinins in group O subjects; anti-B in group A individuals; and anti-A in group B persons; neither anti-A nor anti-B in group AB subjects).

Blood grouping (Figures 7 and 9) is the classification of erythrocytes based on their surface isoantigens. Among the well-known human blood groups are the ABO, Rh and MNS systems.

Plasma is the transparent yellow fluid that constitutes 50–55% of the blood volume. It is 92% fluid and 7% protein. Inorganic salts, hormones, sugars, lipids and gases make up the remaining 1%. Plasma from which fibrinogen and clotting factors have been removed is known as serum.

Blood group antigens are erythrocyte surface molecules that may be detected with antibodies from other individuals, such as the ABO blood group antigens. Various blood group antigen systems, including Rh (rhesus) may be typed in routine blood banking procedures. Other blood group antigen systems may be revealed through cross-matching.

ABO blood group substances are glycopeptides with oligosaccharide side-chains, manifesting ABO epitopes of the same specificity as those present on red blood cells of the individual in whom they are detected. Soluble ABO blood group substances may be found in mucus secretions of man such as saliva, gastric juice, ovarian cyst fluid, etc. Such persons are termed secretors, whereas those without the blood group substances in their secretions are non-secretors.

Natural antibodies are those found in the serum of an individual who has no known previous contact with that antigen, such as by previous immunization or infection with a microorganism containing that antigen. The anti-A and anti-B antibodies related to the ABO blood group system are natural antibodies. Natural antibodies may be a consequence of exposure to cross-reacting antigen(s), e.g. ABO blood group antibodies resulting from exposure to bacterial antigens in the gut. The term also refers to immunoglobulin IgM antibodies produced by B-1 cells specific for microorganisms found in the environment and gastrointestinal tract. There are two kinds of natural antibodies in blood sera. These include: specific, antigen-induced antibodies whose synthesis depends on external antigenic stimuli and corresponds to acquired specificities; a second type that expresses broad specificity, is genetically determined and does not depend on a specific antigenic stimulus. Both kinds of natural antibodies of the IgM, IgG and IgA isotopes specific for many antigens are present in normal sera of humans and other animals. Natural antibodies have a variety of biological functions ranging from physiological to pathological effects.

H substance is a basic carbohydrate of the ABO blood group system structure of man. Most people express this ABO-related antigen. 'Secretors' have soluble H substance in their body fluids.

O antigen In the ABO blood group system, O antigen is an oligosaccharide precursor form of A and B antigens: a fucose-galactose-*N*-acetylglucosamine-glucose.

Immune antibody is a term used to distinguish an antibody induced by transfusion or other immunogenic challenge, in contrast to a natural antibody such as the isohemagglutinins against ABO blood group substances found in humans.

A **hemagglutinin** is a red blood cell-agglutinating substance. Antibodies, lectins and some viral glycoproteins may induce erythrocyte agglutination. In immunology, hemagglutinin usually refers to an antibody that causes red blood cell aggregation in physiological salt solution either at 37°C, in which case they are termed warm hemagglutinins, or at 4°C, in which case they are referred to as cold hemagglutinins.

The **hemagglutination test** is an assay based upon the aggregation of red blood cells into clusters either through the action of antibody specific for their surface epitopes or through the action of a virus that possesses a hemagglutinin as part of its structure and which does not involve antibody.

A **secretor** is an individual who secretes ABH blood group substances into body fluids such as saliva, gastric juice, tears, ovarian cyst fluid, etc. At least 80% of the human population are secretors. The property is genetically determined and requires that the individual be either homozygous (*Se/Se*) or heterozygous (*Se/se*) for the *Se* gene.

A **non-secretor** is an individual whose body secretions such as gastric juice, saliva, tears and ovarian cyst mucin do not contain ABO blood group substances. Non-secretors make up approximately one-fifth of the population and are homozygous for the gene *se*.

The **rhesus blood group system** (Figure 18) comprises rhesus monkey erythrocyte antigens, such as the D antigen, which are found on the red cells of most humans, who are said to be Rh positive. This blood group system was discovered by Landsteiner and associates in the 1940s when they injected rhesus monkey erythrocytes into rabbits and guinea pigs. Subsequent studies showed the system to be quite complex, and the rare Rh alloantigens are still not characterized biochemically (Figure 19). Three closely linked pairs of alleles designated Dd, Cc and Ee are postulated to be at the Rh locus, which is located on chromosome 1. There are several alloantigenic determinants within the Rh system. Clinically, the D antigen is the one of greatest concern, since RhD negative individuals who receive RhD positive erythrocytes by transfusion can develop alloantibodies that may lead to severe reactions with further transfusions of RhD positive blood. The D antigen also poses a problem in RhD negative mothers who bear a child with RhD positive red cells inherited from the father. The entrance of fetal erythrocytes into the maternal circulation at parturition or trauma during the pregnancy (such as in amniocentesis) can lead to alloimmunization against the RhD antigen which may cause hemolytic disease of the newborn in subsequent pregnancies. This is now prevented by the administration of $Rh_o(D)$ immune globulin to these women within 72 h of parturition. Further confusion concerning this system has been caused by the use of separate designations by the Wiener and Fisher systems. Rh antigens are a group of 7–10-kDa, erythrocyte membrane-bound antigens that are independent of phosphatides and proteolipids. Antibodies against Rh antigens do not occur naturally in the serum.

Rhesus antigen refers to an erythrocyte antigen of man that shares epitopes in common with rhesus monkey red blood cells. Rhesus antigens are encoded by allelic genes. D antigen has the greatest clinical significance, as it may stimulate antibodies in subjects not possessing the antigen and induce hemolytic disease of the newborn or cause transfusion incompatibility reactions. Rhesus antibody reacts with rhesus antigen, especially RhD (Figure 20).

Anti-D is an antibody against the Rh blood group D antigen. This antibody is stimulated in RhD negative mothers by fetal RhD positive red blood cells that enter her circulation at parturition. Anti-D antibodies become a problem usually with the third pregnancy, resulting from the booster immune response against the D antigen to which the mother was previously exposed. IgG antibodies pass across the placenta, leading to hemolytic disease of the newborn (erythroblastosis fetalis). Anti-D antibody (Rhogam®) administered up to 72 h following parturition may combine with the RhD positive red blood cells in the mother's circulation, thereby facilitating their removal by the reticuloendothelial system. This prevents maternal immunization against the RhD antigen.

$Rh_o(D)$ immune globulin is prepared from the serum of individuals hyperimmunized against $Rh_o(D)$ antigen. It is used to prevent the immunization of Rh^- mothers by $Rh_o(D)^+$ erythrocytes of the baby, especially at parturition when the baby's red cells enter the maternal circulation in significant quantities, but also at any time during the pregnancy after trauma that might introduce fetal blood into the maternal circulation. This prevents hemolytic disease of the newborn in subsequent pregnancies. The dose used is effective in inhibiting immune reactivity against 15 ml of packed $Rh_o(D)^+$ red blood cells. It should be administered within 72 h of parturition. It may also be used following inadvertent or unavoidable transfusion of RhD^+ blood to RhD^- recipients, especially to a woman of child-bearing age.

Rhogam® refers to $Rh_o(D)$ immune globulin.

Rhesus incompatibility refers to the stimulation of anti-RhD antibodies in a Rh negative mother when challenged by RhD positive red cells of her baby (especially at parturition) that may lead to hemolytic disease of the newborn. The term also refers to the transfusion of RhD positive blood to an Rh negative individual who may form anti-D antibodies against the donor blood, leading to subsequent incompatibility reactions if given future RhD positive blood.

Coombs' test (Figure 22) is an antiglobulin assay that detects immunoglobulin on the surface of a patient's red blood cells. The test was developed in the 1940s by Robin Coombs to demonstrate autoantibodies on the surface of red blood cells that fail to cause agglutination of these red cells. In the direct Coombs' test, rabbit anti-human immunoglobulin is added to a suspension of patient's red cells, and, if they are coated with autoantibody, agglutination results. In the indirect

Coombs' test, the patient's serum can be used to coat erythrocytes, which are then washed, and the anti-immunoglobulin reagent added to produce agglutination if the antibodies in question had been present in the serum sample. The Coombs' test has long been a part of the autoimmune disease evaluation of patients. An incomplete antibody is non-agglutinating and must have a linking agent such as anti-IgG to reveal its presence in an agglutination reaction.

Antiglobulin antibodies are specific for epitopes in the Fc region of immunoglobulin molecules used as immunogen, rendering them capable of agglutinating cells whose surface antigens are combined with Fab regions of IgG molecules whose Fc regions are exposed.

The **direct antiglobulin test** is an assay in which washed erythrocytes are combined with antiglobulin antibody. If the red cells had been coated with non-agglutinating (incomplete) antibody *in vivo*, agglutination would occur. Examples of this in humans include hemolytic disease of the newborn, in which maternal antibodies coat the infant's erythrocytes, and autoimmune hemolytic anemia, in which the subject's red cells are coated with autoantibodies. This is the basis of the direct Coombs' test.

The **indirect antiglobulin test** is a method to detect incomplete (non-agglutinating) antibody in a patient's serum. Following incubation of red blood cells or other cells possessing the antigen for which the incomplete antibodies of interest are specific, rabbit anti-human globulin is added to the antibody-coated cells which have first been washed. If agglutination results, incomplete agglutinating antibody is present in the serum with which the antigen-bearing red cells have been incubated.

Hemolytic disease of the newborn (HDN) (Figure 23) is a condition in which a fetus with RhD positive red blood cells can stimulate an RhD negative mother to produce anti-RhD IgG antibodies that cross the placenta and destroy the fetal red blood cells when a sufficient titer is obtained. This is usually not until the third pregnancy with an Rh positive fetus. At parturition, the RhD positive red blood cells enter the maternal circulation and subsequent pregnancies provide a booster to this response. With the third pregnancy, a sufficient quantity of high-titer antibody crosses the placenta to produce considerable lysis of fetal red blood cells. This may lead to erythroblastosis fetalis (hemolytic disease of the newborn). Seventy per cent of HDN is due to RhD incompatibility between the mother and fetus. Exchange transfusions may be required for treatment. Two other antibodies against erythrocytes that may likewise be a cause for transfusion exchange include anti-Fy^a and Kell. As bilirubin levels rise, the immature blood–brain barrier permits bilirubin to penetrate and deposit on the basal ganglia. Injection of the mother with anti-D antibody following parturition unites with the RhD positive red cells, leading to their elimination by the mononuclear phagocyte system.

P antigen is an ABH blood group-related antigen found on erythrocyte surfaces that comprises the three sugars galactose, *N*-isoacetyl-galactosamine and *n*-acetyl-glucosamine. The P antigens are designated P_1, P_2, P^k and p. P_2 subjects rarely produce anti-P_1 antibody, which may lead to hemolysis in clinical situations. Paroxysmal cold hemagglutinaria patients develop a biphasic autoanti-P antibody that fixes complement in the cold and lyses red blood cells at 37°C.

Donath–Landsteiner antibody is an immunoglobulin specific for P blood group antigens on human erythrocytes. This antibody binds to the patient's red blood cells at cold temperatures and induces hemolysis on warming. It occurs in subjects with paroxysmal cold hemaglobulinemia (PCH). It is also called Donath–Landsteiner cold autoantibody.

The **MNS blood group system** refers to human erythrocyte glycophorin epitopes. There are four distinct sialoglycoproteins (SGPs) on red cell membranes. These include α-SGP (glycophorin A, MN), β-SGP (glycophorin C), γ-SGP (glycophorin D) and δ-SGP (glycophorin B). MN antigens are present on α-SGP and δ-SGP. M and N antigens are present on α-SGP, with an approximately one-half million copies detectable on each erythrocyte. This is a 31-kDa structure that comprises 131 amino acids, with about 60% of the total weight attributable to carbohydrate. This transmembrane molecule has a carboxyl terminus that stretches into the cytoplasm of the erythrocyte, with a 23-amino acid hydrophobic segment embedded in the lipid bilayer. The amino terminal segment extends to the extracellular compartment. Blood group antigen activity is in the external segment. In α-SGP with M antigen activity, the first amino acid is serine and the fifth is glycine. When it carries N antigen activity, leucine and glutamic acid replace serine and glycine at positions 1 and 5, respectively. The Ss antigens are encoded by allelic genes at a locus closely linked to the MN locus. The U antigen is also considered a part of the MNS system. Whereas anti-M and anti-N antibodies may occur without red cell stimulation, antibodies against Ss and U antigens generally follow erythrocyte stimulation. The MN and Ss alleles positioned on chromosome 4 are linked. Antigens of the MNS system may provoke the formation of antibodies that can mediate hemolytic disease of the newborn.

The **Lewis blood group system** is an erythrocyte antigen system that differs from other red cell groups in that the antigen is present in soluble form in the blood and saliva. Lewis antigens are adsorbed from the plasma onto the red cell membrane. The Lewis phenotype expressed is based on whether the individual is a secretor or a non-secretor of the Lewis gene product. Expression of the Lewis phenotype is dependent also on the ABO phenotype. Lewis antigens are carbohydrates chemically. Lewis blood secretors have an increased likelihood of urinary tract infections induced by *Escherichia coli* or other microbes, because of the linkage of carbohydrate residues of glycolipids and glycoproteins on urothelial cells.

Platelet antigens are surface epitopes on thrombocytes that may be immunogenic, leading to platelet antibody formation resulting in such conditions as neonatal alloimmune thrombocytopenia and post-transfusion purpura. The Pl^{A1} antigen may induce platelet antibody formation in Pl^{A1} antigen-negative individuals. Additional platelet antigens associated with purpura include Pl^{A2}, Bak^a, and HLA-A2. Anti-Bak^a is a normal human platelet (thrombocyte) antigen. Anti-Bak^a IgG antibody synthesized by a Bak^a negative female may be passively transferred across the placenta to induce immune thrombocytopenia in the neonate.

Platelets possess surface FcγRII receptors that combine with IgG or immune complexes. The platelet surfaces can become saturated with immune complexes as in autoimmune or idiopathic thrombocytopenic purpura (AITP or ITP). Fab-mediated antibody binding to platelet antigens may be difficult to distinguish from Fc-mediated binding of immune complexes to the surface.

Platelet transfusion is the administration of platelet concentrates prepared by centrifuging a unit of whole blood at low speed to provide 40–70 ml of plasma that contains 3–4×10^{11} platelets. This amount can increase an adult's platelet concentration by $10\,000/\text{mm}^3$. It is best to store platelets at 20–24°C, subjecting them to mild agitation. They must be used within 5 days of collection.

Transfusion describes the transplantation of blood cells, platelets and/or plasma from the blood circulation of one individual to another. Acute blood loss due to hemorrhage or the replacement of deficient cell types due to excess destruction or inadequate formation are indications for blood transfusion. With the description of human blood groups by Landsteiner in 1900, the transfusion of blood from one human being to another became possible. This ushered in the field of transfusion medicine which relates to substitution therapies with human blood, protein deficiencies and blood loss. Peripheral blood cell and plasma collection, processing, storage, compatibility matching and transfusion are routine procedures in medical centers throughout the world. The description of multiple other blood group systems followed the initial description of the ABO types. Modern-day blood group serology and immunohematology laboratories consider all aspects of allo- and autoantibodies against red cells in clinical transfusion. Bloodborne viruses are recognized as critical risk factors in transfusion. In recent years, the rate of viral transmission through transfusions has been greatly diminished with the development of adequate methods of screening for human immunodeficiency virus (HIV), hepatitis viruses and other infectious agents.

A **universal recipient** is an ABO blood group individual whose cells express antigens A and B, but whose serum does not contain anti-A and anti-B antibodies. Thus, red blood cells containing any of the ABO antigens may be transfused to them without inducing a hemolytic transfusion reaction, i.e. from an individual with type A, B, AB or O. It is best if the universal recipient is Rh$^+$, i.e. has the RhD antigen on his erythrocytes, to avoid developing a hemolytic transfusion reaction. However, blood group systems other than ABO may induce hemolytic reactions in a universal recipient. Thus, it is best to use type-specific blood for transfusions.

A **universal donor** is a blood group O RhD$^-$ individual whose erythrocytes express neither A nor B surface antigens. This type of red blood cell fails to elicit a hemolytic transfusion reaction in recipients who are blood group A, B, AB or O. However, group O individuals serving as universal donors may express other blood group antigens on their erythrocytes that will induce hemolysis. It is preferable to use type-specific blood for transfusions, except in cases of disaster or emergency.

Transfusion reaction(s) may be either immune or non-immune reactions that follow the administration of blood. Transfusion reactions with immune causes are considered serious, and occur in 1 in 3000 transfusions. Patients may develop urticaria, itching, fever, chills, chest pains, cyanosis and hemorrhage. The appearance of these symptoms together with an increase in temperature by 1°C signals the need to halt the transfusion. Immune, non-infectious transfusion reactions include allergic urticaria (immediate hypersensitivity); anaphylaxis, as in the administration of blood to IgA-deficient subjects, some of whom develop anti-IgA antibodies of the IgE class; and serum sickness, in which the serum proteins such as immunoglobulins induce the formation of precipitating antibodies that lead to immune complex formation.

REFERENCES

1. Saunders JBdeCM. A conceptual history of transplantation. In Najarian JS, Simmons RL, eds. *Transplantation*. Philadelphia: Lea & Febiger, 1972

2. Zmijewski CM. *Immunohematology*, 3rd edn. New York: Appleton-Century-Crofts, 1978

3. Ehrlich P, Morgenroth J. Uber Hamolysine. *Berl Klin Wschr* 1900;37:453–58, 39:681–7

4. Landsteiner K. Zur Kenntniss der antifermentativen, lytischen und agglutinierenden Wirkungen des Blutserums und der Lymphe. *Zentrabl Bakt* 1900;27:357–62

5. Landsteiner K. Uber Agglutinationserscheinungen normalen menschlichen Blutes. *Wien Klin Woch* 1901;14:1132–4

6. von Decastello A, Sturli A. Uber die Isoagglutininine in Serum gesumder und Kraner Menschen. *Munch Med Wschr* 1902;49:1090–5

7. von Dungern E, Hirszfeld L. Uber Vererbung grupenspecifischer Strukturen des Blutes. III. *Z ImmunForsch* 1910;6:284–92

8. Speiser P, Smekel F. *Karl Landsteiner*. Vienna: Bruder Hollinek, 1975

9. Landsteiner K, Levine P. A new agglutinable factor differentiating individual human bloods. *Proc Soc Exp Biol Med* 1926–27;24:600–02, 24:941–2

10. Landsteiner K, Levine P. On the inheritance of agglutinogens of human blood demonstrable by immune agglutinins. *J Exp Med* 1928;48:731–49

11. Landsteiner K, Wiener AS. An agglutinable factor in human blood recognised by immune sera from rhesus blood. *Proc Soc Exp Biol Med* 1940;42:223–4

12. Landsteiner K, Wiener AS. Studies on an agglutinogen (Rh) in human blood reacting with anti-rhesus sera and with human isoantibodies. *J Exp Med* 1941;74:309–20

13. Dausset J, Nenna A. Presence d'une leuco-agglutinine dans le serum d'un cas d'agranulocytose chronique. *C R Soc Biol* 1952;140:1534–61

14. Dausset J. Iso-leuco-anticorps. *Acta-Haem* 1958;20:156–66

15. Benacerraf B, McDevitt HO. Histocompatibility-linked immune response genes. *Science* 1972;175:273–9

CHAPTER 11

Immunogenetics, immunologic tolerance, transfusion and transplantation

From early times, the practice of medicine was plagued with other problems which had to wait for solution until there was an understanding of the immune mechanisms of the human body. In time of war, in the days of hand-to-hand combat, the loss of a limb was the lot of many soldiers. The patron saints of the surgeons were St Cosmas and St Damian (Figures 1 and 2) who

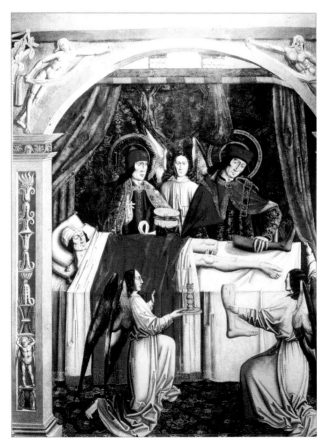

Figure 1 St Cosmas and St Damian transplanting the leg of a Moor onto the stump of a young man who had lost his leg

were said to have transplanted the leg of a Moor onto the stump of a young man whose leg had been amputated. A number of famous artists, including Fra Angelico and Fra Lippi, illustrated some aspects of this popular legend. John Hunter (Figure 3), who was given the title 'father of experimental surgery', was intrigued by the possibility of transplantation, and was successful in replacing a premolar tooth some hours after it had been knocked out. He thought he was successful in transplanting a human tooth into the comb of a cock, a specimen still on view at the Hunterian Museum.

Early understanding of the principles of skin grafting by the Indian physician Sushruta can be found in a Sanskrit text from India dated about 450 BC. Grafts of skin from the forehead, neck and cheek were used to restore mutilations of the nose, ear or lip (Figure 4). Apparently the physicians of the Alexandrian school understood how to repair such defects with skin flaps also, which is documented in the *De medicina* of Celcus. During the 13th and 14th centuries there was a resurgence of surgery practiced in the ancient medical school of Salerno, and in the 15th century mention was made of two skilled practitioners of plastic surgery, Branca de Branca and his son Antonio, who practiced in Catania in Sicily. The next great step in transplantation was the work of Gaspare Tagliacozzi (Figure 5) of Bologna, who published *De curtorum chirurgia per insitionem*, showing in detail his methods and procedure and illustrated with pictures of his instruments and methods of bandaging. He drew analogies from the agricultural practices of grafting in explaining his technique. He understood that xenografts were impossible and allografts were highly unlikely to unite, if only because of the awkwardness of keeping the two parts in close contact

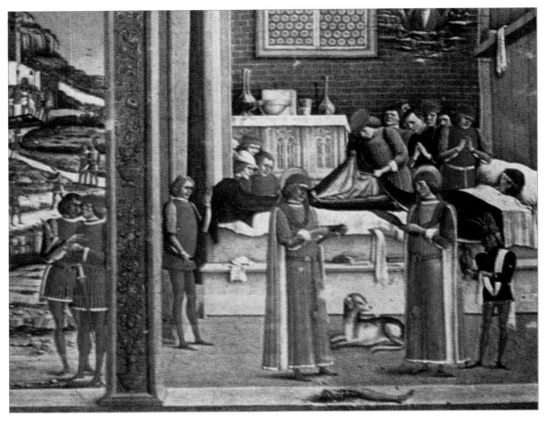

Figure 2 Another artistic rendering of the transplantation of the leg of a Moor onto the stump of a young sacristan who had lost his leg

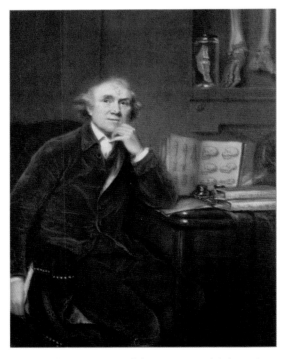

Figure 3 John Hunter, English surgeon and father of experimental surgery, who transplanted a tooth into the comb of a rooster

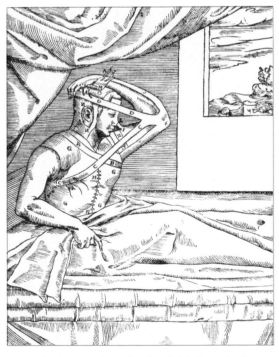

Figure 4 Early depiction of grafts of skin from the forehead, neck and cheek, used to restore mutilations of the nose, ear or lip

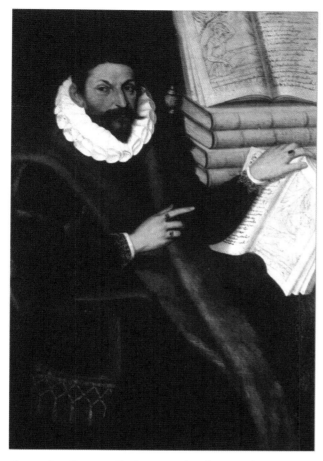

Figure 5 Gaspare Tagliacozzi of Bologna, who wrote a famous book on skin grafting

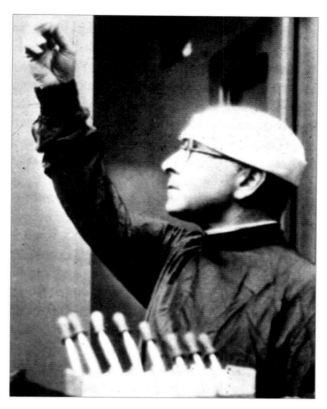

Figure 6 Alexis Carrel, French surgeon working at the Rockefeller Institute for Medical Research in New York City, who first successfully sewed blood vessels together after approximating their ends by triangulation suture. This technique earned him the Nobel Prize in Medicine and made organ and tissue grafts surgically possible

so that the graft could take. In spite of the excellence of Tagliacozzi's book, the technique of skin grafting did not progress further until the 19th century when interest revived. A number of surgeons tried making free grafts in animals and also attempts were made in humans, although, without the refinements of aseptic technique and anesthesia and since the principles of immunology were not yet known, not much progress was made[1].

Alexis Carrel (1873–1944) (Figure 6), French surgeon who received the Nobel Prize in Medicine or Physiology for successfully joining blood vessels by end-to-end anastomosis with triangulation sutures, thereby permitting the rapid re-establishment of blood circulation to a transplanted organ.

Alexis Carrel was born in 1873 in Sainte-Foy near Lyon, France. In 1900 he graduated as Doctor of Medicine at Lyon, and departed for America in 1904 to work in the Physiology Department at the University of Chicago. In 1906, he joined the Rockefeller Institute for Medical Research in New York City as an Associate Member, achieving Full Membership in 1912.

Becoming interested in tissue culture devised by Yale University researcher Ross G. Harrison, Carrel sent his colleague, M. T. Burrows, to learn the technique from Harrison. Their aim was to grow cells from warm-blooded animals, although this had already been accomplished in 1908 by Margaret Reid in Berlin. Carrel and Burrows claimed to have devised a method that employed a simple surgical technique, freshly sterilized glassware and instruments. They transformed the simple technology of tissue culture into an elaborate laboratory ritual. Carrel and Burrows worked in two separate suites of rooms consisting of animal preparation rooms, scrub room and culture/operating room fitted with built-in sprays used to cause dust to settle by spraying with water prior to commencing work. He required technicians, including Charles Lindbergh, of subsequent aviation fame, to dress somewhat theatrically in black, full-length gowns fitted with hoods.

Carrel stated that 'the technique [of tissue culture] is delicate and in untrained hands, the experimental errors are of such magnitude as to render the results worthless'. This caused other investigators to shy away from research involving tissue culture because of its apparent complexity, the cost of laboratory equipment and space. Critics termed this Carrel's 'mumbo jumbo' that stalled medical progress for years.

He developed the technique of end-to-end anastomosis of blood vessels in 1902. This technical advance permitted him to transplant organs successfully 6 years later. Continuing the work on organ transplantation begun by Emerich Ullmann in Vienna, Alexis Carrel became the first researcher in America to win the Nobel Prize in Medicine or Physiology by devising a skillful technique of approximating the ends of blood vessels to be anastomosed through triangulation sutures. He also successfully perfected surgical techniques to suture small vessels. In 1905, together with his colleague, Charles Guthrie, Carrel successfully performed a kidney autotransplant in a dog even though the animal died after the kidney failed.

He demonstrated that blood vessels could be maintained in the cold for 'prolonged periods' before use for transplantation. Carrel and Burrows used Harrison's technique to grow sarcoma cells successfully in culture in 1910. Together with Tuffier, Carrel performed a number of successful experimental valvotomies. In World War I, he and Dakin developed a treatment for wounds that was used extensively.

A positive accomplishment in his tissue culture research was the 'Carrel flask' which reduced bacterial contamination that had been a principal cause of failure of tissue cultures before the discovery of antibiotics in the 1940s. He also claimed to have developed an immortal cell line of chick embryo heart cultures that was begun in 1912 and supposedly maintained by him and a colleague, A. H. Ebeling, until 1942. How this was accomplished remains an enigma, as cells are now known to have a finite longevity. In 1938, Carrel retired from the Rockefeller Institute and returned to France, where he set up an Institute for the Study of Human Problems in Paris. The Vichy French Government assisted him during World War II and he negotiated with the Germans. In August 1944, following the liberation, Carrel was accused of collaborating with the enemy, but died before he could be arrested.

Further reading

Carrel A. Rejuvenation of cultures of tissues. *J Am Med Assoc* 1911;57:1611

Carrel A, Burrows MT. Cultures de sarcome en dehors de l'organisme. *C R Soc Biol (Paris)* 1910;69:332–4

Carrel A. La technique operatoire des anastomoses vasculaires et la transplantation des viscres. *Lyon Med* 1902;98:859–64

Carrel A. The surgery of blood vessels. *Johns Hopkins Hosp Bull* 1907;18:18–28

Carrel A. Results of the transplantation of blood vessels, organs and limbs. *J Am Med Assoc* 1908;51:I 662–7

Carrel A. Latent life of arteries. *J Exp Med* 1910;12:460–86

Carrel A. Transplantation in mass of the kidneys. *J Exp Med* 1908;10:98–140

Carrel A. Traitement abortif de l'infection des plaies. *Bull Acad Med (Paris)* 1915;74:361–8

Garrison FH. *An Introduction to the History of Medicine*. Philadelphia: WB Saunders Co, 1929

Lyons AS, Petrucelli RJ II. *Medicine: An Illustrated History*. New York: Harry N Abrams, 1987

When Professor M. R. Irwin (Figure 7) of the University of Wisconsin in Madison coined the term 'immunogenetics' in 1933 to describe an uncertain association between immunology and genetics[2], no one could have predicted that revelations of histocompatibility genes and antigens and of immune response (Ir) genes would lead to the award of a Nobel Prize in Medicine in 1980 to George Snell, Baruj Benacerraf and Jean Dausset for immunogenetics research.

The studies of Jensen[3] and Loeb[4], working independently with inbred strains of mice, at the turn of the century, demonstrated that the genetic similarity between a tumor transplant and the host into which it was inoculated governed the success or failure of the tumor allograft. These findings were confirmed and expanded by Tyzzer in 1909[5]. Little (1914) suggested

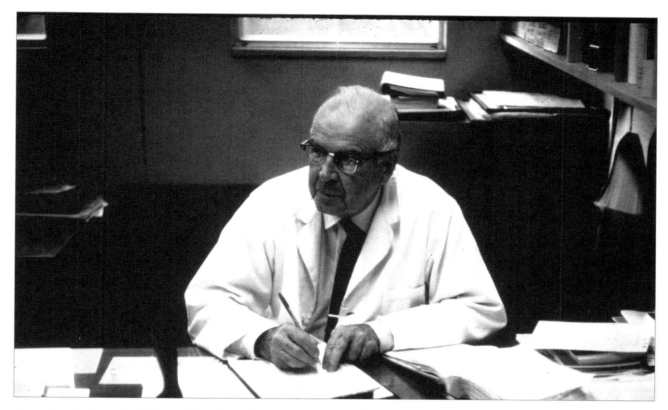

Figure 7   Professor M. R. Irwin of the University of Wisconsin who first coined the term 'immunogenetics'

that dominant genes govern susceptibility to tumor allografts[6]. This line of research led to the development of more inbred strains of mice which became a valuable tool in biomedical research. Several investigators sought antibodies to tumor-specific antigens in animals making an immune response against transplanted tumors, but without success. It was Haldane in 1933 who pointed out that a tumor retains many of the alloantigens of the tissue from which it arises[7]. He further postulated that these alloantigens, rather than tumor-specific antigens, stimulate an immune response in a transplant recipient lacking them. For such a hypothesis to have credibility, it would be necessary to demonstrate blood group antigenic differences among various strains of mice. Regrettably, such information was not available. Peter Gorer (Figure 8), father of modern histocompatibility testing, described four blood group antigens in mice which he designated I, II, III and IV (1936–38)[8–11]. To examine whether an association existed between genes controlling blood groups and those predicted to govern tumor susceptibility, Gorer inoculated A strain carcinoma into A and C57BI mice, their hybrids and back-crosses. He concluded that tumor susceptibility was governed by two or three

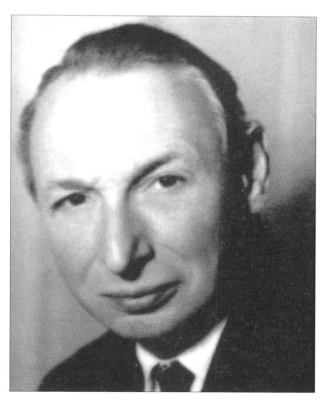

Figure 8   Peter A. Gorer, MD, British pathologist who became father of modern histocompatibility testing based on his description of four blood group antigens in mice

genes, and that one of these was the same as the blood group gene encoding antigen II. This finding led him to the belief that tumor regression in these animals had an immunological basis. The blood sera from animals rejecting the tumor allotransplant contained hemagglutinins specific for red blood cells derived from A strain mice. Thus, antibodies against blood group antigen I represented strong evidence that the tumor tissue expresses antigen II in common with normal tissues. Thus, Gorer's research showed that genes governing susceptibility to tumor allotransplants were the same as those encoding alloantigens. His demonstration that alloantibodies were produced by mice rejecting tumor transplants proved that this process had an immunological basis. Gorer's tissue transplantation concept proposed that both normal and tumor tissues contain genetically determined isoantigens, and that the host makes an immune response against those isoantigens in grafted tissue which the host does not possess.

Peter Alfred Gorer (1907–61) (Figure 6), British pathologist who was professor at Guy's Hospital Medical School, London, where he made major discoveries in transplantation genetics. With Snell, he discovered the H-2 murine histocompatibility complex. Most of his work was in transplantation genetics. He identified antigen II and described its association with tumor rejection. *The Gorer Symposium*. Oxford: Blackwell, 1985.

Medawar (1944–46) and associates (Figures 9 and 10) provided the first convincing proof that the rejection of grafts between individuals who are not related to one another, i.e. allografts or homografts, has an immunological basis[12]. He showed that allogeneic skin grafts heal-in and appear healthy. After several days, however, host lymphoid cells may infiltrate the skin graft and undergo blastogenesis. Twelve days later the allograft may appear necrotic, representing first-set rejection. A second graft of the same donor specificity is rejected at an accelerated rate, i.e. within 6–10 days. This is termed second-set rejection, which represents host sensitivity to transplantation antigens of the graft. During this same period, Ray Owen (Figures 11 and 12) described dizygotic cattle twins in which blood cells of one twin were tolerated immunologically by the other, i.e. they were chimeras[13].

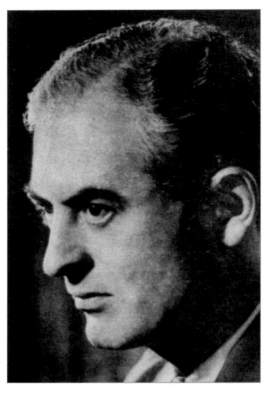

Figure 9 Sir Peter B. Medawar, Nobel Laureate in Medicine or Physiology for his research on immunologic tolerance

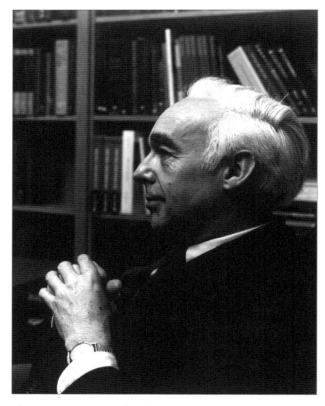

Figure 10 Rupert Billingham, colleague of P. B. Medawar, who also was a pioneer in immunologic tolerance

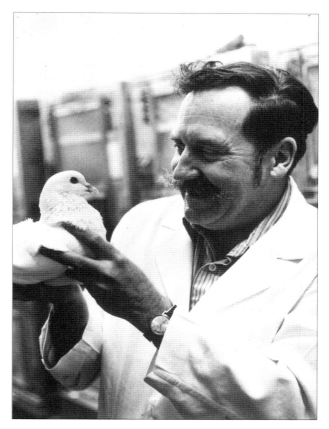

Figure 11 Dr Ray Owen of the University of Wisconsin, who described dizygotic cattle twins in which blood cells of one twin were tolerated immunologically by the other, i.e. they were chimeras

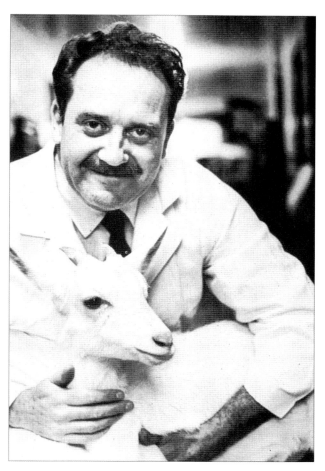

Figure 12 A second view of Dr Owen at work

Ray David Owen (1915–) (Figures 9 and 10), American geneticist who described erythrocyte mosaicism in dizygotic cattle twins. This discovery of reciprocal erythrocyte tolerance contributed to the concept of immunological tolerance. This observation that cattle twins that shared a common fetal circulation were chimeras and could not reject transplants of each other's tissues later in life provided the groundwork for Burnet's ideas about tolerance and Medawar's work in transplantation.

Medawar, Billingham and Brent went on to conduct grafting experiments in which tissues and cells from one strain of mouse were successfully transplanted in recipients of a different strain that had been administered cells bearing donor antigen prior to birth[14]. Their classic paper on acquired immunological tolerance, which was published in *Nature* in 1953[15], demonstrated that sensitization could be transferred passively with specifically sensitized lymphoid cells.

Peter Brian Medawar (1915–87) (Figure 7), British transplantation biologist who received his PhD at Oxford, 1935, where he served as lecturer in zoology. He was subsequently a Professor of Zoology at Birmingham (1947) and at University College, London, 1951. He became Director of the Medical Research Council, 1962 and of the Clinical Research Center at Northwick Park, 1971. Together with Billingham and Brent, he made seminal discoveries in transplantation and immunobiology and described immunological tolerance and its importance for tissue transplantation. He shared the 1960 Nobel Prize in Medicine or Physiology with Sir Frank Macfarlane Burnet.

Although serologically identifiable antibodies are produced in animals rejecting allografts, the demonstration of round cell infiltration (i.e. lymphocytes) in the graft bed suggested to Mitchison that graft rejection was dependent upon lymphoid cells rather than serum antibodies. By taking lymphoid cells from animals rejecting a tumor and injecting them into a recipient never before exposed to the graft, he showed that sensitization against graft antigens could be transferred with specifically immune lymphoid cells but not with serum. Mitchison termed this procedure adoptive immunization[16]. Those investigators who could not accept the idea that lymphoid cells rather than humoral antibodies were responsible for graft rejection postulated that cytophilic antibodies in the serum adsorb to lymphoid cells and confer specific reactivity on them. This subject was explored by Boyden and Sorkin in the 1960s[17].

Meanwhile, Burnet and Fenner, at the Walter and Eliza Hall Institute, were beginning to take a view of antibody production different from that proposed by chemists adhering to the template theory of antibody synthesis.

Their first monograph on *The Production of Antibodies* was published in 1941 and the second edition appeared in 1949[18]. Modifying their views through various explanations that included a self-marker hypothesis to explain antibody production, Burnet noted with interest that Jerne had proposed a selective theory of antibody formation in 1955[19]. Whereas Jerne discussed various antibody populations, Burnet (Figures 13 and 14) applied this natural selection concept, which was the first selective or genetically based theory of immunity since the time of Ehrlich, to a new hypothesis, which he termed the clonal selection theory of acquired immunity, in 1959[20]. The template theory of antibody production, which had been popular with the chemists for so many years could no longer explain these new biological revelations that included immunological tolerance, and it had never explained the secondary (or anamnestic) immune response. Burnet proposed precursor cells with a limited range of specificity for interaction with antigens. Upon stimulation, the precursor cell would proliferate into a clone of cells producing antibody of that specificity. Since that time, various modifications of the clonal selection hypothesis have been offered. Dreyer and Bennett offered a germ line theory[21]. Smithies proposed a half gene concept to explain antibody diversity[22] and Tonegawa won the Nobel Prize for his elegant studies and explanation of the generation of diversity in antibody synthesis[23].

Snell (Figures 15 and 16) in 1948, introduced the term histocompatibility antigens to designate the

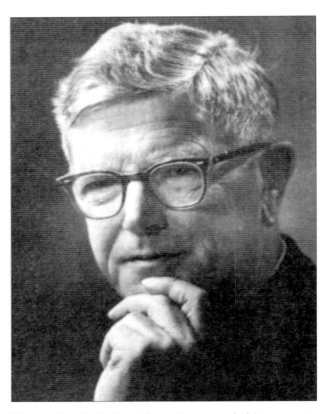

Figure 13 Sir F. Macfarlane Burnet, Nobel Laureate in Medicine, who described the clonal selection theory of acquired immunity

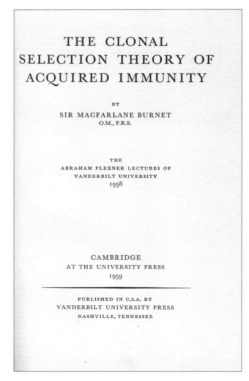

Figure 14 Dr Burnet's famous book describing clonal selection, for which he was awarded the Nobel Prize in Medicine

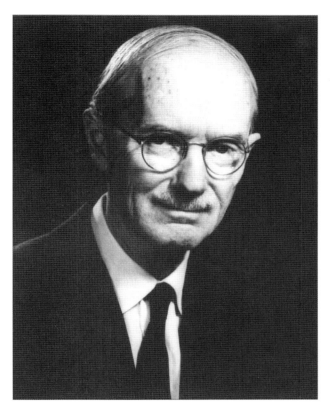

Figure 15 Dr George D. Snell, senior scientist at the Jackson Laboratory, Bar Harbor, ME, who received the Nobel Prize in Medicine for his work on histocompatibility genes, elucidation of complex histocompatibility loci and his development of congenic strains of mice

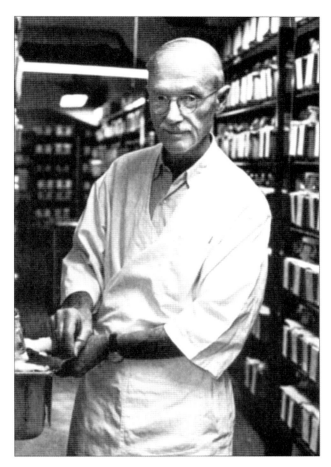

Figure 16 Dr Snell at work in his laboratory

antigenic specificities that confer tissue compatibility[24]. He stated that histocompatibility genes (or H genes) determine these antigens. Snell went on to develop the sophisticated genetic methods required to unravel the mystery of histocompatibility loci. He developed coisogenic (or congenic) strains of mice showing only one H difference. Snell's development of the congenic lines of mice was the most significant event in transplantation biology since the introduction of inbred strains. His careful development of the congenic lines made the mouse the prototype animal in transplantation genetics and immunology[25]. He went on to discover the existence of major (strong) and minor (weak) H genes in mice. The major histocompatibility locus of the mouse was designated H-2 by Snell and co-workers[26]. With the demonstration that more than one gene is present at the H-2 locus, it was called the major histocompatibility complex (MHC) in the mouse. Snell was subsequently awarded the Nobel Prize for his work. Following the success of Snell's histogenetic methods, Gorer in England proceeded to characterize antibodies to H-2

products by serological methods. He and his co-workers employed hemagglutination and cytotoxicity tests[27,28]. Among the group of investigators gathered around Gorer at Guy's Hospital Medical School in London during the 1950s were Bernard Amos, Z. B. Mikulska, O'Gorman, Gustavo Hoecker and Nathan Kaliss, who later made important contributions in immunological enhancement of tumor allografts.

George Davis Snell (1903–) *(*Figures 15 and 16), American geneticist who shared the 1980 Nobel Prize with Jean Dausset and Baruj Benacerraf, 'For their work on genetically determined structures of the cell surface that regulate immunologic reactions'. Snell's major contributions were in the field of mouse genetics, including discovery of the H-2 locus (together with Gorer) and the development of congenic mice. He made many seminal contributions to transplantation genetics and received the Gairdner Award in 1976. *Histocompatibility* (with Dausset and Nathenson), 1976.

Although conceded by all to have attracted a group of brilliant investigators and to represent exquisite scientific methodology and results, the H-2 system was considered by many to be an esoteric topic in biology and medicine. Studies designed to decipher the H-2 system were aimed at clarifying the two-locus model, i.e. H-2K and H-2D, and elucidating the nature and function of I-regions, among others, in the major histocompatibility complex of the mouse[29].

With the discovery of histocompatibility antigens of human leukocytes in 1958 by Dausset[30] (Figure 17) and Rapaport, all of the valuable data garnered by the mouse H-2 researchers took on a new significance. The remarkable similarity between the H-2 of the mouse and the human leukocyte antigen (HLA) of man, and the numerous cross-reactions between the two, provided researchers on human histocompatibility testing with a head start in their attempt to define the immunogenetics of human HLA. A major difference between human and mouse histocompatibility was the need to study large groups of unrelated human subjects, in striking contrast to the inbred strains of mice where numerous genetically identical individuals of a single strain could be tested. Using the leukoagglutination technique, Dausset described the first HLA antigen, designated Mac, which was subsequently identified on platelets by complement fixation[31]. The fortunate demonstration that multiparous women produce antibodies against lymphocytes provided a major source of antibodies for tissue-typing trays used in clinical histocompatibility testing[32]. Dausset's work encouraged Rose Payne to undertake studies of human histocompatibility and immunogenetics in the US. With advances in DNA technology, molecular typing is supplanting serological assays.

Jean Baptiste Gabriel Dausset (1916–) (Figure 17), French physician and investigator. He pioneered research on the HLA system and the immunogenetics of histocompatibility. For this work, he shared a Nobel Prize with Benacerraf and Snell in 1980. He made numerous discoveries in immunogenetics and transplantation biology. *Immunohematologie Biologique et Clinique*, 1956; *HLA and Disease* (with Svejaard), 1977.

Rose Payne (1909–99) (Figure 18), earned her PhD in bacteriology at the University of Washington,

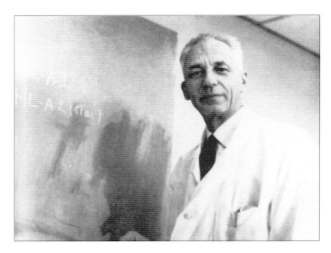

Figure 17 Professor Jean Dausset, who discovered that human leukocyte antigens represented histocompatibility antigens, which serve as a basis for tissue transplantation

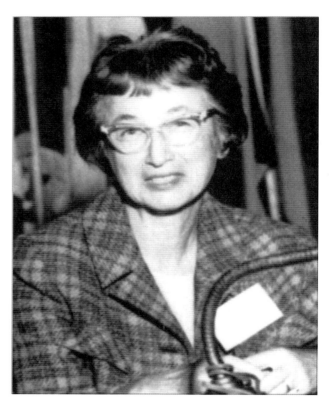

Figure 18 Dr Rose Payne, a pioneer in human histocompatibility

Seattle. She spent her professional career at Stanford where she co-authored an important paper on Evans syndrome, a combination of autoimmune hemolytic anemia and thrombocytopenic purpura. She became an authority on red cell and platelet autoantibodies, and in 1957 found that chill-fever transfusion

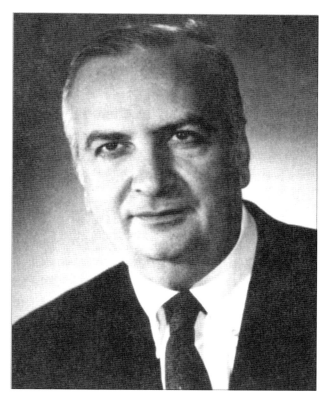
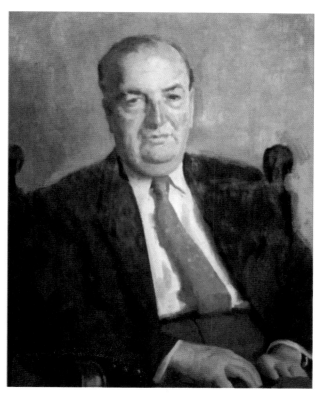

Figure 19   Professor Baruj Benacerraf, Nobel Laureate for his work in immunogenetics

reactions were attributable to patient alloantibodies to donor leukocytes. She also discovered an association between previous pregnancies and the presence of leukoagglutinins, which prompted her to begin an extensive program of serum collection searching for potential typing sera. She and Emanuel Hackel showed that the leukocyte antigens were inherited. Payne and Walter Bodmer identified two alleles from a single locus: LA-1 and LA-2 (HLA-A1 and HLA-A2). Subsequently they reported a third allele at the LA locus (LA-3 or HLA-A3), and additional new antigens. Further definition of HLA antibodies was achieved through International Histocompatibility Workshops.

Baruj Benacerraf (1920–) (Figure 19), American immunologist born in Caracas, Venezuela. Beginning his scientific career studying hypersensitivity mechanisms in Elvin Kabat's laboratory at Columbia, he moved to Paris to investigate reticuloendothelial function in relation to immunity. On returning to the USA, he joined the Pathology faculty at New York University where he resumed experiments on hypersensitivity mechanisms. He investigated cellular hypersensitivity, immune complex disease, anaphylactic hypersensitivity, tumor-specific immunity and the structure of antibodies, in relation to their specificity. He mentored a host of gifted fellows and students at NYU. He initiated immunogenetics studies that led to the observation that random bred animals immunized with antigens with restricted heterogeneity, such as hapten conjugates of poly-L-lysine, distribute themselves into two groups, responders and non-responders. Benacerraf determined that responsiveness to these antigens is controlled by dominant autosomal genes termed immune response (Ir) genes, located in the major histocompatibility complex of mammals. His studies led to understanding of the manner in which these genes exercise their function and determine immune responsiveness. His subsequent work at the National Institutes of Health and at Harvard concerned the role of immune response genes in the regulation of specific immunity and the control of immune suppression, among other investigations. His multiple contributions include the carrier effect in delayed hypersensitivity, lymphocyte subsets, MHC and Ir immunogenetics, for which he shared the

Nobel Prize in 1980 with Jean Dausset and George Snell. Benacerraff and colleagues showed that many of the genes within the MHC control the immune response to various immunogens. Using synthetic polypeptides as antigens, Benacerraf, McDevitt and co-workers demonstrated that immune response Ir genes control an animal's response to a given antigen. These genes were localized in the I region of the MHC. (Benacerraf B, Unanue ER. *Textbook of Immunology*. Baltimore, MD: Williams & Wilkins, 1979.)

In 1964, Bernard Amos (Figure 20) invited a group of HLA researchers to gather for the first workshop on histocompatibility testing in Durham, North Carolina[33]. Although concerned that their methods were contradictory, the international group met again in 1965 in Leiden at the invitation of J. J. van Rood (Figure 21)[34]. Using improved techniques they demonstrated that different human tissue types do indeed exist. Ceppelini organized the third workshop held in Turin, Italy in 1967, where genetic studies using Italian families demonstrated classic Mendelian inheritance of tissue specificities[35]. The fourth workshop organized by Paul Terasaki (Figure 22) was held in Los Angeles in 1970, where the major histocompatibility system of man was clearly established as a result of serological investigations of 300 families[36].

Paul Terasaki (1929–) American immunologist, who began his career in transplantation immunology as a postdoctoral research fellow under Peter Medawar in London in 1957. On returning to UCLA in 1959, he perfected the microcytotoxicity test which was important in identification of the HLA system. He established the usefulness of HLA in cross-matching and detection of presensitization in organ grafting. The principal theme of his research has concerned evaluation of the role of HLA matching in transplantation. His more recent work has been in establishing the role of HLA antibodies in chronic rejection. Terasaki has played a significant international role in tissue typing as Director of Tissue Typing at UCLA and of the Regional Organ Procurement Agency of Southern California. He is one of the world's leading researchers in HLA and transplantation. The company he founded, One Lambda, Inc., has made key contributions to HLA technology.

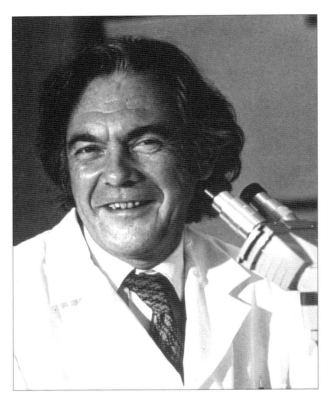

Figure 20 Dr D. Bernard Amos, pioneer in human histocompatibility

J. J. van Rood, of The Netherlands, wrote his MD thesis on leukocyte grouping and techniques. He reported the first two allele systems, which he called 4a and 4b. The 4a and 4b antigens were difficult to define, public antigens shared by many molecules. By testing leukocyte alloantibodies obtained from the sera of a large number of women during pregnancy against leukocytes from 100 unrelated donors, a systematic approach was developed to decipher the complexity of the HLA system. van Rood and associates described nine HLA antigens and a diallelic system not linked to HLA (the group Five system). Balner and van Rood showed that leukocyte antigens were transplantation antigens. Dr van Rood's contributions to HLA research are legion.

Fifty-four human populations studied over the vast reaches of the earth constituted the subject of the fifth workshop sponsored by Dausset in France in 1972[37]. They found that the same genetic laws govern tissue types among divergent populations from remote areas as the ones they had described previously in national or ethnic populations. Kissmeyer-Nielsen (Figure 23) sponsored the sixth histocompatibility or transplantation

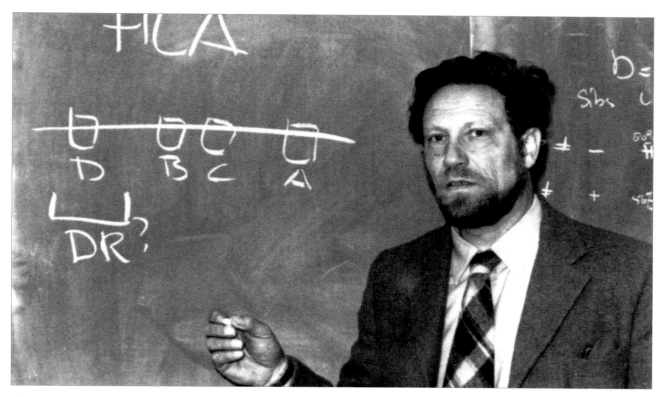

Figure 21   Dr J. J. van Rood, of The Netherlands, pioneer in human histocompatibility genetics

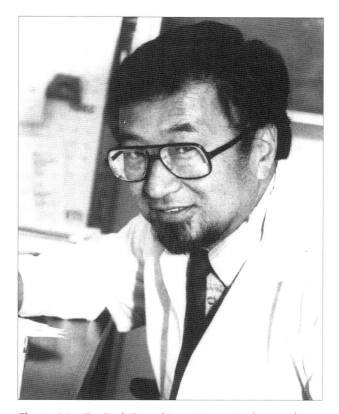

Figure 22   Dr Paul Terasaki, a pioneer in human histocompatibility

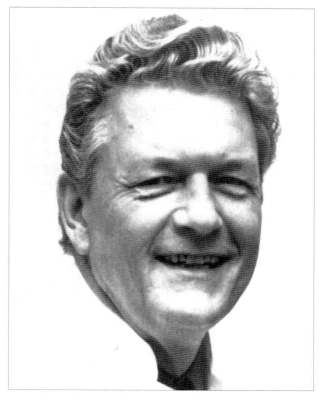

Figure 23   Dr F. Kissmeyer-Nielsen of Aarhus, Denmark, pioneer in genetics of the human leukocyte antigen (HLA) system

workshop in 1975, where six HLA-D alleles were described and the HLA-C locus was demonstrated[38]. Besides genes coding for histocompatibility or transplantation antigens, the major histocompatibility complex in man (i.e. HLA) contains genes that govern specific immunological responsiveness, T and B lymphocyte cooperation and complement components. A seventh workshop was held in Oxford in September 1977, the main theme being the serological investigation and genetics of the Ia determinants and serological studies of specificities of HLA-A, -B and -C loci[39]. Subsequent international workshops have addressed equally important topics in HLA. The eleventh was held in Japan. In addition to the use of clinical histocompatibility testing to predict the success of organ and bone marrrow grafts, many human diseases were found to be associated with certain HLA antigenic specificities. Notable among these associations was the finding that some B-27 positive individuals suffer from ankylosing spondylitis. HLA testing has also found wide application in resolving cases of disputed paternity.

E. Donnall Thomas (1920–) and Joseph E. Murray (1919–)

(Figure 24), recipients of the 1990 Nobel Prize for Medicine or Physiology for their work during the 1950s and 1960s on reducing the risk of organ rejection by the body's immune system. Murray performed the first successful organ transplant in the world, which was a kidney from one identical twin to another, at the Peter Bent Brigham Hospital in 1954. Two years later, Thomas was the first to perform a successful transplant of bone marrow, which he achieved by administering a drug that prevented rejection. The two doctors have made significant discoveries that 'have enabled the development of organ and cell transplantation into a method for the treatment of human disease', said the Nobel Assembly in its citation for the prize.

In subsequent years other organ and tissue transplants were pioneered. Dr James D. Hardy, of the University of Mississippi Medical Center successfully performed the first human lung transplant in 1963. The following year he transplanted a chimpanzee heart, which functioned successfully for 90 minutes, into the chest of a dying man with advanced heart failure. Dr Christian Barnard of South Africa went on to transplant a healthy human heart into a dentist with heart failure. Dr Thomas Starzl of Pittsburgh

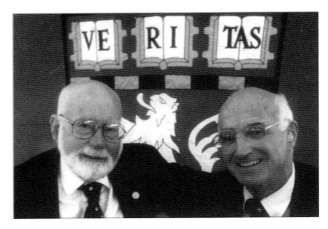

Figure 24 Dr E. Donnall Thomas (left), Nobel Laureate in Medicine for his perfection of bone marrow transplantation, and Dr Joseph Murray, Nobel Lauteate in Medicine for performing the first successful kidney transplant from one identical twin to another

pioneered liver transplantation in 1963. Dr Paul Lacy and colleagues of Washington University in St. Louis perfected islet cell transplantation in the BB rat model of diabetes mellitus.

Rolf Zinkernagel (1944–) and Peter Doherty (1940–)

(Figure 25), recipients of the 1996 Nobel Prize for Medicine or Physiology for their demonstration of MHC restriction. In an investigation of how T lymphocytes protect mice against lymphocytic choriomeningitis virus (LCMV) infection, they found that T cells from mice infected by the virus killed only infected target cells expressing the same major histocompatibility complex (MHC) class I antigens but not those expressing a different MHC allele. In their study, murine cytotoxic T cells (CTLs) would only lyse virus-infected target cells if the effector and target cells were H-2 compatible. This significant finding had broad implications, demonstrating that T cells did not recognize the virus directly but only in conjunction with MHC molecules.

The finding that repeated blood transfusions prior to grafting actually improved the survival of kidney allotransplants, possibly through tolerance induction, led to deliberate transfusions prior to grafting. This assumed lesser importance with the introduction of cyclosporine for immunosuppressive therapy[40]. The best transplant results guaranteeing long-term graft survival were with

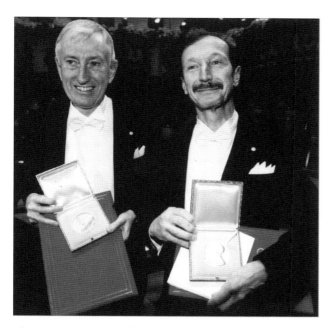

Figure 25 Peter Doherty and Rolf Zinkernagel, Nobel Laureates in Medicine for their work on major histocompatibility complex (MHC) restriction

HLA-A, -B, -DR matching in addition to cyclosporine and subsequent immunosuppressive drug therapy[41].

Immunoregulation refers to control of the immune response usually by its own products, such as the idiotypic network of antibody regulation described by Niels Jerne, feedback inhibition of antibody formation by antibody molecules, T cell receptor interaction with antibodies specific for them, and the effect of immunosuppressive and immunoenhancing cytokines on the immune response, in addition to other mechanisms. It refers to control of both humoral and cellular limbs of the immune response by mechanisms such as antibody feedback inhibition, the immunoglobulin idiotype anti-idiotype network, and helper and suppressor T cells and cytokines. Results of these immunoregulatory interactions may lead to either suppression or potentiation of one or the other limb of the immune response.

Immunological unresponsiveness is characterized by failure to form antibodies or develop a lymphoid cell-mediated response following exposure to immunogen (antigen). Immunosuppression that is specific for only one antigen with no interference with the response to all other antigens is termed immunological tolerance. By contrast, the administration of powerful immunosuppressive agents such as azathioprine, cyclosporine or total body irradiation causes generalized immunological unresponsiveness to essentially all immunogens to which the host is exposed.

Immunological inertia refers to specific immunosuppression related to paternal histocompatibility antigens during pregnancy, such as suppression of maternal immune reactivity against fetal histocompatibility antigens.

Tolerance is an active state of unresponsiveness by lymphoid cells to a particular antigen (tolerogen) as a result of the cells' interaction with that antigen. The immune response to all other immunogens is unaffected. Thus, this is an acquired non-responsiveness to a specific antigen. When inoculated into a fetus or a newborn, an antigenic substance will be tolerated by the recipient in a manner that will prevent manifestations of immunity when the same individual is challenged with this antigen as an adult. This treatment has no suppressive effect on the response to other unrelated antigens. Immunologic tolerance is much more difficult to induce in an adult whose immune system is fully developed. However, it can be accomplished by administering repetitive minute doses of protein antigens or by administering them in large quantities. Mechanisms of tolerance induction have been the subject of numerous investigations, and clonal deletion is one of these mechanisms. Either helper T or B lymphocytes may be inactivated, or suppressor T lymphocytes may be activated, in the process of tolerance induction. In addition to clonal deletion, clonal anergy and clonal balance are among the complex mechanisms proposed to account for self-tolerance in which the animal body accepts its own tissue antigens as self and does not reject them. Nevertheless, certain autoantibodies form under physiologic conditions and are not pathogenic. However, autoimmune phenomena may emerge under disease conditions and play a significant role in the pathogenesis of autoimmune disease.

An immunological adaptation to a specific antigen is distinct from unresponsiveness, which is the genetic or pathologic inability to mount a measurable immune response. Tolerance involves lymphocytes as individual cells, whereas unresponsiveness is an attribute of the whole organism. The humoral or cell-mediated response may be affected individually or at the same time. The genetic form of unresponsiveness has been demonstrated with the immune response to synthetic antigens and has led to characterization of the immune response (Ir) locus of the major histocompatibility complex. The immune response of experimental animals, which are classified as high, intermediate or non-responders, is not defective, but is not reactive to the particular antigen. In some cases, suppressor cells prevent the development of an appropriate response. Unresponsiveness may also be the result of immunodeficiency states, some with clinical expression, or may be induced by immunosuppressive therapy such as that following X-irradiation, chemotherapeutic agents or antilymphocyte sera. Tolerance, as the term is currently used, has a broader connotation and is intended to represent all instances in which an immune response to a given antigen is not demonstrable. Immunologic tolerance refers to a lack of response as a result of prior exposure to antigen.

The **Brester–Cohn theory** maintains that self–notself discrimination occurs at any stage of lymphoreticular development. The concept is based on three principles: engagement of the lymphocyte receptor by antigen provides signal (1), and signal (1) alone is a tolerogenic signal for the lymphocyte; provision of signal (1) in conjunction with signal (2), a costimulatory signal, results in lymphocyte induction; and delivery of signal (2) requires associative recognition of two distinct epitopes on the antigen molecule. The requirement for associative recognition blocks the development of autoimmunity in an immune system where diversity is generated randomly throughout an individual's lifetime.

Immunologic tolerance is an active but carefully regulated response of lymphocytes to self antigens. Autoantibodies are formed against a variety of selfantigens. Maintenance of self-tolerance is a quantitative process. When comparing the case with which T and B cell tolerance may be induced, it was found that T cell tolerance is induced more rapidly and is longer lasting than B cell tolerance. For example, T cell tolerance may be induced in a single day, whereas B cells may require 10 days for induction. In addition, 100 times more tolerogen may be required for B cell tolerance than for T cell tolerance.

Adoptive tolerance is the passive transfer of immunologic tolerance with lymphoid cells from an animal tolerant to that antigen to a previously non-tolerant and irradiated recipient host animal.

Tolerogen is an antigen that is able to induce immunologic tolerance. The production of tolerance rather than immunity in response to antigen depends on such variables as physical state of the antigen, i.e. soluble or particulate, route of administration, level of maturation of the recipient's immune system or immunologic competence. For example, soluble antigens administered intravenously will favor tolerance in many situations, as opposed to particulate antigens injected into the skin which might favor immunity. Immunologic tolerance with cells is easier to induce in the fetus or neonate than it is in adult animals, who would be more likely to develop immunity rather than tolerance.

Self-tolerance is a term used to describe the body's acceptance of its own epitopes as self antigens (Figure 26). The body is tolerant to these autoantigens, which are exposed to the lymphoid cells of the host immune system. Tolerance to self antigens is developed during fetal life. Thus, the host is immunologically tolerant to self- or autoantigens. Self-tolerance is due mainly to inactivation or killing of self-reactive lymphocytes induced by exposure to selfantigens. Failure of self-tolerance in the normal immune system may lead to autoimmune diseases (refer also to tolerance and to immunologic tolerance).

Clonal deletion (negative selection) refers to the elimination of self-reactive T lymphocyte in the thymus during the development of natural self-tolerance. T cells recognize self antigens only in the context of major histocompatibility complex (MHC) molecules. Autoreactive thymocytes are eliminated following contact with self antigens expressed in the thymus before maturation is completed. The majority of CD4[+] T lymphocytes in the blood circulation that survived clonal deletion in the thymus failed to respond to any stimulus. This reveals that clonal anergy participates in suppression of autoimmunity. Clonal deletion represents a critical mechanism to rid the body of autoreactive T lymphocytes. This is brought about by minor lymphocyte stimulation (mls) antigens that interact with the T cell receptor's Vβ

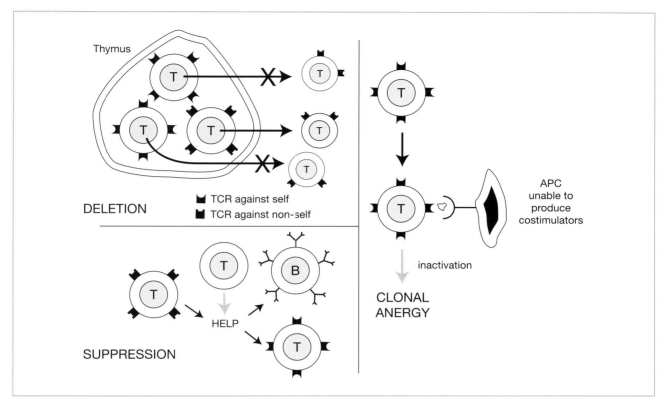

Figure 26   Schematic representation of the mechanism of self-tolerance. TCR, T cell receptor; APC, antigen-presenting cell

region of the T lymphocyte receptor, thereby mimicking the action of bacterial superantigen. Intrathymic and peripheral tolerance in T lymphocytes can be accounted for by clonal deletion and functional inactivation of T cells reactive against self.

Acquired tolerance is induced by the inoculation of a neonate or fetus *in utero* with allogeneic cells prior to maturation of the recipient's immune response (Figure 27). The inoculated antigens are accepted as self. Immunologic tolerance may be induced to some soluble antigens by low-dose injections of neonates with the antigen, or to older animals by larger doses, the so-called low-dose and high-dose tolerance, respectively.

High-dose tolerance is specific immunologic unresponsiveness induced in immunocompetent adult animals by the repeated administration of large doses of antigen (tolerogen), if the substance is a protein. A massive single dose is administered if the substance is a polysaccharide. Although no precise inducing dose of antigen can be defined, in high-dose tolerance the antigen (Ag) level usually exceeds

10^{-4} mol Ag per kilogram of body weight. This is also called high-zone tolerance.

High-zone tolerance is antigen-induced specific immunosuppression with relatively large doses of protein antigens (tolerogens). B cell tolerance usually requires high antigen doses. High-zone tolerance is relatively short-lived. It is also called high-dose tolerance (refer to high-dose tolerance).

Low-dose (or low-zone) tolerance is an antigen-specific immunosuppression induced by the administration of antigen in a suboptimal dose. Low-dose tolerance is achieved easily in the neonatal period, in which the lymphoid cells of the animal are not sufficiently mature to mount an antibody or cell-mediated immune response. This renders helper T lymphocytes tolerant, thereby inhibiting them from signaling B lymphocytes to respond to immunogenic challenge. Although no precise inducing dose of antigen can be defined, in low-dose tolerance 10^{-8} mol Ag per kilogram of body weight is usually effective. Low-dose tolerance is relatively long-lasting. This is also called low-zone tolerance.

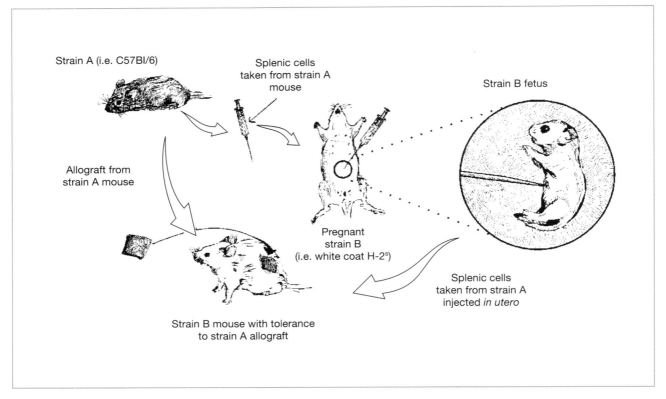

Strain A (i.e. C57Bl/6)

Splenic cells taken from strain A mouse

Strain B fetus

Allograft from strain A mouse

Pregnant strain B (i.e. white coat H-2^s)

Splenic cells taken from strain A injected *in utero*

Strain B mouse with tolerance to strain A allograft

Figure 27   Acquired immunologic tolerance

Central tolerance is the mechanism involved in the functional inactivation of cells requisite for the initiation of an immune response. Central tolerance affects the afferent limb of the immune response, which is concerned with sensitization and cell proliferation. It is established in lymphocytes developing in central lymphoid organs, and prevents the emergence of lymphocytes with high-affinity receptors for self antigens present in bone marrow or thymus.

Peripheral tolerance is involved in the inhibition of expression of the immune response. The cells delivering the actual response are functionally impaired, but not defective. Peripheral tolerance affects the efferent limb of the immune response which is concerned with the generation of effector cells.

Mechanisms that interfere with maturation or stimulation of lymphocytes with the potential for reacting with self include self-tolerance, which is acquired and not inherited. Lymphocytes reactive with self may either be inhibited from responding to self or inactivated upon combination with self antigens. Self-tolerance may involve both central and peripheral tolerance. In central tolerance, immature lymphocytes

capable of reacting with self encounter self antigen producing tolerance instead of activation. By contrast, peripheral tolerance involves the interaction of mature self-reactive lymphocytes with self antigens in peripheral tissues if the lymphocytes are under conditions that promote tolerance instead of activation. Clonal deletion and clonal anergy are also principal mechanisms of tolerance in clones of lymphocytes reactive with self antigens.

Control tolerance refers to the mechanism that involves the absence or functional inactivation of cells requisite for the initiation of an immune response. These cells are defective or inactivated. Control tolerance affects the afferent limb of the immune response, which is concerned with sensitization and cell proliferation.

Clonal ignorance may also play a role that is yet ill-defined. Tolerance of T or B lymphocytes reactive with self antigen may also contribute to tolerance to self proteins. Properties of self antigens that render them tolerogenic and govern their ability to induce central or peripheral tolerance include self-antigen concentration and persistence in the formative lymphoid organs, the type and strength of signals that self antigens activate in lymphocytes and the ability to recognize antigens in the absence of costimulators.

T cell tolerance to self antigens involves the processing and presentation of self proteins complexed with major histocompatibility complex (MHC) molecules on antigen-presenting cells of the thymus. The interaction of immature T cells in the thymus with self-peptide–MHC molecules leads to either clonal deletion or clonal anergy. Through this mechanism of negative selection, the T lymphocytes exiting the thymus are tolerant to self antigens. Tolerance of T cells to tissue antigens not represented in the thymus is maintained by peripheral tolerance. It is attributable to clonal anergy in which antigen-presenting cells recognize antigen in the absence of costimulation. Thus, cytokines are not activated to stimulate a T cell response. The activation of T lymphocytes by high antigen concentration may lead to their death through Fas-mediated apoptosis. Regulatory T lymphocytes may also suppress the reactivity of T lymphocytes specific for self antigens. Interleukin (IL)-10 or transforming growth factor (TGF)-β or some other immunosuppressive cytokine produced by T lymphocytes reactive with self may facilitate tolerance. Clonal ignorance may also be important in preventing autoimmune reactivity to self.

B cell tolerance is manifested as a decreased number of antibody-secreting cells following antigenic stimulation, compared with a normal response. Hapten-specific tolerance can be induced by inoculation of deaggregated haptenated gamma globulins (Ig). Induction of tolerance requires membrane Ig cross-linking. Tolerance may have a duration of 2 months in B cells of the bone marrow and 6–8 months in T cells. Whereas prostaglandin E enhances tolerance induction, IL-1, lipopolysaccharide (LPS), or 8-bromoguanosine block tolerance instead of an immunogenic signal. Tolerant mice carry a normal complement of hapten-specific B cells. Tolerance is not attributable to a diminished number or isotype of antigen receptors. It has also been shown that the six normal activation events related to membrane Ig turnover and expression do not occur in tolerant B cells. Whereas tolerant B cells possess a limited capacity to proliferate, they fail to do so in response to antigen. Antigenic challenge of tolerant B cells induces them to enlarge and increase expression, yet they are apparently deficient in a physiologic signal requisite for progression into a proliferative stage.

Much of the understanding of B cell tolerance to self has been developed through models that permit the investigation of B cell development and function following exposure to self antigen in the absence of T cell help. Both central and peripheral mechanisms may be involved in B lymphocyte tolerance to self-antigens. The amount and valence of antigens in the bone marrow control the fate of immature B lymphocytes specific for these self antigens. Concentrated antigens that are multivalent may cause death of B lymphocytes. Other B cells specific for self antigens may survive to maturity following interaction with specific antigen, but are permanently barred from migration to lymphoid follicles in the peripheral lymphoid tissues. Therefore, they do not respond to antigen in peripheral lymphoid sites. Soluble self antigens in lower concentrations may interact with B cells to produce anergy, which could be attributable to diminished membrane Ig receptor expression on B lymphocytes or a failure in transmission of activation signals following interaction of antigen with its receptor. Thus, the power of the signal induced by antigen may determine the fate. In brief, larger concentrations of multivalent antigen may lead to unresponsiveness.

If specific helper T lymphocytes are absent in peripheral lymphoid tissues, mature B cells may interact with self antigen there to become tolerant. Following interaction with antigen, some B lymphocytes may be unable to activate tyrosine kinases and others may diminish their antigen receptor expression after they have interacted with self antigen. Exposure to self antigen fails to cause self-reactive B lymphocyte proliferation or increased expression of costimulators. These B cells also fail to become activated when aided by T cells. Other B cells may become blocked from terminal differentiation into antibody-forming cells following reaction with self antigens. B cells capable of reacting with self may remain inactive in the absence of helper T cell activity.

B lymphocyte tolerance refers to immunologic non-reactivity of B lymphocytes induced by relatively large doses of antigen. It has a relatively short duration. By contrast, T cell tolerance requires less antigen and is of a longer duration. Exclusive B cell tolerance leaves T cells immunoreactive and unaffected.

Lymphocyte anergy refers to the failure of clones of T or B lymphocytes to react to antigen and may represent a mechanism to maintain immunologic tolerance to self. It is also called clonal anergy. Antigen stimulation of a lymphocyte without costimulation leads to tolerance.

Clonal anergy is the interaction of immune system cells with an antigen, without a second antigen signal, of the type usually needed for a response to an immunogen. This leads to functional inactivation of the immune system cells in contrast to the development of antibody formation or cell-mediated immunity. Clonal ignorance refers to lymphocytes that survive the principal mechanisms of self-tolerance and remain functionally competent but are unresponsive to self antigens and do not cause autoimmune reactions.

It is convenient to describe **clonal balance** as an alteration in the helper/suppressor ratio with a slight predominance of helper activity. Factors that influence the balance of helper/suppressor cells include aging, steroid hormones, viruses and chemicals. The genetic constitution of the host and the mechanism of antigen presentation are the two most significant factors that govern clonal balance. Immune response genes associated with MHC determine class II MHC antigen expression on cells presenting antigen to helper CD4$^+$ lymphocytes. Thus, the MHC class II genotype may affect susceptibility to autoimmune disease. Other genes may be active as well. Antigen presentation exerts a major influence on the generation of an autoimmune response. Whereas a soluble antigen administered intravenously with an appropriate immunologic adjuvant may induce an autoimmune response leading to immunopathologic injury, the same antigen administered intravenously without the adjuvant may induce no detectable response. Animals rendered tolerant to foreign antigens possess suppressor T lymphocytes associated with the induced unresponsiveness. Thus, self-tolerance could be due, in part, to the induction of suppressor T cells. This concept is called clonal balance rather than clonal deletion. Self antigens are considered normally to induce mostly suppressor rather than helper T cells leading to a negative suppressor balance in the animal body. Three factors with the potential to suppress immune reactivity against self include non-antigen-specific suppressor T cells, antigen-specific suppressor T cells and anti-idiotypic antibodies. Suppressor T lymphocytes may leave the thymus slightly before the corresponding helper T cells. Suppressor T cells specific for self antigens are postulated to be continuously stimulated and usually in greater numbers than the corresponding helper T cells.

Sulzberger–Chase phenomenon refers to the induction of immunological unresponsiveness to skin-sensitizing chemicals such as picryl chloride by feeding an animal (e.g. guinea pig) the chemical in question prior to application to the skin. Intravenous administration of the chemical may also block the development of delayed-type hypersensitivity when the same chemical is later applied to the skin. Simple chemicals such as picryl chloride may induce contact hypersensitivity when applied to the skin of guinea pigs. The unresponsiveness may be abrogated by adoptive immunization of a tolerant guinea pig with lymphocytes from one that has been sensitized by application of the chemical to the skin without prior oral feeding.

Anergy refers to diminished or absent delayed-type hypersensitivity, i.e. type IV hypersensitivity, as revealed by lack of responsiveness to commonly used skin test antigens including purified protein derivative (PPD), histoplasmin, candidin, etc. Decreased skin test reactivity may be associated with uncontrolled infection, tumor, Hodgkin's disease, sarcoidosis, etc. There is decreased capacity of T lymphocytes to secrete lymphokines when their T cell receptors interact with a specific antigen. Anergy describes non-responsiveness to antigen. Individuals are anergic when they cannot develop a delayed-type hypersensitivity reaction following challenge with an antigen. T and B lymphocytes are anergic when they cannot respond to their specific antigen.

Immunological ignorance is a type of tolerance to self in which a target antigen and lymphocytes capable of reacting with it are both present simultaneously in an individual without an autoimmune reaction occurring. The abrogation of immunologic ignorance may lead to autoimmune disease.

Immunologic (or immune) paralysis is an immunologic unresponsiveness induced by the injection of large doses of pneumococcal polysaccharide into mice, where it is metabolized slowly. Any antibody that is formed is consumed and not detectable. The pneumococcal polysaccharide antigen remained in tissues of the recipient for months, during which time the animals produced no immune response to the antigen. Immunologic paralysis is much easier to induce with polysaccharide than with protein antigens. It is highly specific for the antigen used for its induction. Felton's first observation of immunologic paralysis preceded the demonstration of acquired immunologic tolerance by Medawar and associates.

Infectious tolerance was described in the 1970s. Animals rendered tolerant to foreign antigens were found to possess suppressor T lymphocytes associated with the induced unresponsiveness. Thus, self tolerance was postulated to be based on the induction of suppressor T cells. Rose has referred to this concept as clonal balance rather than clonal deletion. Self antigens are considered normally to induce mostly suppressor rather than helper T cells, leading to a negative suppressor balance in the animal body. Three factors with the potential to suppress immune reactivity against self include non-antigen-specific suppressor T cells, antigen-specific suppressor T cells and anti-idiotypic antibodies. Rose suggested that suppressor T lymphocytes leave the thymus slightly before the corresponding helper T cells. Suppressor T cells specific for self antigens are postulated to be continuously stimulated and usually in greater numbers than the corresponding helper T cells.

Immunosuppression describes either the deliberate administration of drugs such as cyclosporine, azathioprine, corticosteroids, FK506 or rapamycin; the administration of specific antibody; the use of irradiation to depress immune reactivity in recipients of organ or bone marrow allotransplants; and the profound depression of the immune response that occurs in patients with certain diseases such as acquired immunodeficiency syndrome in which the helper/inducer (CD4$^+$) T lymphocytes are destroyed by human immunodeficiency virus type 1 (HIV-1). In addition to these examples of non-specific immunosuppression, antigen-induced specific immunosuppression is associated with immunologic tolerance.

Immunosuppressive agents include drugs such as cyclosporine, FK506, rapamycin, azathioprine or corticosteroids; antibodies such as antilymphocyte globulin; and irradiation. These produce mild to profound depression of a host's ability to respond to an immunogen (antigen), as in the conditioning of an organ allotransplant recipient. Substances that inhibit adaptive immune responses may be used also to treat autoimmune diseases.

Cyclosporine (cyclosporin A) (ciclosporin) is a cyclic endecapeptide of 11 amino acid residues isolated from soil fungi, which has revolutionized organ transplantation (Figure 28). Rather than acting as a cytotoxic agent, which defines the activity of a number of currently available immmunosuppressive drugs, cyclosporine (CSA) produces an immunomodulatory effect principally on the helper/inducer (CD4) lymphocytes which orchestrate the generation of an immune response. A cyclic polypeptide, CSA blocks T cell help for both humoral and cellular immunity. A primary mechanism of action is its ability to suppress interleukin-2 (IL-2) synthesis. It fails to block activation of antigen-specific suppressor T cells, and thereby assists development of antigen-specific tolerance. Side-effects include nephrotoxicity and hepatotoxicity, with a possible increase in B cell lymphomas. Some individuals may also develop hypertension. CSA's mechanism of action appears to include inhibition of the synthesis and release of lymphokines and alteration of expression of MHC gene products on the cell surface. CSA inhibits IL-2 mRNA formation. This does not affect IL-2 receptor expression on the cell surface. Although CSA may diminish the number of low-affinity binding sites, it does not appear to alter high-affinity binding sites on the cell surface. CSA inhibits the early increase in cytosolic-free calcium, which occurs in beginning activation of normal T lymphocytes. It appears to produce its effect in the cytoplasm rather than on the cell surface of a lymphocyte. This could be due to its ability to dissolve in the

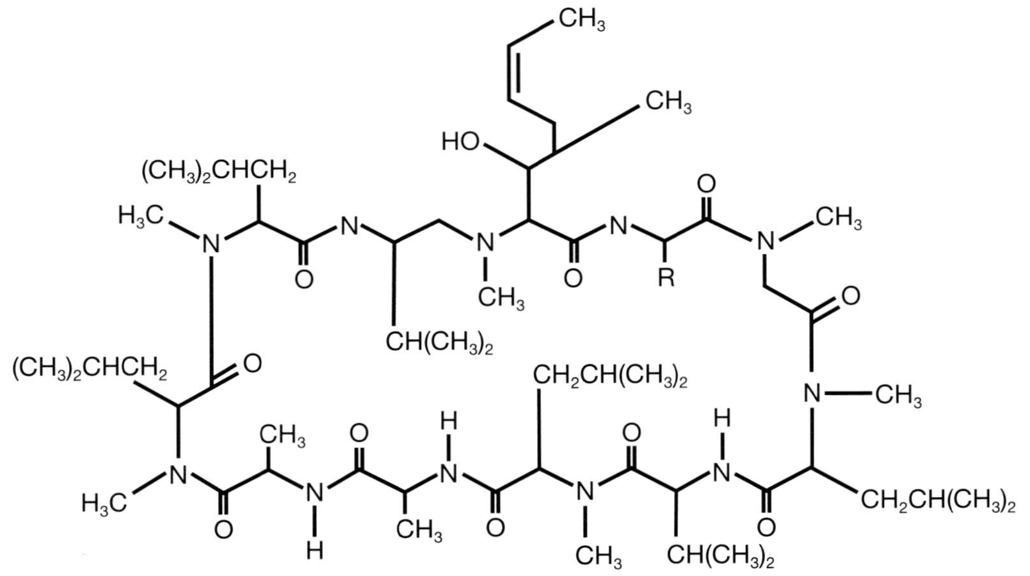

Figure 28 Structure of cyclosporine

plasma membrane lipid bilayer. CSA's cytosolic site of action may involve calmodulin and/or cyclophilin, a protein kinase.

Although immunosuppressive action cannot be explained based upon CSA–calmodulin interaction, this association closely parallels the immunosuppressive effect. CSA produces a greater suppressive effect upon class II than upon class I antigen expression in at least some experiments. While decreasing T helper lymphocytes, the T suppressor cells appear to be spared following CSA therapy. Not only sparing, but amplification of T lymphocyte suppression has been reported during CSA therapy. This is a powerful immunosuppressant that selectively affects $CD4^+$ helper T cells without altering the activity of suppressor T cells, B cells, granulocytes and macrophages. It alters lymphocyte function, but it does not destroy the cells. CSA's principal immunosuppressive action is to inhibit IL-2 production and secretion. Thus, the suppression of IL-2 impairs the development of suppressor and cytotoxic T lymphocytes that are antigen specific. It has a synergistic immunosuppressive action with corticosteroids. Corticosteroids interfere with IL-2 synthesis by inhibiting IL-1 release from monocytes and macrophages. Cyclosporine, although water insoluble, has been successfully employed as a clinical immunosuppressive agent principally in preventing rejection of organ and tissue allotransplants including kidney, heart, lung, pancreas and bone marrow. It has also been successful in preventing graft-versus-host reactions. The drug has some nephrotoxic properties, which may be kept to a minimum by dose reduction. As with other long-term immunosuppressive agents, there may be an increased risk of lymphoma development such as Epstein–Barr virus (EBV) associated B cell lymphomas.

Immunophilins are high-affinity receptor proteins in the cytoplasm that combine with such immunosuppressants as cyclosporine A, FK-506 and rapamycin. They prevent the activity of rotamase by blocking conversion between *cis-* and *trans-*rotamers of the peptide and protein substrate peptidyl–prolylamide bond. Immunophilins are important in transducing signals from the cell surface to the nucleus. Immunosuppressants have been postulated to prevent signal transduction mediated by T lymphocyte receptors, which blocks nuclear factor activation in activated T lymphocytes. Cyclophilin- and FK506-binding proteins represent immunophilins. Drug-immunophilin complexes are implicated in the mechanism of action of the immunosuppressant drugs, cyclosporine, FK506 and rapamycin.

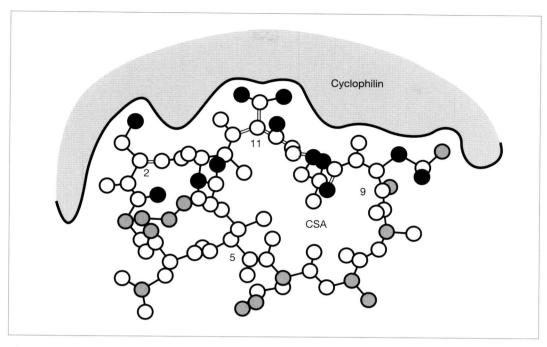

Figure 29   Cyclosporine (CSA) bound to cyclophilin

Cyclophilin is an 18-kDa protein in the cytoplasm that has peptidyl–prolyl isomerase functions. It has a unique and conserved amino acid sequence that has a broad phylogenetic distribution. It represents a protein kinase with a postulated critical role in cellular activation. It serves as a catalyst in *cis-trans*-rotamer interconversion. It catalyzes phosphorylation of a substrate, which then serves as a cytoplasmic messenger associated with gene activation. Genes encoding the synthesis of lymphokines would be activated in helper T lymphocyte responsiveness. Cyclophilin has a high affinity for cyclosporine (CSA), which accounts for the drug's immunosuppressive action (Figure 29). Inhibition of cyclophilin-mediated activities as a consequence of CSA–cyclophilin interaction could lead to inhibition of the synthesis and release of lymphokines. CSA not only inhibits primary immunization, but may halt an ongoing immune response. This has been postulated to occur through inhibition of continued lymphokine release and by suppression of continued effector cell activation and recruitment.

Tacrolimus   Refer to FK506.

FK506 (Figure 30) is a powerful immunosuppressive agent synthesized by *Streptomyces tsukubaensis*. Its principal use is for immunosuppression to prevent transplant rejection. FK506 has been used experimentally in liver transplant recipients. It interferes with the synthesis and binding of IL-2 and resembles cyclosporine, with which it may be used synergistically. Its immunosuppressive properties are 50 times greater than those of cyclosporine. It has been used in renal allotransplantation, but like cyclosporine also produces nephrotoxicity. It also has some neurotoxic effects and may have diabetogenic potential. The drug continues to be under investigation and is awaiting Food and Drug Administration (FDA) approval. It is also called tacrolimus.

FKBP (FK-binding proteins) is a protein that binds FK506. It is a rotamase enzyme with an amino acid sequence that closely resembles that of protein kinase C. It serves as a receptor for both FK506 and rapamycin. Cyclophilins that bind tacrolimus (FK506) are FK-binding proteins.

Rapamycin (Figure 31) is a powerful immunosuppressive drug derived from a soil fungus on Rapa Nui on Easter Island. It resembles FK506 in structure, but it has a different mechanism of action. Rapamycin suppresses B and T lymphocyte proliferation, lymphokine synthesis and T cell responsiveness to IL-2. To achieve clinical immunosuppression, rapamycin

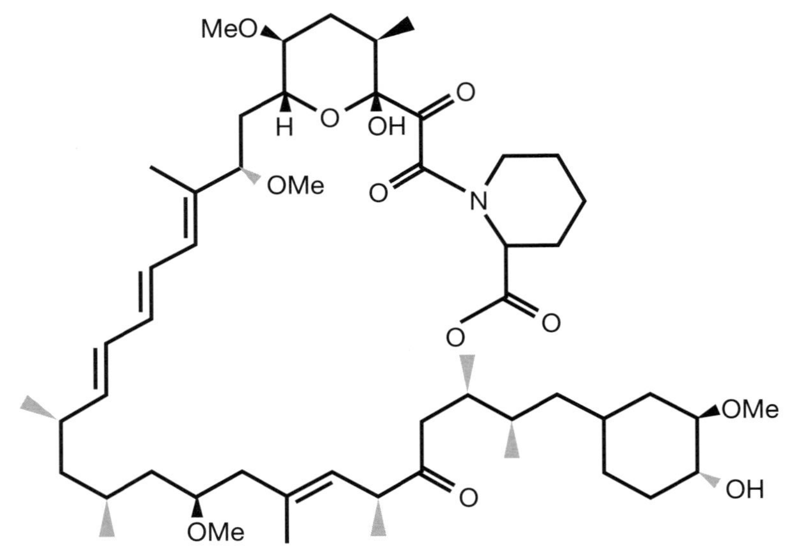

Figure 30 Structure of FK506

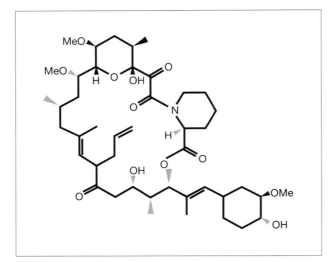

Figure 31 Structure of rapamycin

is effective at concentrations one-eighth of those required for FK506 and at 1% of the levels required for cyclosporine.

Sirolimus is the drug name for rapamycin.

Mycophenolate mofetil (Figure 32) is a new immunosuppressive drug that induces reversible antiproliferative effects specifically on lymphocytes, but does not induce renal, hepatic and neurologic toxi-

city. Its action is based on the fact that adequate amounts of guanosine and deoxyguanosine nucleotides are requisite for lymphocytes to proliferate following antigenic stimulation. Thus, an agent that reversibly inhibits the final steps in purine synthesis, leading to a depletion of guanosine and deoxyguanosine nucleotides, could induce effective immunosuppression. Mycophenolate mofeteil was found to produce these effects. It is the morpholinoethyl ester of mycophenolic acid. *In vivo*, it is hydrolyzed to the active form, mycophenolic acid, which the liver converts to mycophenolic acid glucuronide that is biologically inactive and is excreted in the urine. Mycophenolate blocks proliferation of peripheral blood mononuclear cells of humans to both B and T cell mitogens. It also blocks antibody formation, as evidenced by the inhibition of a recall response by human cells challenged with tetanus toxoid. Its ability to block glycosylation of adhesion molecules that facilitate leukocyte attachment to endothelial cells and target cells probably diminishes recruitment of lymphocytes and monocytes to sites of rejection or chronic inflammation. It does not affect neutrophil chemotaxis, microbicidal activity or supraoxide production. *In vivo*, mycophenolate prevents cytotoxic T cell generation and rejection of allergeneic cells. It inhibits antibody formation in a dose-dependent

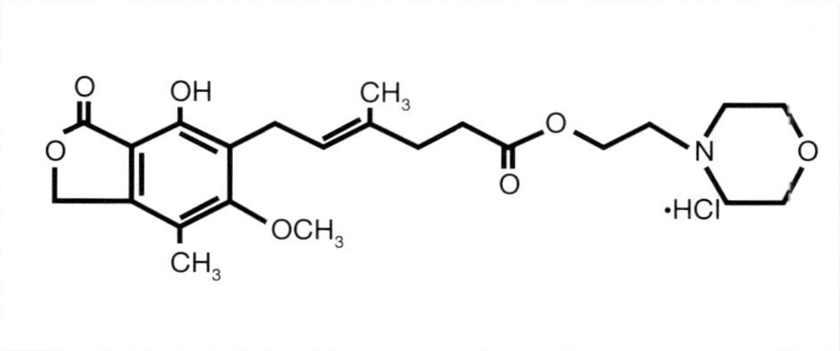

Figure 32 Structure of mycophenolate mofetil

manner and effectively prevents allograft rejection in animal models, especially when used in conjunction with cyclosporine. Current data suggest that the use of mycophenolate, together with cyclosporine and prednisone, leads to less allograft rejection than is achieved with combinations of these drugs without mycophenolate.

Antithymocyte globulin (ATG) is the globulin fraction of serum containing antibodies generated through immunization of animals such as rabbits or horses with human thymocytes. It has been used clinically to treat rejection episodes in organ transplant recipients.

Muromonab® OKT®3 (Orthoclone OKT®3) is a commercial mouse monoclonal antibody against the T cell surface marker CD3 (Figure 33). It may be used therapeutically to diminish T cell reactivity in organ allotransplant recipients experiencing a rejection episode; OKT3 may act in concert with the complement system to induce T cell lysis, or may act as an opsonin, rendering T cells susceptible to phagocytosis. Rarely, recirculating T lymphocytes are removed in patients experiencing rejection crisis by thoracic duct drainage or extracorporeal irradiation of the blood. Plasma exchange is useful for temporary reduction in circulating antibody levels in selective diseases, such as hemolytic disease of the newborn, myasthenia gravis or Goodpasture's syndrome. Immunosuppressive drugs act on all of the T and B cell maturation processes.

Transplantation is the replacement of an organ or other tissue, such as bone marrow, with organs or tissues derived ordinarily from a non-self source such as an allogeneic donor. Organs include kidney, liver, heart, lung, pancreas (including pancreatic islets),

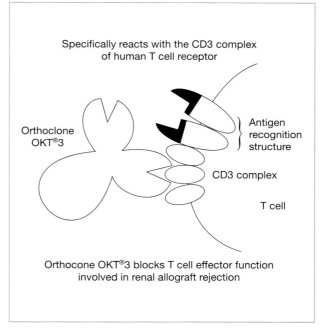

Figure 33 OKT®3 bound to the CD3 complex of a T cell receptor

intestine or skin. In addition, bone matrix and cardiac valves have been transplanted. Bone marrow transplants are given for non-malignant conditions such as aplastic anemia, as well as to treat certain leukemias and other malignant diseases.

Transplantation immunology is the study of immunologic reactivity of a recipient to transplanted organs or tissues from a histoincompatible recipient. Effector mechanisms of transplantation rejection or transplantation immunity consist of cell-mediated immunity and/or humoral antibody immunity, depending upon the category of rejection. For example, hyperacute rejection of an organ such as a renal allograft is mediated by preformed antibodies and takes place soon after the vascular anastomosis is completed in transplantation. By contrast, acute allograft rejection is mediated principally by T lymphocytes and occurs during the first week after transplantation. There are instances of humoral vascular rejection mediated by antibodies as a part of the acute rejection in response. Chronic rejection is mediated by a cellular response.

Histocompatibility is tissue compatibility, as in the transplantation of tissues or organs from one member to another of the same species, an allograft, or from one species to another, a xenograft. The genes that encode antigens which should match if a tissue or organ graft is to survive in the recipient are located in the major histocompatibility complex (MHC) region. This is located on the short arm of chromosome 6 in man (Figures 34 and 35) and of chromosome 17 in the mouse (Figure 36). Class I and class II MHC antigens are important in tissue transplantation. The greater is the match between donor and recipient, the more likely the transplant is to survive. For example, a six-antigen match implies sharing of two HLA-A antigens, two HLA-B antigens and two HLA-DR antigens between donor and recipient. Even though antigenically dissimilar grafts may survive when a powerful immunosuppressive drug such as cyclosporine is used, the longevity of the graft is still improved by having as many antigens match as possible.

A **histocompatibility locus** is a specific site on a chromosome where the histocompatibility genes that encode histocompatibility antigens are located. There are major histocompatibility loci such as HLA in man and H-2 in the mouse, across which incompatible grafts are rejected within 1–2 weeks. There are also several minor histocompatibility loci, with more subtle antigenic differences, across which only slow, low-level graft rejection reactions occur.

Histocompatibility antigen is one of a group of genetically encoded antigens present on tissue cells of an animal that provoke a rejection response if the tissue containing them is transplanted to a genetically dissimilar recipient. These antigens are detected by typing lymphocytes on which they are expressed. They are encoded in man by genes at the HLA locus on the short arm of chromosome 6. In the mouse, they are encoded by genes at the H-2 locus on chromosome 17.

The **minor histocompatibility locus** is a chromosomal site of genes that encode minor histocompatibility antigens that stimulate immune responses against grafts containing these antigens.

Minor histocompatibility antigens are molecules expressed on cell surfaces that are encoded by the minor histocompatibility loci, not the major histocompatibility

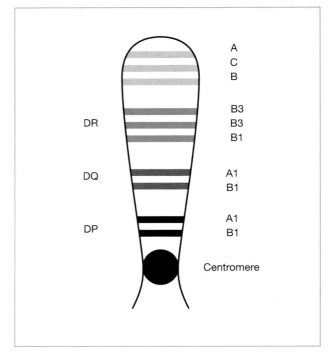

Figure 34 Human chromosome 6

locus. They represent weak transplantation antigens by comparison with the major histocompatibilty antigens. However, they are multiple, and their cumulative effect may contribute considerably to organ or tissue graft rejection. Graft rejection based on a minor histocompatibility difference between donor and recipient requires several weeks, compared with the 7–10 days required for a major histocompatibility difference. Minor histocompatibility antigens may be difficult to identify by serological methods.

Histocompatibility testing is a determination of the MHC class I and class II tissue type of both donor and recipient prior to organ or tissue transplantation. In man, HLA-A, HLA-B and HLA-DR types are determined, followed by cross-matching donor lymphocytes with recipient serum prior to transplantation. A mixed lymphocyte culture (MLC) was formerly used in bone marrow transplantation, but has now been replaced by molecular DNA typing. The MLC may also be requested in living related organ transplants. As in renal allotransplantation, organ recipients have their serum samples tested for percentage reactive antibodies, which reveals whether or not they have been presensitized against HLA of an organ for which they may be the recipient.

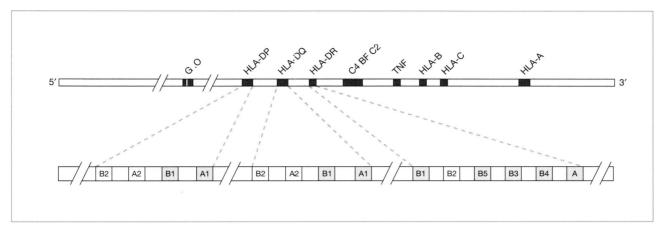

Figure 35   Short arm of human chromosome 6

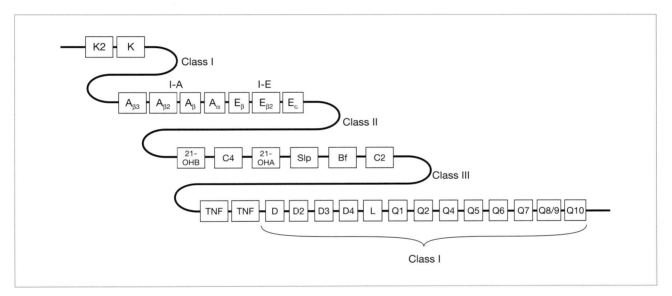

Figure 36   H-2 complex on chromosome 17 of a mouse

Human leukocyte antigen (HLA) is the product of the major histocompatibility complex in humans that contains the genes that encode the polymorphic MHC class I and class II molecules as well as other important genes.

HLA is an abbreviation for human leukocyte antigen. The HLA histocompatibility system in humans represents a complex of MHC class I molecules, distributed on essentially all nucleated cells of the body, and MHC class II molecules that are distributed on B lymphocytes, macrophages and a few other cell types. These are encoded by genes at the major histocompatibility complex. In humans the HLA locus is found on the short arm of chromosome 6. This has now been well defined, and in addition to encoding surface isoantigens, genes at the HLA locus also encode immune response (*Ir*) genes. The class I region consists of HLA-A, HLA-B and HLA-C loci and the class II region consists of the D region, which is subdivided into HLA-DP, HLA-DQ and HLA-DR subregions. Class II molecules play an important role in the induction of an immune response, since antigen-presenting cells must complex an antigen with class II molecules to present it in the presence of interleukin-1 to CD4+ T lymphocytes. Class I molecules are important in presentation of intracellular antigen to CD8+ T lymphocytes as well as for effector functions of target cells. Class III molecules encoded by genes located between those that encode class I and class II molecules include C2, BF, C4a and C4b. Class I and class II molecules play an important role in the transplantation of organs and tissues. The microlymphocytotoxicity assay is used for HLA-A, -B, -C, -DR and -DQ typing. The primed lymphocyte test is used for DP typing. Upper case letters designate individual HLA loci, such as HLA-B, and alleles are designated by numbers such as in HLA-B*0701.

HLA-A is a class I histocompatibility antigen in humans. It is expressed on nucleated cells of the body. Tissue typing to identify an individual's HLA-A antigens employs lymphocytes.

HLA-B is a class I histocompatibility antigen in humans which is expressed on nucleated cells of the body. Tissue typing to define an individual's HLA-B antigens employs lymphocytes.

HLA-C is a class I histocompatibility antigen in humans which is expressed on nucleated cells of the body. Lymphocytes are employed for tissue typing to determine HLA-C antigens. HLA-C antigens play little or no role in graft rejection.

The human MHC class II region is the **HLA-D region** which comprises three subregions designated DR, DQ and DP. Multiple genetic loci are present in each of these. DN (previously DZ) and DO subregions each consist of one genetic locus. Each class II HLA molecule comprises one α and one β chain that constitute a heterodimer. Genes within each subregion encode a particular class II molecule's α and β chains. Class II genes that encode α chains are designated A, whereas class II genes that encode β chains are designated B. A number is used following A or B if a particular subregion contains two or more A or B genes.

The **HLA-DP subregion** is the site of two sets of genes designated HLA-DPA1 and HLA-DPB1 and the pseudogenes HLA-DPA2 and HLA-DPB2. DP α and DP β chains encoded by the corresponding genes DPA1 and DPB1 unite to produce the DPαβ molecule. DP antigen or type is determined principally by the very polymorphic DPβ chain, in contrast to the much less polymorphic DPα chain. DP molecules carry DPw1–DPw6 antigens.

The **HLA-DQ subregion** consists of two sets of genes designated DQA1 and DQB1, and DQA2 and DQB2. DQA2 and DRB2 are pseudogenes. DQα and DQβ chains, encoded by DQA1 and DQB1 genes, unite to produce the DQαβ molecule. Although both DQα and DQβ chains are polymorphic, the DQβ chain is the principal factor in determining the DQ antigen or type. DQαβ molecules carry DQw1–DQw9 specificities.

The **HLA-DR subregion** is the site of one HLA-DRA gene. Although DRB gene number varies with DR type, there are usually three DRB genes, termed DRB1, DRB2 and DRB3 (or DRB4). The DRB2 pseudogene is not expressed. The DR α chain, encoded by the DRA gene, can unite with products of DRB1 and DRB3 (or DRB4) genes which are the DR β-1 and DR β-3 (or DR β-4) chains. This yields two separate DR molecules, DRαβ-1 and DRαβ-3 (or DR αβ-4). The DR β chain determines the DR antigen (DR type) since it is very polymorphic, whereas the DR α chain is not. DR αβ-1 molecules carry DR specificities DR1–DRw18. Yet, DRαβ-3 molecules carry the DRw52, and DRαβ-4 molecules carry the DRw53 specificity.

HLA-DR antigenic specificities are epitopes on DR gene products. Selected specificities have been mapped to defined loci. HLA serologic typing requires the identification of a prescribed antigenic determinant on a particular HLA molecular product. One typing specificity can be present on many different molecules. Different alleles at the same locus may encode these various HLA molecules. Monoclonal antibodies are now used to recognize certain antigenic determinants shared by various molecules bearing the same HLA typing specificity. Monoclonal antibodies have been employed to recognize specific class II alleles with disease associations.

HLA-DM facilitates the loading of antigenic peptides onto MHC class II molecules. As a result of proteolysis of the invariant chain, a small fragment called the class II-associated invariant chain peptide, or CLIP, remains bound to the MHC class II molecule. CLIP is replaced by antigenic peptides, but in the absence of HLA-DM this does not occur. The

HLA-DM molecule must therefore play some part in removal of the CLIP and in the loading of antigenic peptides.

HLA-G is a polymorphic class I HLA antigen with extensive variability in the α-2 domain. It is found on trophoblasts, i.e. placenta cells and trophoblastic neoplasms. HLA-G is expressed only on cells such as placental extravillous cytotrophoblasts and choriocarcinoma that fail to express HLA-A, -B and -C antigens. HLA-G expression is most pronounced during the first trimester of pregnancy. Trophoblast cells expressing HLA-G at the maternal–fetal junction may protect the semiallogeneic fetus from 'rejection'. Prominent HLA-G expression suggests maternal immune tolerance.

HLA-H is a pseudogene found in the MHC class I region that is structurally similar to HLA-A, but is non-functional due to the absence of a cysteine residue at position 164 in its protein product and the deletion of the codon 227 nucleotide.

HLA non-classical class I genes are located within the MHC class I region that encode products that can associate with β2 microglobulin. However, their function and tissue distribution are different from those of HLA-A, -B and -C molecules. Examples include HLA-E, -F and -G. Of these, only HLA-G is expressed on the cell surface. It is uncertain whether or not these HLA molecules are involved in peptide binding and presentation like classical class I molecules.

An **extended haplotype** consists of linked alleles in positive linkage disequilibrium situated between and including HLA-DR and HLA-B of the major histocompatibility complex of man. Examples of extended haplotypes include the association of B8/DR3/SCO1/GLO2 with membranoproliferative glomerulonephritis and of A25/B18/DR2 with complement C2 deficiency. Extended haplotypes may be a consequence of crossover suppression through environmental influences together with selected HLA types, leading to autoimmune conditions. The B27 relationship to *Klebsiella* is an example. Polymerase chain reaction (PCR) amplification and direct sequencing help to identify a large number of allelic differences

and specific associations of extended haplotypes with disease. Extended haplotypes are more informative than single polymorphisms. Some diseases associated with extended haplotypes include Graves' disease, pemphigus vulgaris, type I (juvenile onset) insulin-dependent diabetes mellitus, celiac disease, psoriasis and autoimmune hepatitis.

Linkage disequilibrium refers to the appearance of HLA genes on the same chromosome with greater frequency than would be expected by chance. This has been demonstrated by detailed studies in both populations and families, employing outbred groups where numerous different haplotypes are present. With respect to the HLA-A, -B and -C loci, a possible explanation for linkage disequilibrium is that there has not been sufficient time for the genes to reach equilibrium. However, this possibility is remote for HLA-A, -B and -D linkage disequilibrium. Natural selection has been suggested to maintain linkage disequilibrium that is advantageous. If products of two histocompatibility loci play a role in the immune response and appear on the same chromosome, they might reinforce one another and represent an advantageous association. An example of linkage disequilibrium in the HLA system of man is the occurrence on the same chromosome of HLA-A3 and HLA-B7 in the Caucasian American population.

HLA disease association Certain HLA alleles occur in a higher frequency in individuals with particular diseases than in the general population. These type of data permit estimation of the 'relative risk' of developing a disease with every known HLA allele. For example, there is a strong association between ankylosing spondylitis, which is an autoimmune disorder involving the vertebral joints, and the class I MHC allele, HLA-B27. There is a strong association between products of the polymorphic class II alleles HLA-DR and -DQ and certain autoimmune diseases, since class II MHC molecules are of great importance in the selection and activation of CD4$^+$ T lymphocytes which regulate the immune responses against protein antigens. For example, 95% of Caucasians with insulin-dependent (type I) diabetes mellitus have HLA-DR3 or HLA-DR4 or both. There is also a strong association of HLA-DR4 with rheumatoid arthritis. Numerous other examples exist and are the

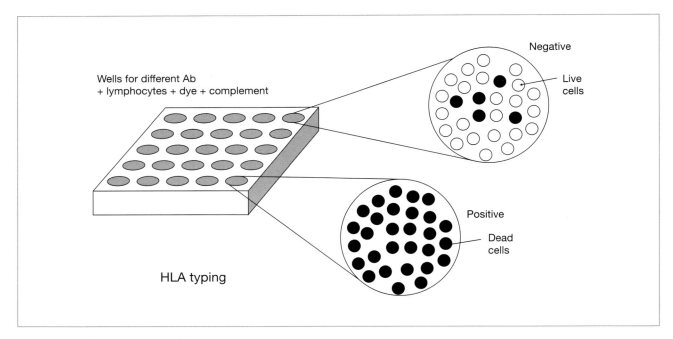

Figure 37   HLA tissue typing. Ab, antibody

targets of current investigations, especially in extended studies employing DNA probes.

HLA tissue typing (Figure 37) is the identification of major histocompatibility complex class I and class II antigens on lymphocytes by serological and cellular techniques. The principal serological assay is microlymphocytotoxicity, using a microtiter plate containing predispensed antibodies against HLA specificities to which lymphocytes of unknown specificity plus rabbit complement and vital dye are added. Following incubation, the wells are scored according to the relative proportion of cells killed. This method is employed for organ transplants such as renal allotransplants. For bone marrow transplants, mixed lymphocyte reaction procedures are performed to determine the relative degree of histocompatibility or histoincompatibility between donor and recipient. Serological tests are largely being replaced by DNA typing procedures employing polymerase chain reaction (PCR) methodology and DNA or oligonucleotide probes, especially for MHC class II typing.

Class I typing involves reactions between lymphocytes to be typed with HLA antisera of known specificity in the presence of complement. Cell lysis is detected by phase or fluorescence microscopy. This is important in parentage testing, disease association, transfusion practices and transplantation. HLA-A, -B and -C antigens should be defined by at least one of the following:

(1)   At least two different sera if both are monospecfic;

(2)   One monospecific and two multispecific antisera;

(3)   At least three multispecific antisera if all multispecific are used.

Class II typing detects HLA-DR antigens using purified B cell preparations. It is based on antibody-specific, complement-dependent disruption of the cell membrane of lymphocytes. Cell death is demonstrated by penetration of dye into the membrane. Class II typing is more difficult than type I methods and complement toxicity. At least three antisera must be used if all are monospecific; at least three antisera must be used if all are monospecific; at least five antisera must be used for multispecifc sera.

Antibody screening   Candidates for organ transplants, especially renal allografts, are monitored with relative frequency for changes in their percentage reactive antibody (PRA) levels. Obviously, those with relatively high PRA values are considered to be less favorable candidates for renal allotransplants than are those in whom the PRA values are low. PRA determinations may vary according to the composition of the cell panel. If the size of the panel is inadequate, it may affect the relative frequency of common histocompatibility antigens found in the population.

Molecular (DNA) typing Sequence specific priming (SSP) is a method that employs a primer with a single mismatch in the 3'-end that cannot be employed efficiently to extend a DNA strand because the enzyme Taq polymerase, during the PCR reaction, and especially in the first PCR cycles which are very critical, does not manifest 3'–5' proofreading endonuclease activity to remove the mismatched nucleotide. If primer pairs are designed to have perfectly matched 3'-ends with only a single allele, or a single group of alleles, and the PCR reaction is initiated under stringent conditions, a perfectly matched primer pair results in an amplification product, whereas a mismatch at the 3'-end primer pair will not provide any amplification product. A positive result, i.e. amplification, defines the specificity of the DNA sample. In this method, the PCR amplification step provides the basis for identifying polymorphism. The postamplification processing of the sample consists only of simple agarose gel electrophoresis to detect the presence or absence of amplified product. DNA amplified fragments are visualized by ethidium bromide staining and exposure to ultraviolet (UV) light. A separate technique detects amplified product by color fluorescence. The primer pairs are selected in such a manner that each allele should have a unique reactivity pattern with the panel of primer pairs employed. Appropriate controls must be maintained (Figure 38).

Haplotype designates those phenotypic characteristics encoded by closely linked genes on one chromosome inherited from one parent. It frequently describes several major histocompatibility complex (MHC) alleles on a single chromosome. Selected haplotypes are in strong linkage disequilibrium between alleles of different loci. According to Mendelian genetics, 25% of siblings will share both haplotypes.

Phenotype designates observable features of a cell or organism that are a consequence of interaction between the genotype and the environment. The phenotype represents those genetically encoded

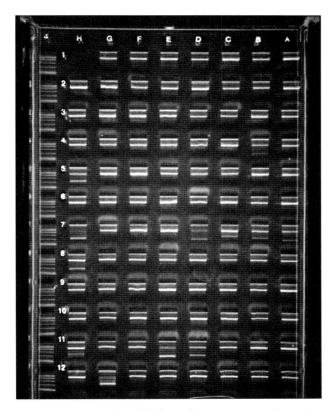

Figure 38 Example of high-resolution DRB1 typing using sequence-specific primer methodology. Molecular weight ladder of known base pairs is in the far left column for base pair sizing

characteristics that are expressed. Phenotype may also refer to a group of organisms with the same physical appearance and the same detectable characteristics.

Cross-match testing is an assay used in blood typing and histocompatibility testing to ascertain whether or not donor and recipient have antibodies against each other's cells that might lead to transfusion reaction or transplant rejection. Cross-matching reduces the chances of graft rejection by preformed antibodies against donor cell surface antigens which are usually MHC antigens. Donor lymphocytes are mixed with recipient serum, complement is added and the preparation observed for cell lysis.

Flow cytometry can also be used to perform the cross-matching procedure. This method is highly sensitive (considerably more sensitive than the direct cytotoxicity method). Flow cross-matching is also faster and can distinguish antibodies according to class (IgG vs. IgM) and target cell specificity (T cells from B cells). It is a valuable procedure in organ and bone marrow transplantation and is particularly suitable to measuring antibodies against HLA class I antigens on donor T cells. False positives are rare, and most errors are due to low sensitivity (lower antibody concentration). Flow cross-matching has the potential to be standardized and automated. The flow cytometry cross-matching method commonly utilizes F(ab′)$_2$ antihuman IgG conjugated to fluorescein, and anti-CD3 versus IgG is generated. A positive flow cross-match is defined as median channel shift values > 40.

Splits are human leukocyte antigen (HLA) subtypes. For example, the base antigen HLA-B12 can be subdivided into the splits HLA-B44 and HLA-B45. The term 'split' is used to designate an HLA antigen that was first believed to be a private antigen, but later was shown to be a public antigen. The former designation can be placed in parentheses following its new designation, e.g. HLA-B44(12).

A **private antigen** (Figure 39) is:

(1) An antigen confined to one major histocompatibility complex (MHC) molecule;

(2) An antigenic specificity restricted to a few individuals;

(3) A tumor antigen restricted to a specific chemically induced tumor;

(4) A low-frequency epitope present on red blood cells of fewer than 0.1% of the population, e.g. Pt^a, By, Bp^a, etc.;

(5) HLA antigen encoded by one allele such as HLA-B27.

A **public antigen (supratypic antigen)** is an epitope which several distinct or private antigens have in common (Figure 39). A public antigen such as a blood group antigen is one that is present in greater than 99.9% of a population. It is detected by the indirect antiglobulin (Coombs' test). Examples include Ve, Ge, Jr, Gy^a and Ok^a. Antigens that occur frequently but are not public antigens include Mns, Lewis, Duffy, P, etc. In blood banking, there is a problem finding a suitable unit of blood for a transfusion to recipients who have developed antibodies against public antigens.

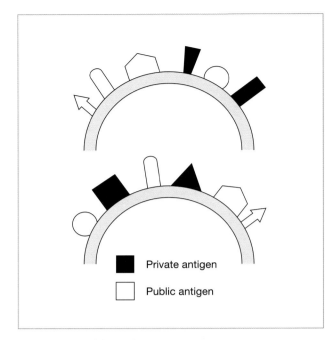

Figure 39 Public and private antigens

Heart–lung transplantation is a procedure that has proved effective for the treatment of primary respiratory disease with dysfunction of gas exchange and alveolar mechanics, together with a secondary elevation in pulmonary vascular resistance, and in primary high-resistance circulatory disorder associated with pulmonary vascular disease.

Immunologically privileged sites are certain anatomical sites within the animal body that provide an immunologically privileged environment which favors the prolonged survival of alien grafts. The potential for development of a blood and lymphatic vascular supply connecting graft and host may be a determining factor in the qualification of an anatomical site as an area which provides an environment favorable to the prolonged survival of a foreign graft. Immunologically privileged areas include:

(1) The anterior chamber of the eye;

(2) The substantia propria of the cornea;

(3) The meninges of the brain;

(4) The testis;

(5) The cheek pouch of the Syrian hamster.

Foreign grafts implanted in these sites show a diminished ability to induce transplantation immunity in the host. These immunologically privileged sites usually fail to protect alien grafts from the immune rejection mechanism in hosts previously or simultaneously sensitized with donor tissues. The capacity of cells expressing Fas ligand to cause deletion of activated lymphocytes provides a possible explanation for the phenomenon of immune privilege. Animals with a deficiency in either Fas ligand or the Fas receptor fail to manifest significant immune privilege. Both epithelial cells of the eye and Sertoli cells of the testes express Fas ligand. Immune privilege is a consequence not only of the lack of an inflammatory response but also from immune consequences of the accumulation of apoptotic immune cells within a tissue. Immune cell apoptosis may be a signal to terminate inflammation. Apoptotic cell accumulation during an immune response could activate the development of cells that function to downregulate or suppress further immune activation.

Immunologic enhancement is the prolonged survival, conversely the delayed rejection, of a tumor allograft in a host as a consequence of contact with specific antibody. Both the peripheral and central mechanisms have been postulated. In the past, coating of tumor cells with antibody was presumed to interfere with the ability of specifically reactive lymphocytes to destroy them, but today a central effect in suppressing cell-mediated immunity, perhaps through suppressor T lymphocytes, is also possible.

Fetus allograft Success of the haplo-non-identical fetus as an allograft was suggested in the 1950s by Medawar, Brent and Billingham to rely on four possibilities. This proposal suggested that:

(1) The conceptus might not be immunogenic;

(2) Pregnancy might alter the immune response;

(3) The uterus might be an immunologically privileged site;

(4) The placenta might represent an effective immunological barrier between mother and fetus.

Further studies have shown that transplantation privilege afforded the fetal–placental unit in pregnancy depends on intrauterine mechanisms. The pregnant uterus has been shown not to be an immunologically privileged site. Pregnancies are usually successful in maternal hosts with high levels of pre-existing alloim-

munity. The temporary status has focused on specialized features of fetal trophoblastic cells that facilitate transplantation protection. Fetal trophoblast protects itself from maternal cytotoxic attack by failing to express on placental villous cytotrophoblast and syncytiotrophoblast any classical polymorphic class I or II histocompatibility complex (MHC) antigens. Constitutive HLA expression is also not induced by known upregulators such as interferon γ. Thus, classical MHC antigens are not expressed throughout gestation. Extravillous cytotrophoblast cells selectively express HLA-G, a non-classical class I MHC antigen which has limited genetic polymorphism. HLA-G might protect the cytotrophoblast population from MHC-non-restricted natural killer (NK) cell attack. The trophoblast also protects itself from maternal cytotoxicity during gestation by expressing a high level of complement regulatory proteins on its surface, such as membrane cofactor protein (MCP; CD46), decay accelerating factor (DAF; CD55) and membrane attack complex inhibitory factor (CD59). The maternal immune system recognizes pregnancy, i.e. the fetal trophoblast, in a manner that results in cellular, antibody and cytokine responses that protect the fetal allograft. CD56-positive large granular lymphocytes may be regulated by hormones in the endometrium that control their function. They have been suggested to be a form of NK cell in arrested maturation possibly due to persistent expression of HLA-G on target invasive cytotrophoblast. Contemporary studies have addressed cytokine interactions at the fetal–maternal tissue interface in pregnancy. HLA-G or other fetal trophoblast antigens have been postulated possibly to stimulate maternal lymphocytes in endometrial tissue, to synthesize cytokines and growth factors that act in a paracrine manner beneficial to trophoblast growth and differentiation. This has been called the immunotrophism hypothesis. Other cytokines released into decidual tissue include colony stimulating factors (CSFs), tumor necrosis factor-α (TNF-α), interleukin-6 (IL-6) and transforming growth factor (TGF-β). Fetal syncytiotrophoblast has numerous growth factor receptors. Thus, an extensive cytokine network is preset within the uteroplacental tissue that offers both immunosuppressive and growth-promoting signals. In humans, IgG is selectively transported across the placenta into the fetal circulation following combination with transporting Fcγ receptors on the placenta.

This transfer takes place during the 20th to the 22nd week of gestation. Maternal HLA-specific alloantibody that is specific for the fetal HLA type is bound by non-trophoblastic cells expressing fetal HLA antigens. These include macrophages, fibroblasts and endothelium within the villous mesenchyme of placental tissue, thereby preventing these antibodies from reaching the fetal circulation. Maternal antibodies against any other antigen of the fetus will likewise be bound within the placental tissues to a cell expressing that antigen. The placenta acts as a sponge to absorb potentially harmful antibodies. Exceptions to placental trapping of deleterious maternal IgG antibodies include maternal IgG antibodies against RhD antigen and certain maternal organ-specific autoantibodies.

An **allograft** is an organ, tissue or cell transplant from one individual or strain to a genetically different individual or strain within the same species. Allografts are also called homografts (Figure 40).

Homograft is the earlier term for allograft, i.e. an organ or tissue graft from a donor to a recipient of the same species.

A **xenograft** is a tissue or organ graft from a member of one species, i.e. the donor, to a member of a different species, i.e. the recipient. It is also called a heterograft. Antibodies and cytotoxic T cells reject xenografts several days following transplantation.

A **syngraft** is a transplant from one individual to another within the same strain. Syngrafts are also called isografts.

Syngeneic is an adjective that implies genetic identity between identical twins in humans or among members of an inbred strain of mice or other species. It is used principally to refer to transplants between genetically identical members of a species.

An **isograft** is a tissue transplant from a donor to an isogenic recipient. Grafts exchanged between members of an inbred strain of laboratory animals such as mice are syngeneic rather than isogenic.

Isogeneic (isogenic) is an adjective implying genetic identity, such as identical twins. Although used as a

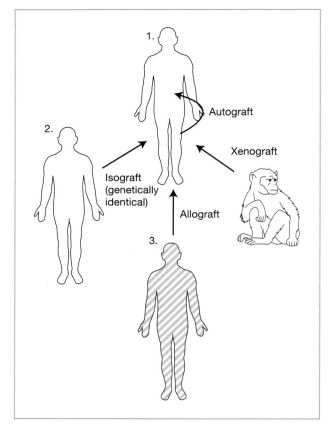

Figure 40 Types of grafts

synonym for syngeneic when referring to the genetic relationship between members of an inbred strain (of mice), the inbred animals never show the absolute identity, i.e. identical genotypes, observed in identical twins.

Isologous means derived from the same species, also called isogeneic or syngeneic.

An antigen found in a member of a species that induces an immune response if injected into a genetically dissimilar member of the same species is termed an **isoantigen**.

Isoantibody is an antibody that is specific for an antigen present in other members of the species in which it occurs. Thus, it is an antibody against an isoantigen (also called alloantibody).

A **donor** is one who offers whole blood, blood products, bone marrow or an organ to be given to another individual. Individuals who are drug addicts or test positively for certain diseases such as HIV-1 infection or hepatitis B, for example, are not suitable as donors. There are various other reasons for donor rejection not listed here. To be a blood donor, an individual must meet certain criteria which include blood pressure, temperature, hematocrit, pulse and history. There are many reasons for donor rejection, including low hematocrit, skin lesions, surgery, drugs or positive donor blood tests.

An **organ bank** is a site where selected tissues for transplantation, such as acellular bone fragments, corneas and bone marrow, may be stored for relatively long periods until needed for transplantation. Several hospitals often share such a facility. Organs such as kidneys, liver, heart, lung and pancreatic islets must be transplanted within 48–72 h and are not suitable for storage in an organ bank.

Organ brokerage, or the selling of an organ such as a kidney from a living related donor to the transplant recipient is practiced in certain parts of the world, but is considered unethical and is illegal in the USA, as it is in violation of the National Organ Transplant Act (Public Law 98-507,3 USC).

Adoptive immunity is the term assigned by Billingham, Brent and Medawar (1955) to transplantation immunity induced by the passive transfer of specifically immune lymph node cells from an actively immunized animal to a normal (previously non-immune) syngeneic recipient host.

Adoptive immunization is the passive transfer of immunity by the injection of lymphoid cells from a specifically immune individual to a previously non-immune recipient host. The resulting recipient is said to have adoptive immunity.

A **skin graft** uses skin from the same individual (autologous graft) or donor skin that is applied to areas of the body surface that have undergone third-degree burns. A patient's keratinocytes may be cultured into confluent sheets that can be applied to the affected areas, although these may not 'take' because of the absence of type IV collagen 7S basement membrane sites for binding and fibrils to anchor the graft.

A **split thickness graft** is a skin graft that is only 0.25–0.35 mm thick that consists of epidermis and a small layer of dermis. These grafts vascularize rapidly and last longer than do regular grafts. They are especially useful for skin burns, contaminated skin areas and sites that are poorly vascularized. Thick split thickness grafts are further resistant to trauma, produce minimal contraction and permit some amount of sensation, but graft survival is poor.

Pancreatic transplantation is a treatment for diabetes. Either a whole pancreas or a large segment of it, obtained from cadavers, may be transplanted together with kidneys into the same diabetic patient. It is important for the patient to be clinically stable and for there to be as close a tissue (HLA antigen) match as possible. Graft survival is 50–80% at 1 year.

Islet cell transplantation is an experimental method aimed at treatment of type I diabetes mellitus. The technique has been successful in rats, but less so in man. It requires sufficient functioning islets from a minimum of two cadaveric donors that have been purified, cultured and shown to produce insulin. The islet cells are administered into the portal vein. The liver serves as the host organ in the recipient who is treated with FK506 or other immunosuppressant drugs.

Bone marrow transplantation is a procedure used to treat both non-neoplastic and neoplastic conditions not amenable to other forms of therapy. It has been especially used in cases of aplastic anemia, acute lymphocytic leukemia and acute non-lymphocytic leukemia. Bone marrow (750 ml) is removed from the iliac crest of an HLA-matched donor. Following appropriate treatment of the marrow to remove bone spicules, the cell suspension is infused intravenously into an appropriately immunosuppressed recipient who has received whole body irradiation and immunosuppressive drug therapy. Graft-versus-host episodes, acute graft-versus-host disease or chronic graft-versus-host disease may follow bone marrow transplantation in selected subjects. The immunosuppressed patients are highly susceptible to opportunistic infections

An **autograft** is a graft of tissue taken from one area of the body and placed in a different site on the body of the same individual, e.g. grafts of skin from un-affected areas to burned areas in the same individual.

Autologous bone marrow transplantation (ABMT) Leukemia patients in relapse may donate marrow which can be stored and readministered to them following a relapse. Leukemic cells are removed from the bone marrow, which is cryopreserved until needed. Prior to reinfusion of the bone marrow, the patient receives supralethal chemoradiotherapy. This mode of therapy has improved considerably the survival rate of some leukemia patients.

Allogeneic (or allogenic) is an adjective that describes genetic variations or differences among members or strains of the same species. The term refers to organ or tissue grafts between genetically dissimilar humans or unrelated members of other species.

Allogeneic bone marrow transplantation Hematopoietic cell transplants are performed in patients with hematologic malignancies, certain non-hematologic neoplasms, aplastic anemias and certain immunodeficiency states. In allogeneic bone marrow transplantation the recipient is irradiated with lethal doses either to destroy malignant cells or to create a graft bed. The problems that arise include graft-versus-host disease (GVHD) and transplant rejection. GVHD disease occurs when immunologically competent cells or their precursors are transplanted into immunologically crippled recipients. Acute GVHD occurs within days to weeks after allogeneic bone marrow transplantation and primarily affects the immune system and epithelia of the skin, liver and intestines. Rejection of allogeneic bone marrow transplants appears to be mediated by natural killer (NK) cells and T cells that survive in the irradiated host. NK cells react against allogeneic stem cells that are lacking self-major histocompatibility complex (MHC) class I molecules and therefore fail to deliver the inhibitory signal to NK cells. Host T cells react against donor MHC antigens in a manner resembling their reaction against solid tissue grafts.

Immunotoxin The linkage of an antibody specific for target cell antigens with a cytotoxic substance such as the toxin ricin yields an immunotoxin. Upon parenteral injection, its antibody portion directs the immunotoxin to the target and its toxic portion destroys target cells on contact. Among its uses is the purging of T cells from hematopoietic cell preparations used for bone marrow transplantation.

Immunotoxin is a substance produced by the union of a monoclonal antibody or one of its fractions to a toxic molecule such as a radioisotope, a bacterial or plant toxin, or a chemotherapeutic agent. The antibody portion is intended to direct the molecule to antigens on a target cell, such as those of a malignant tumor, and the toxic portion of the molecule is for the purpose of destroying the target cell. Contemporary methods of recombinant DNA technology have permitted the preparation of specific hybrid molecules for use in immunotoxin therapy. Immunotoxins may have difficulty reaching the intended target tumor, may be quickly metabolized and may stimulate the development of anti-immunotoxin antibodies. Cross-linking proteins may likewise be unstable. Immunotoxins have potential for antitumor therapy and as immunosuppressive agents.

Hematopoietic stem cell (HSC) transplants are used to reconstitute hematopoietic cell lineages and to treat neoplastic diseases. Twenty-five per cent of allogeneic marrow transplants in 1995 were performed using hematopoietic stem cells obtained from unrelated donors. Since only 30% of patients requiring an allogeneic marrow transplant have a sibling who is HLA-genotypically identical, it became necessary to identify related or unrelated potential marrow donors. It became apparent that complete HLA compatibility between donor and recipient is not absolutely necessary to reconstitute patients immunologically. Transplantation of unrelated marrow is accompanied by an increased incidence of graft-versus-host disease (GVHD). Removal of mature T lymphocytes from marrow grafts decreases the severity of GVHD but often increases the incidence of graft failure and disease relapse. HLA-phenotypically identical marrow transplants among relatives are often successful. HSC transplantation provides a method to reconstitute hematopoietic cell lineages with normal cells capable of continuous self-renewal. The principal complications of HSC transplantation are GVHD, graft rejection, graft failure, prolonged immunodeficiency, toxicity from radiochemotherapy given pre- and post-transplantation, and GVHD prophylaxis.

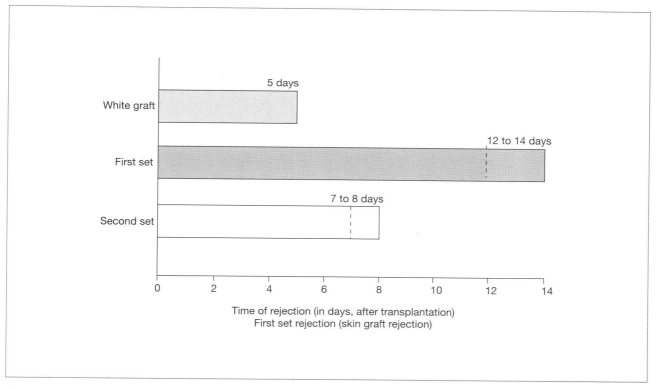

Figure 41 Types of skin graft rejection

Methotrexate and cyclosporine A are given to help prevent acute GVHD. Chronic GVHD may also be a serious complication involving the skin, gut and liver and an associated sicca syndrome. Allogenic HSC transplantation often involves older individuals and unrelated donors. Thus, blood stem cell transplantation represents an effective method for the treatment of patients with hematologic and non-hematologic malignancies and various types of immunodeficiencies. The *in vitro* expansion of a small number of CD34$^+$ cells stimulated by various combinations of cytokines appears to give hematopoietic reconstitution when reinfused after a high-dose therapy. Recombinant human hematopoietic growth factors (HGFs) (cytokines) may be given to counteract chemotherapy treatment-related myelotoxicity. HGFs increase the number of circulating progenitor and stem cells, which is important for the support of high-dose therapy in autologous as well as allogeneic HSC transplantation.

Hematopoietic chimerism A successful bone marrow transplant leads to a state of hematological and/or immunological chimerism in which donor type blood cells coexist permanently with host type tissues, without manifesting alloreactivity to each other. Usually incomplete or mixed hematopoietic chimerism is generated following bone marrow transplantation, in which both host type and donor type blood cells can be detected in the recipient. In bone marrow transplantation, not only is immune reactivity against donor type cells an obstacle to bone marrow engraftment, there is also the problem of GVHD mediated by donor T cells reactive against host antigens (refer to chimera).

A **take** is the successful grafting of skin that adheres to the recipient graft site 3–5 days following application. This is accompanied by neovascularization as indicated by a pink appearance. Thin grafts are more likely to 'take' than thicker grafts, but the thin graft must contain some dermis to be successful. The term 'take' also refers to an organ allotransplant that has survived hyperacute and chronic rejection.

Engraftment is the phase during which transplanted bone marrow manufactures new blood cells.

Graft rejection (Figure 41) is an immunologic destruction of transplanted tissues or organs between two members or strains of a species differing at the major histocompatibility complex for that species (i.e. HLA in man and H-2 in the mouse). The rejection is based upon both cell-mediated and antibody-mediated immunity against cells of the graft by the histoincompatible recipient. First-set rejection usually occurs within 2 weeks after transplantation. The placement of a second graft with the same antigenic specificity as the first in the same host leads to rejection within 1 week and is termed second-set rejection. This demonstrates the presence of immunological memory learned from the first experience with the histocompatibility antigens of the graft. When the donor and recipient differ only at minor histocompatibility loci, rejection of the transplanted tissue may be delayed, depending upon the relative strength of the minor loci in which they differ.

Immunofluorescent 'staining' of C4d in peritubular capillaries of renal allograft biopsies reveals a humoral component of rejection (Figure 42).

First-set rejection is an acute form of allograft rejection in a non-sensitized recipient. It is usually completed in 12–14 days. It is mediated by type IV (delayed-type) hypersensitivity to graft antigens.

Rejection is an immune response to an organ allograft such as a kidney transplant. **Hyperacute rejection** is due to preformed antibodies and is apparent within minutes following transplantation (Figures 43 and 44). Antibodies reacting with endothelial cells cause complement to be fixed, which attracts polymorphonuclear neutrophils, resulting in denuding of the endothelial lining of the vascular walls. This causes platelets and fibrin plugs to block the blood flow to the transplanted organ, which becomes cyanotic, undergoes infarction and must be removed. Only a few drops of bloody urine are usually produced. Segmental thrombosis, necrosis and fibrin thrombi form in the glomerular tufts. There is hemorrhage in the interstitium, and mesangial cell swelling; IgG, IgM and C3 may be deposited in arteriole walls. **Acute rejection** occurs within days to weeks following transplantation and is characterized by extensive cellular infiltration of the interstitium (Figures 45 and 46). These cells are largely mononuclear cells and include plasma cells,

lymphocytes, immunoblasts and macrophages, as well as some neutrophils. Tubules become separated, and the tubular epithelium undergoes necrosis. Endothelial cells are swollen and vacuolated. There is vascular edema, bleeding with inflammation, renal tubular necrosis and sclerosed glomeruli. **Chronic rejection** occurs after more than 60 days following transplantation and may be characterized by structural changes such as interstitial fibrosis, sclerosed glomeruli, mesangial proliferative glomerulonephritis, crescent formation and various other changes (Figures 47 and 48).

Second-set rejection is rejection of an organ or tissue graft by a host who is already immune to the histocompatibility antigens of the graft as a consequence of rejection of a previous transplant of the same antigenic specificity as the second, or as a consequence of immunization against antigens of the donor graft. The accelerated second-set rejection compared with rejection of a first graft is reminiscent of a classic secondary or booster immune response.

Indirect antigen presentation In organ or tissue transplantation, this is the mechanism whereby donor allogeneic MHC molecules present microbial proteins. The recipient professional antigen-presenting cells process allogeneic MHC proteins. The resulting allogeneic MHC peptides are presented, in association with recipient (self) MHC molecules to host T lymphocytes. By contrast, recipient T cells recognize unprocessed allogeneic MHC molecules on the surface of the graft cells in direct antigen presentation.

Muromonab® Orthoclone OKT3 is a commercial antibody against the T cell surface marker CD3. It may be used therapeutically to diminish T cell reactivity in organ allotransplant recipients experiencing a rejection episode; OKT3 may act in concert with the complement system to induce T cell lysis, or may act as an opsonin, rendering T cells susceptible to phagocytosis. Rarely, recirculating T lymphocytes are removed in patients experiencing rejection crisis by thoracic duct drainage or extracorporeal irradiation of the blood. Plasma exchange is useful for temporary reduction in circulating antibody levels in selective diseases, such as hemolytic disease of the newborn, myasthenia gravis or Goodpasture's syndrome. Immunosuppressive drugs act on all of the T and B cell maturation processes.

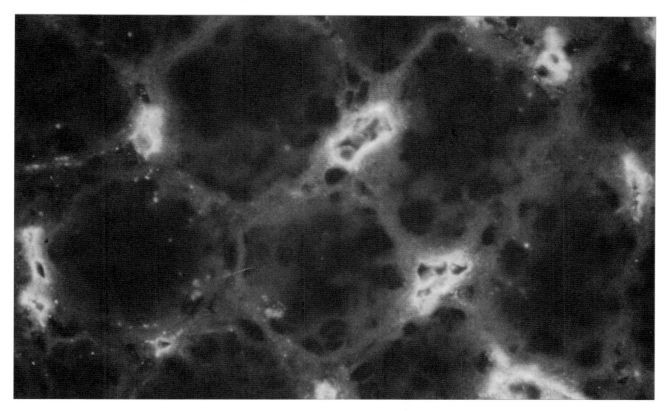

Figure 42 Immunofluorescent 'staining' of C4d in peritubular capillaries in acute renal allograft rejection

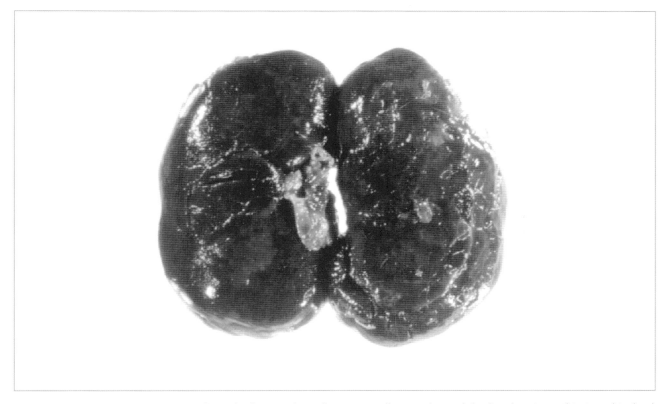

Figure 43 Hyperacute rejection of renal allotransplant showing swelling and purplish discoloration. This is a bivalved transplanted kidney. The allograft was removed within a few hours following transplantation

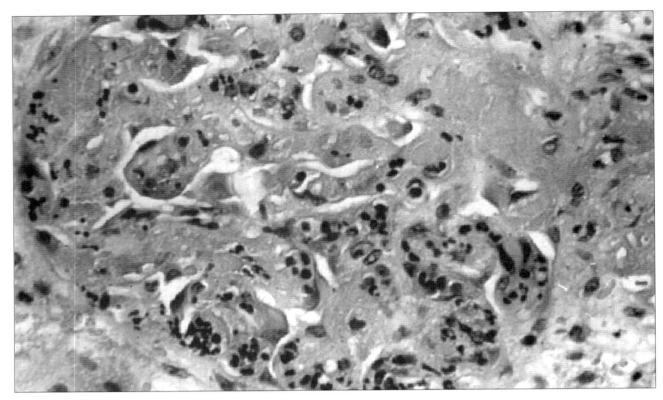

Figure 44 Microscopic view of hyperacute rejection showing a necrotic glomerulus infiltrated with numerous polymorphonuclear leukocytes. Hematoxylin and eosin (H&E) stained section. ×250 magnification

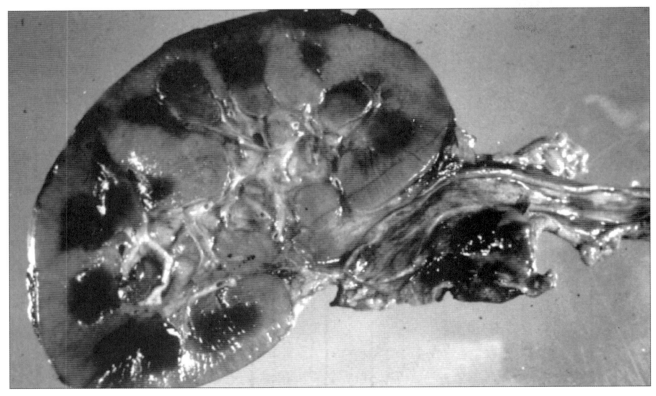

Figure 45 Acute rejection in a bivalved kidney. The cut surface bulges and is variably hemorrhagic and shows fatty degeneration of the cortex

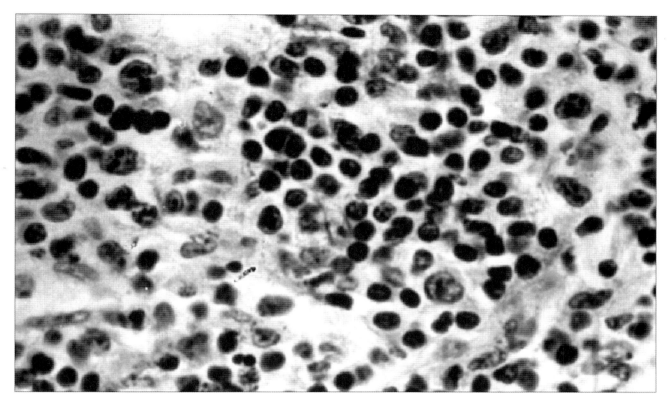

Figure 46   Microscopic view of the interstitium revealing predominantly cellular acute rejection. There is an infiltrate of variably sized lymphocytes. There is also an infiltrate of eosinophils. ×400 magnification

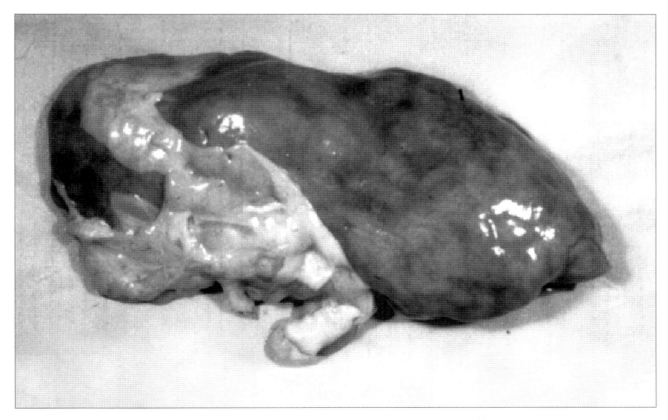

Figure 47   Renal allotransplant showing chronic rejection. The kidney is shrunken and malformed

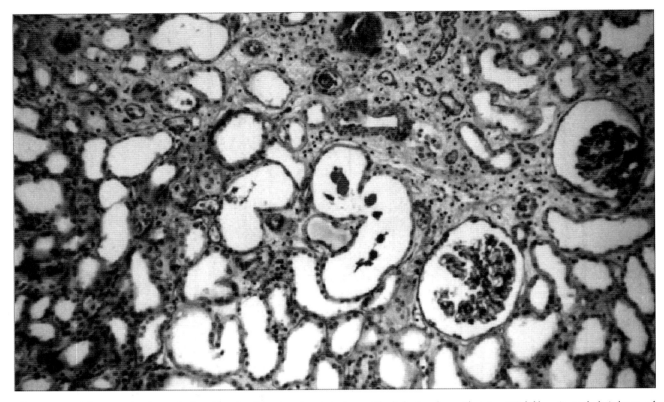

Figure 48   Microscopic view of chronic rejection showing tubular epithelial atrophy with interstitial fibrosis and shrinkage of glomerular capillary tufts. ×100 magnification

The **graft-versus-host reaction (GVHR)** is the reaction of a graft containing immunocompetent cells against the genetically dissimilar tissues of an immunosuppressed recipient. Criteria requisite for a GVHR include:

(1)   Histoincompatibility between the donor and recipient;

(2)   Passively transferred immunologically reactive cells;

(3)   A recipient host who has been either naturally immunosuppressed because of immaturity or genetic defect, or deliberately immunosuppresed by irradiation or drugs.

The immunocompetent grafted cells are especially reactive against rapidly dividing cells. Target organs include the skin, gastrointestinal tract (including the gastric mucosa) and liver, as well as the lymphoid tissues. Patients often develop skin rashes and hepatosplenomegaly and may have aplasia of the bone marrow. GVHR usually develops within 7–30 days following the transplant or infusion of the lymphocytes. Prevention of the GVHR is an important procedural step in several forms of transplantation and may be accomplished by irradiating the transplant. The clinical course of GVHR may take a hyperacute, acute or chronic form as seen in graft rejection.

REFERENCES

1.   Saunders JB. A conceptual history of transplantation. In Najarian JS, Simmons RL, eds. *Transplantation*. Philadelphia: Lea & Febiger, 1972

2.   Irwin MR, Cole LJ. Immunogenic studies of species and of species hybrids in doves, and the separation of species-specific substances in the backcross. *J Exp Zool* 1936;73:83–108

3.   Jensen CD. Experimentelle Untersuchungen über Krebs bei Mausen. *Zentralbl Bakteriol Parasitenk Infekt* 1903;34:28

4.   Loeb L. Uber die Entstehung eines Sarkoms nach Transplantation eines Adenocarcinoma einer japanischen Maus. *Z Krebsforschung* 1908;7:80

5. Tyzzer EE. A study of inheritance in mice with reference to their susceptibility to transplantable tumors. *Med Res* 1909;21:519

6. Little CC. A possible Mendelian explanation for a type of inheritance apparently non-Medelian in nature. *Science* 1914;40:904–6

7. Haldane JBS. The genetics of cancer. *Nature (London)* 1933;132:265

8. Gorer PA. The detection of a hereditary antigenic difference in the blood of mice by means of human blood group A serum. *J Genet* 1938;32:17–31

9. Gorer PA. The detection of antigenic differences in mouse erythrocytes by the employment of immune sera. *Br J Exp Pathol* 1936;17:42–50

10. Gorer PA. The genetic and antigenic basis of tumour transplantation. *J Pathol Bacteriol* 1937;44:691–7

11. Gorer PA. Further studies on antigenic differences in mouse erythrocytes. *Br J Exp Pathol* 1937;18:31–6

12. Medawar PB. The behavior and fate of skin autografts and skin homografts in rabbits. *J Anat (London)* 1944;78:176–99

13. Owen RD. Immunogenetic consequences of vascular anastomoses between bovine twins. *Science* 1945;102:400–1

14. Billingham RE, Brent L, Medawar P. Quantitative studies on tissue transplantation immunity: actively acquired tolerance. *Philos Trans R Soc (London)* 1956;B239:357–414

15. Billingham RE, Brent L, Medawar PB. 'Actively acquired tolerance' of foreign cells. *Nature (London)* 1953;172:603–6

16. Mitchison NA. Passive transfer of transplantation immunity. *Proc R Soc London B* 1954;142:72–87

17. Boyden SV, Sorkin E. The absorption of antigen by spleen cells previously treated with antiserum *in vitro*. *Immunology* 1960;3:272–83

18. Burnet FM, Fenner F. *The Production of Antibodies*, 2nd edn. Melbourne: Macmillan, 1949 (Monograph of the Walter and Eliza Hall Institute, Melbourne)

19. Jerne NK. The natural selection theory of antibody formation. *Proc Natl Acad Sci USA* 1955;41:849–57

20. Burnet FM. *The Clonal Selection Theory of Acquired Immunity*. London: Cambridge University Press, 1959

21. Dreyer WJ, Bennett JC. The molecular basis of antibody formation: a paradox. *Proc Natl Acad Sci USA* 1965;54:864

22. Smithies O. Antibody variability. Somatic recombination between the elements of 'antibody gene pairs' may explain antibody variability. *Science* 1967;157:267–73

23. Tonegawa S. Somatic generation of antibody diversity. *Nature (London)* 1983;302:575

24. Snell GD. Methods for the study of histocompatibility genes. *J Genet* 1948;49:87–108

25. Klein J. *Biology of the Mouse Histocompatibility-2 Complex.* New York: Springer-Verlag, 1975:9

26. Snell GD, Smith P, Gabrielson F. Analysis of the histocompatibility-2 locus in the mouse. *J Natl Cancer Inst* 1953;14:457–80

27. Gorer PA, Mikulska ZB. The antibody response to tumor inoculation. Improved methods for antibody detection. *Cancer Res* 1954;14:651–5

28. Gorer PA, O'Gorman P. The cytotoxic activity of isoantibodies in mice. *Transpl Bull* 1956;3:142–3

29. Neauport-Sautes C, Lilly F, Silvestre G, Kourilsky FM. Independence of H-2K and H-2D antigenic determinants on the surface of mouse lymphocytes. *J Exp Med* 1973;137:511–26

30. Dausset J. Iso-leuco-anticorps. *Acta Haematol* 1958;20:156–66

31. Shulman NR, Aster RH, Pearson HA, Hiller MC. Immuno-reactions involving platelets. VI. Reactions of maternal isoantibodies responsible for neonatal purpura. Differentiation of a second platelet antigen system. *J Clin Invest* 1962;61:1059–69

32. Dausset J, Colombani J, Legrand L, *et al.* Genetic and biological aspects of the HL-A system of human histocompatibility. *Blood* 1970;35:591–612

33. Amos DB, Russell PS, eds. *Histocompatibility Testing, Report of a Conference and Workshop.* Conference on Histocompatibility Testing Washington, DC. Sponsored by the Division of Medical Sciences National Academy of Science, 7–12 June, 1964. Washington: National Academy of Sciences, National Research Council, 1965

34. Russell PS, eds. *Histocompatibility testing, 1965.* Baltimore: Williams & Wilkins, 1965

35. Curtoni ES, PL Mattiuz, RM Tosi, eds. *Histocompatibility Testing, 1967.* Baltimore: Williams & Wilkins, 1967

36. Terasaki PI, ed. *Histocompatibility Testing, 1970.* Copenhagen: Munksgaard, 1970

37. Dausset J, Colombani J, eds. *Histocompatibility Testing, 1972.* Copenhagen: Munksgaard, 1973

38. Kissmeyer-Nielsen F, ed. *Histocompatibility Testing, 1975.* Copenhagen: Munksgaard, 1978

39. Bodmer WF, *et al.* eds. *Histocompatibility Testing, 1977.* Copenhagen: Munksgaard, 1978

40. Fauchet R, Genetet B, Campion JP, *et al.* Occurrence and specificity of anti-B lymphocyte antibodies in renal allograft recipients. *Transplantation* 1980;30:114–17

41. Cruse JM, Lewis RE. *Atlas of Immunology*, 2nd edn. Boca Raton, FL: CRC Press, 2004

CHAPTER 12

Immunization against infectious diseases; interferon; congenital immunodeficiencies; AIDS

IMMUNIZATION AGAINST INFECTIOUS DISEASES

Edward Jenner (Chapter 1, Figure 4) induced a mild disease, cowpox, to protect against a more serious infection (namely smallpox) caused by the antigenically related variola virus. Nearly a century later, Pasteur

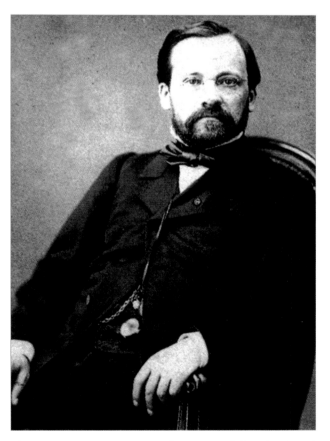

Figure 1 Louis Pasteur, who successfully developed vaccines for chicken cholera, anthrax and rabies

(Figure 1) and associates used attenuated microorganisms to induce a state of protective immunity against chicken cholera.

Subsequently, killed bacterial vaccines were developed to induce immunity against other diseases, such as anthrax. There was a great ferment among medical investigators during the latter half of the 19th and early 20th centuries to confer immunoprophylaxis through the use of vaccines, to protect the population against all sorts of infectious diseases. In addition to vaccines, antitoxin and toxoids were developed for diseases induced by exotoxins, i.e. diphtheria and tetanus. Ehrlich's (Chapter 2, Figures 28 and 35) venture into the development of a chemotherapeutic agent for the treatment of syphilis, which he termed Salvarsan, an arsenical compound, signaled the beginning of diminished emphasis on the preparation of new bacterial vaccines. With the discovery of the sulfonamides in the mid-1930s by Gerhard Gomagk, and the subsequent use of penicillin and other antibiotic agents, interest in vaccines was confined principally to those directed against virus diseases, which could not be treated successfully by chemotherapy or antibiotics. As bacterial strains resistant to antibiotic agents appeared, there was renewed interest in bacterial vaccines. Typhoid and pertussis vaccines proved highly effective, and an attenuated strain of bovine tubercle bacillus called bacillus Calmette–Guérin (BCG) (Figure 2) produced limited success in immunization against tuberculosis during the first third of the 20th century. In later years this vaccine found another use as adjunct therapy in reawakening the subdued immune response in cancer victims, apparently by producing a generalized activation of the cells involved in the immune response.

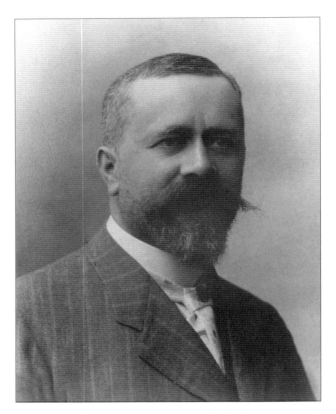

Figure 2 Albert Calmette, who with Guérin, developed BCG vaccine for immunization against tuberculosis

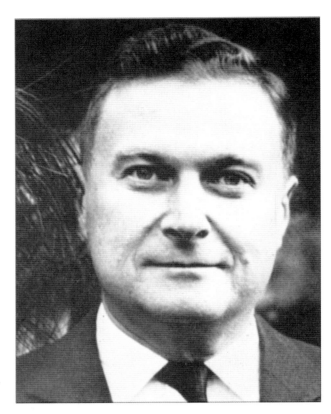

Figure 3 Hilary Koprowski, who developed a superior rabies vaccine from virus grown in human embryonic cell cultures

Nevertheless, the major accomplishments in immunoprophylaxis were associated with the development of viral and rickettsial vaccines. Pasteur was the first to treat a case of human rabies successfully by repeated injections of a vaccine prepared from the spinal cords of rabbits challenged with the virus. Since that time, rabies vaccines prepared from hen and duck embryos infected with the virus have been used with some success. But in the 1960s, Martin Kaplan and Hilary Koprowski (Figure 3) prepared a highly potent vaccine from virus grown in normal human embryonic cell cultures. It had the advantage of requiring fewer injections than the Pasteur treatment, and eliminated the possibility of allergy to duct embryo antigens.

The chick embryo and the mouse have proved highly beneficial for the development of viral and rickettsial vaccines. One of the more important of these was the production of a highly effective yellow fever vaccine from the attenuated 17D strain of the virus, which led to the award of a Nobel Prize to Max Theiler (Figure 4), its discoverer. John Enders (Figure 5), F. C. Robbins and T. H. Weller of Harvard Medical School found in 1949 that polio viruses could be successfully propagated in human embryonic and adult non-nervous tissue cultures. They were awarded the Nobel Prize in 1954 for this work.

Dr John F. Enders (1897–1985), American microbiologist, shared the 1954 Nobel Prize in Medicine with T.H. Weller and F.C. Robbins for discovering that many viruses (specifically poliomyelitis virus) can be grown in tissue culture and thereby studied and isolated, making possible the production of vaccines.

Jonas Salk (Figure 6), at the University of Pittsburgh, prepared a vaccine including all three types of polio virus, inactivated by formaldehyde, which proved safe and effective and was used in 650 000 children in 1954. Employing the principles of local immunization established by Besredka at the Pasteur Institute during the early part of the 20th century, Albert Sabin (Figure 7) developed a live attenuated oral vaccine for poliomyelitis, which produced local immunity in the intestine. Later, Enders and associates isolated the measles virus, grew it in tissue culture and developed highly effective vaccines. This was followed by the

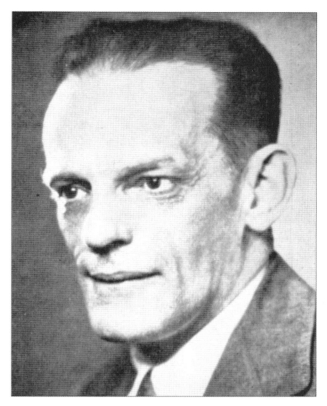

Figure 4   Max Theiler, Nobel Laureate, who perfected the 17D strain of yellow fever vaccine

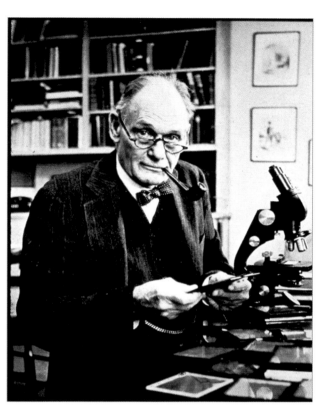

Figure 5   John F. Enders

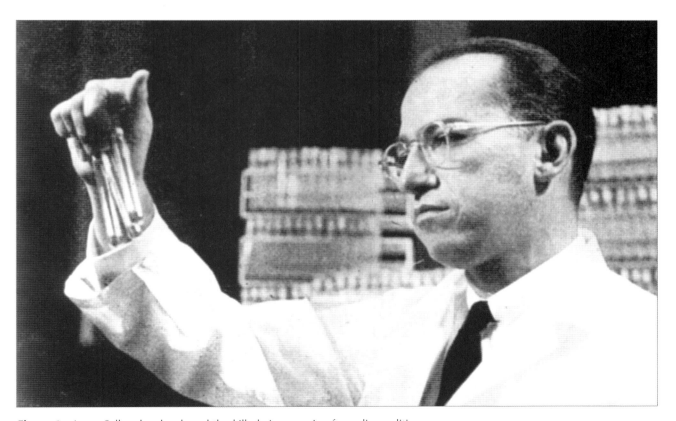

Figure 6   Jonas Salk, who developed the killed virus vaccine for poliomyelitis

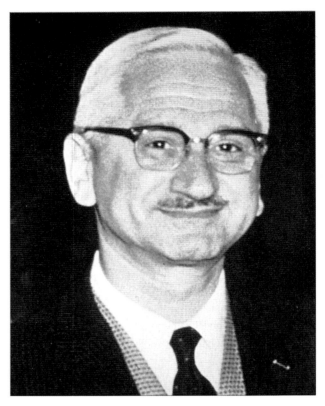

Figure 7 Albert Sabin, who developed the oral attenuated polio virus vaccine

isolation of rubella virus in 1962 by Weller and Parkman, and a successful vaccine was developed. A live mumps vaccine was introduced for general use in 1967, and is generally given with measles and rubella at age 15 months. Other vaccines developed include one against arboviruses, which infect domestic animals, meningococcal polysaccharide vaccines, adenovirus, herpes virus and some others, such as a rickettsial vaccine for typhus. Later a vaccine was developed for B viral hepatitis that is carried in the blood and other bodily fluids of some 200 million humans. A team led by Wolf Szmuness of the New York Blood Center in 1980 concluded a large field trial on a preparation developed from work begun in 1963, when the Australia antigen was first recognized by Baruch Blumberg in Philadelphia. Saul Krugman of New York University and Maurice Hilleman of the Merck Institute contributed to the research that led to hepatitis B vaccine.

Some attempts at vaccination have been disappointing. Although strains A, B and C, as well as A2, which causes Asian influenza, have been known for many years, the ability of influenza viruses to vary their antigenic patterns makes immunization difficult. Once a variant strain with a new antigenic structure develops against which the host does not have antibodies, the disease results. Much attention has been devoted to the development of protozoal vaccines. Vaccines for malaria have received top priority. There is great hope for the production of effective vaccines against other protozoan infections, which could be effectively used in the underdeveloped countries of the world. Immunoprophylaxis is not without hazard. For example, the use of live virus vaccines can prove fatal in children with T cell immunodeficiencies or in adults who have been deliberately immunosuppressed by drugs. Smallpox vaccination was sometimes followed by encephalitis or progressive vaccinia, both of which could lead to death. Yellow fever vaccination can lead to encephalitis. Live measles vaccine may produce convulsions. There is always the chance that live polio virus vaccine can lead to paralytic poliomyelitis. A live virus might penetrate the placenta, leading to infection of the fetus. Viruses contaminating tissue culture materials may cause problems. SV40 virus was found in live polio virus vaccine, and fowl leukosis viruses were discovered in yellow fever vaccine preparations. Viruses oncogenetic for one species could hybridize with a human virus, thereby passing on its oncogenic potential. In recent years, conjugate vaccines have proven especially valuable in the protection of very young children against *Haemophilus influenzae* and related infections.

Max Theiler (1899–1972), South African virologist who received the Nobel Prize in 1951 'for his development of vaccines against yellow fever'.

INTERFERON

While studying the phenomenon of viral interference, i.e. the resistance shown by cells infected by one virus to simultaneous infection by another, Alick Isaacs (Figure 8) and Jean Lindenmann discovered a substance which they named interferon. In these experiments, chick cells infected with influenza viruses were resistant to infection with other viruses. Healthy chick cells treated with an extract prepared from the growth medium were resistant to infection when challenged with a live virus preparation. Thus, it was clear that the virus-infected cells had produced a substance which

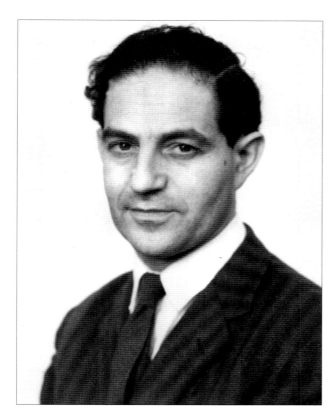

Figure 8 Alick Isaacs, discoverer, with Lindenmann, of interferon

interfered with the infection of other cells by viruses. The substance was soon shown to be cell- or species-specific and not-virus specific. This was all the more reason to pin great hopes on a substance that might aid the animal in resisting a cadre of viruses associated with various types of infectious diseases. Although impressive at first, interest began to wane because living cells produced only minute amounts, and interferon was technically difficult to purify and the process expensive. Kari Cantell, a Finnish virologist, produced interferon from leukocytes collected from 500–800 pints of blood collected each day from donors at the Finnish Red Cross. After infecting leukocytes with Sendai virus, he incubated the cells and then extracted interferon. His interferon was used in clinical trials throughout the world, not only to protect individuals against potentially devastating virus diseases, but it also proved effective in the treatment of some forms of cancer, apparently through the activation of natural killer (NK) cells.

Recombinant DNA technology and cDNA cloning techniques have revolutionized our understanding of complex molecules, such as interleukin-2 (IL-2) and other lymphokines, produced in picomolar quantities by immune system cells but made available for analysis in milligram quantities by the marvels of genetic engineering technology and the polymerase chain reaction.

CONGENITAL IMMUNODEFICIENCIES

In 1952, Bruton described hereditary sex-linked agammaglobulinemia in young boys who had only trace amounts of immunoglobulins in the blood, but their T cell immune function remained intact. This represented a classic defect of B cells. By contrast, DiGeorge syndrome, characterized by defective T cell immunity, was described later and attributed to failure of the thymus to develop. On the other hand, the severe combined form (Swiss type) of immunodeficiency represented a failure of both B and T cell limbs of the immune response. Robert Good, Donnall Thomas and others instituted widespread clinical application of bone marrow transplants for treatment of these unfortunate children with defective immunity. Richard Hong at Wisconsin successfully treated selected T cell and combined immunodeficient children with fetal tissue thymus transplants.

Adenosine deaminase-deficient patients have been successfully treated by 'gene therapy' at the National Institutes of Health (USA) as a consequence of phenomenal advances in genetic engineering and gene transfection technology.

ACQUIRED IMMUNE DEFICIENCY SYNDROME

In mid-1981, five young homosexual males in Los Angeles contracted *Pneumocystis carinii* pneumonia, and two died. This heralded the beginning of what became known as the AIDS (acquired immune deficiency syndrome) epidemic. An intensive research program was launched that led to rapid advances, with the discovery in 1984 of a retrovirus as the etiologic agent of the disease. Luc Montagnier and associates, at the Institut Pasteur in Paris, discovered LAV (lymphadenopathy-associated virus), which was subsequently named HIV (human immunodeficiency virus), the causative agent of AIDS. This was followed by the development of an antibody test to protect the blood supply. In spite of phenomenal advances in unraveling the molecular biology of AIDS, development of an effective vaccine has proved elusive thus far. The infection, which was first described in the USA but was subsequently found in countries around the world, is characterized by profound immunosuppression as the virus targets CD4 lymphocytes. This renders patients susceptible to a litany of opportunistic microbial agents, secondary neoplasms and neurologic manifestations. Although first described in homosexual and bisexual males, it also afflicts intravenous drug abusers, and recipients of HIV-infected blood and blood products. In Africa it is a heterosexual disease. Controlling the AIDS epidemic is one of the most challenging public health problems in the world today.

Vaccines and immunization

A **vaccine** may contain live attenuated or killed microorganisms, or parts or products from them, capable of stimulating a specific immune response comprising protective antibodies and T cell immunity. A vaccine should stimulate a sufficient number of memory T and B lymphocytes to yield effector T cells and antibody-producing B cells from memory cells. Viral vaccine should also be able to stimulate high titers of neutralizing antibodies. Injection of a vaccine into a non-immune subject induces active immunity against the modified pathogens.

Other than macromolecular components, a vaccine may consist of a plasmid that contains a cDNA encoding an antigen of a microorganism. Other vaccines include anti-insect vector vaccines, fertility-control vaccines, peptide-based preparations, anti-idiotype preparations and DNA vaccines, among others. There is no anti-parasite vaccine manufactured by conventional technology in use at present. Vaccines can be prepared from weakened or killed microorganisms; inactivated toxins; toxoids derived from microorganisms; or immunologically active surface markers extracted from microorganisms. They can be administered intramuscularly, subcutaneously, intradermally, orally or intranasally, as single agents or in combination. An ideal vaccine should be effective, well tolerated, easy and inexpensive to produce, easy to administer and convenient to store. Vaccine side-effects include fever, muscle aches and injection site pain, but these are usually mild. Reportable adverse reactions to vaccines include anaphylaxis, shock, seizures, active infection and death.

Vaccination is immunization against infectious disease through the administration of vaccines for the production of active (protective) immunity in man or other animals.

To **attenuate** is the process of diminishing the virulence of a pathogenic microorganism, rendering it incapable of causing disease. Attenuated bacteria or viruses may be used in vaccines to induce better protective immunity than would have been induced with a killed vaccine.

Hyperimmunization is the successive administration of an immunogen to an animal to induce the synthesis of antibody in relatively large amounts. This procedure is followed in the preparation of therapeutic antisera by repeatedly immunizing animals to render them 'hyperimmune'.

A **live vaccine** is an immunogen for protective immunization that contains an attenuated strain of the causative agent, an attenuated strain of a related microorganism that cross-protects against the pathogen of interest, or the introduction of a disease agent through an avenue other than its normal portal of entry or in combination with an antiserum.

A **killed vaccine** is an immunizing preparation composed of microorganisms, either bacterial or viral, that are dead, but retain their antigenicity, making them capable of inducing a protective immune response with the formation of antibodies and/or stimulation of cell-mediated immunity. Killed vaccines do not induce even a mild case of the disease, which is sometimes observed with attenuated (greatly weakened, but still living) vaccines. Although the first killed vaccines contained intact dead microorganisms, some modern preparations contain subunits or parts of microorganisms to be used for immunization. Killed microorganisms may be combined with toxoids, as in the case of the DPT (diphtheria–pertussis–tetanus) preparations administered to children.

Live attenuated vaccine is an immunizing preparation consisting of microorganisms whose disease-producing capacity has been weakened deliberately in order that they may be used as immunizing agents. Response to a live attenuated vaccine more closely resembles a natural infection than does the immune response stimulated by killed vaccines. The microorganisms in the live vaccine are actually dividing to increase the dose of immunogen, whereas the microorganisms in the killed vaccines are not reproducing, and the amount of injected immunogen remains unchanged. Thus, in general, the protective immunity conferred by the response to live attenuated vaccines is superior to that conferred by the response to killed vaccines. Examples of live attenuated vaccines include those used to protect against measles, mumps, polio and rubella. Live attenuated virus vaccines contain live viruses in which accumulated mutations impede their growth in human cells and their disease-causing capacity.

Live attenuated measles (rubeola) virus vaccine is an immunizing preparation that contains live measles virus strains. It is the preferred form except in patients with lymphoma, leukemia or other generalized malignancies; radiation therapy; pregnancy; active tuberculosis; egg sensitivity; prolonged drug treatment that suppresses the immune response, such as corticosteroids or antimetabolites; or administration of gammaglobulin, blood or plasma. Persons in these groups should be administered immune globulin immediately following exposure.

Live measles virus vaccine is a standardized attenuated virus immunizing preparation used to protect against measles.

Live measles and mumps virus vaccine is a standardized immunizing preparation that contains attenuated measles and mumps viruses.

Live measles and rubella virus vaccine is a standardized immunizing preparation that contains attenuated measles and rubella viruses.

Live oral polio virus vaccine is an immunizing preparation prepared from three types of live attenuated polio viruses. An advisory panel to the Centers for Disease Control and Prevention recommended in 1999 that its routine use be discontinued. It contains a live yet weakened virus that has led to eight to ten cases of polio each year. Now that the polio epidemic has been eliminated in the United States, this risk is no longer acceptable. It is also called Sabin vaccine.

Live rubella virus vaccine is an attenuated virus immunizing preparation employed to protect against rubella (German measles). All non-pregnant susceptible women of child-bearing age should be provided with this vaccine to prevent fetal infection and the congenital rubella syndrome, i.e. possible fetal death, prematurity, impaired hearing, cataract, mental retardation and other serious consequences.

Tetanus antitoxin is an antibody raised by immunizing horses against *Clostridium tetani* exotoxin. It is a therapeutic agent to treat or prevent tetanus in individuals with contaminated lesions. Anaphylaxis or serum sickness (type III hypersensitivity) may occur in individuals receiving second injections because of sensitization to horse serum proteins following initial exposure to horse antitoxin. One solution to this has been the use of human antitetanus toxin of high titer. Treatment of the immunoglobulin G (IgG) fraction yields $F(ab')_2$ fragments which retain all of the toxi-neutralizing capacity but with diminished antigenicity of the antitoxin preparation.

A **toxoid** is formed by treating a microbial toxin with formaldehyde to inactivate toxicity, but leave the immunogenicity (antigenicity) of the preparation intact. Toxoids are prepared from exotoxins produced in diphtheria and tetanus. These are used to induce protective immunization against adverse effects of the exotoxins in question.

DTaP vaccine is an acellular preparation used for protective immunization, comprising diphtheria and tetanus toxoids and acellular pertussis proteins, that is used to induce protective immunity in children against diphtheria, tetanus and pertussis. Children should receive DTaP vaccine at the ages of 2, 4, 6 and 15 months, with a booster given at 4–6 years of age. The tetanus and diphtheria toxoids should be repeated at 14–16 years of age. The vaccine is contraindicated in individuals who have shown prior allergic reactions to DTaP or in subjects with acute or developing neurologic disease. DTaP vaccine is effective in preventing most cases of the disease it addresses.

Polyvalent pneumococcal vaccine is an immunizing preparation that contains 23 of the known 83 pneumococcal capsular polysaccharides. It induces immunity for a duration of 3–5 years. The vaccine is believed to protect against 90% of the pneumococcal types that induce serious illness in patients over 2 years of age. Children at high risk can be vaccinated at 6 months of age and reinoculated at 2 years of age. It is especially indicated in high-risk patients such as those with sickle cell disease, chronic debilitating disease and immunological defects and the elderly. Vaccination against pneumococcal disease is of increasing significance as *Streptococcus pneumoniae* becomes increasingly resistant to antibiotics.

Rabies vaccine In humans, significant levels of neutralizing antibody can be generated by immunization with a virus grown in tissue culture in diploid human embryo lung cells. A rabies vaccine adapted to chick embryos, especially egg passage material, is used for prophylaxis in animals prior to exposure. The 'historical' vaccine originally prepared by Pasteur made use of rabbit spinal cord preparations to which the virus had become adapted. However, they were discontinued because of the risk of inducing post-rabies vaccination encephalomyelitis.

Typhoid vaccine Two forms of immunizing preparation are currently in use. One is a live, attenuated *Salmonella typhi* strain Ty2la that is used as an oral vaccine administered in four doses to adults and children over 6 years of age. It affords protection for 5 years. This vaccine is contraindicated in patients taking antimicrobial drugs and in AIDS patients. A second type of the vaccine, which is for parenteral use, is prepared from the capsular polysaccharide of *S. typhi*. It is administered to 6-month-old children, divided into two doses spaced 4 weeks apart. It is effective 55–75% of the time and lasts for 3 years.

Yellow fever vaccine is a lyophilized attenuated vaccine prepared from the 17D strain of liver-attenuated yellow fever virus grown in chick embryos. A single injection may confer immunity that persists for a decade.

Salk vaccine is an injectable poliomyelitis virus vaccine, killed by formalin, that was used for prophylactic immunization against poliomyelitis prior to development of the Sabin oral polio vaccine.

Poliomyelitis vaccines A live attenuated oral poliomyelitis vaccine combining the three strains of poliomyelitis virus was first introduced by Sabin. Replication in the gastrointestinal tract stimulates effective local immunity associated with IgA antibody synthesis. Individuals to be immunized receive three oral doses of the vaccine. This largely replaces the Salk vaccine, which was introduced in the early 1950s as a vaccine comprising the three strains of polio virus that had been killed with formalin. This preparation must be administered subcutaneously.

Influenza virus vaccine is a purified and inactivated immunizing preparation made from viruses grown in eggs. It cannot lead to infection. It contains H1N1 and H3N2 type A strains and one type B strain. These are the strains considered most likely to cause influenza in the United States. Whole virus and split virus preparations are available. Children tolerate the split virus preparation better than the whole virus vaccine. The polyvalent immunizing preparation contains inactivated antigenic variants of the influenza virus (types A and B) either individually or combined for annual use. It protects against epidemic disease and the morbidity and mortality induced by influenza virus, especially in the aged and chronically ill. The vaccine is reconstituted each year to protect against the strains of influenza virus present in the population.

BCG (bacillus Calmette–Guérin) is a *Mycobacterium bovis* strain maintained for more than 75 years on potato and bile glycerine agar, which preserves the immunogenicity, but dissipates the virulence of the microorganism. It has long been used in Europe as a vaccine against tuberculosis, although it never gained popularity in the United States. It has also been used in tumor immunotherapy to activate non-specifically the immune response in selected tumor-bearing patients, such as those with melanoma or bladder cancer. It has been suggested as a possible vector for genes that determine HIV proteins such as *gag*, *pol*, *env*, gp20, gp40, reverse transcriptase and tetanus toxin. In certain countries with a high incidence of tuberculosis, BCG provides effective immunity against the disease, diminishing the risk of infection by approximately 75%. The vaccine has a disadvantage of rendering skin testing for tuberculosis inaccurate, especially in the first 5 years after inoculation, because it induces hypersensitivity to tuberculin.

Tuberculosis immunization requires the induction of protective immunity through injection of an attenuated vaccine containing bacillus Calmette–Guérin (BCG). This vaccine was more widely used in Europe than in the USA in an attempt to provide protection against development of tuberculosis. A local papule develops several weeks after injection in individuals who were previously tuberculin negative, as it is not administered to positive individuals. It is claimed to protect against development of tuberculosis, although not all authorities agree on its efficacy for this purpose. In recent years, oncologists have used BCG vaccine to reactivate the cellular immune system of patients bearing neoplasms, in the hope of facilitating anti-tumor immunity.

Measles vaccine is an attenuated virus vaccine administered as a single injection to children at 2 years of age or between 1 and 10 years old. Contra-indications include a history of allergy or convulsions. Puppies may be protected against canine distemper in the neonatal period by the administration of attenuated measles virus, which represents a heterologous vaccine. Passive immunity from the mother precludes

early immunization of puppies with live canine distemper vaccine.

Mumps vaccine is an attenuated virus vaccine prepared from virus generated in chick embryo cell cultures. It is a live attenuated immunizing preparation employed to prevent mumps. It should be administered under the same guidelines and restrictions that apply to live attenuated measles virus vaccine.

Rubella vaccine is an attenuated virus vaccine used to immunize girls 10–14 years of age. It is used in the MMR (measles, mumps and rubella) combination, or used alone to immunize seronegative women of child-bearing age, but it is not to be used during pregnancy.

Hepatitis vaccine (Figure 9) is a vaccine used to immunize subjects actively against hepatitis B virus and contains purified hepatitis B surface antigen. Current practice uses an immunogen prepared by recombinant DNA technology referred to as Recombivax®. The antigen preparation is administered in three sequential intramuscular injections to individuals such as physicians, nurses and other medical personnel who are at risk. Temporary

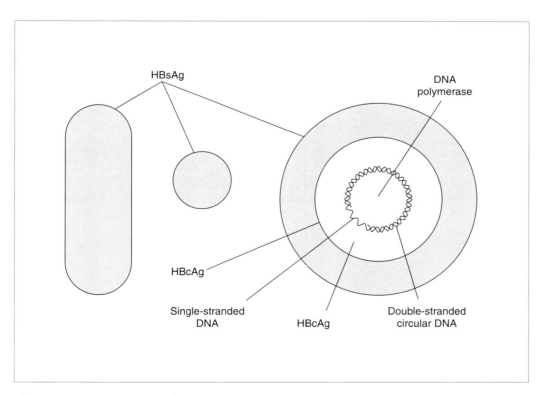

Figure 9 Hepatitis B virus and its antigens (Ag)

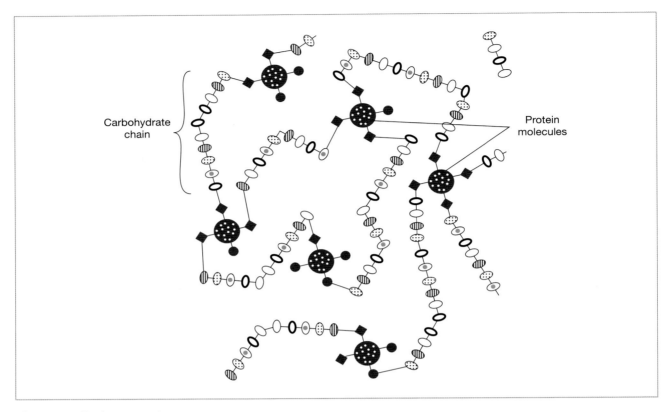

Carbohydrate chain

Protein molecules

Figure 10 Conjugate vaccine

protection against hepatitis A is induced by the passive administration of pooled normal human serum immunoglobulin which protects against hepatitis A virus for a brief time. Antibody for passive protection against hepatitis must be derived from the blood sera of specifically immune individuals.

Hepatitis B vaccine Human plasma-derived hepatitis B vaccine (Heptavax-B®), which was developed in the 1980s, was unpopular because of the fear of AIDS related to any product for injection derived from human plasma. It was replaced by a recombinant DNA vaccine (Recombivax®) prepared in yeast (*Saccharomyces cervesiae*). It is very effective in inducing protective antibodies in most recipients. Non-responders are often successfully immunized by intracutaneous vaccination. The immunizing preparation contains hepatitis B protein antigen produced by genetically engineered yeast.

Conjugate vaccine (Figure 10) is an immunogen comprising polysaccharide bound covalently to proteins. The conjugation of weakly immunogenic, bacterial polysaccharide antigens with protein carrier

molecules considerably enhances their immunogenicity. Conjugate vaccines have reduced morbidity and mortality for a number of bacterial diseases in vulnerable populations, such as the very young or adults with immunodeficiencies. An example of a conjugate vaccine is *Haemophilus influenzae* six-polysaccharide polyribosyl–ribitol–phosphate vaccine.

Haemophilus influenzae **type b vaccine (HB)** is an immunizing preparation that contains purified polysaccharide antigen from *H. influenzae* microorganisms and a carrier protein. It diminishes the risks of epiglottitis, meningitis and other *H. influenzae*-induced diseases during childhood.

Malaria vaccine Although there is no effective vaccine against malaria (Figure 11), several vaccine candidates are under investigation, including an immunogenic but non-pathogenic *Plasmodium* sporozoite that has been attenuated by radiation. Circumsporozoite proteins combined with sporozoite surface protein 2 (SSP-2) are immunogenic. Murine studies have shown the development of transmission-blocking antibodies following immunization with

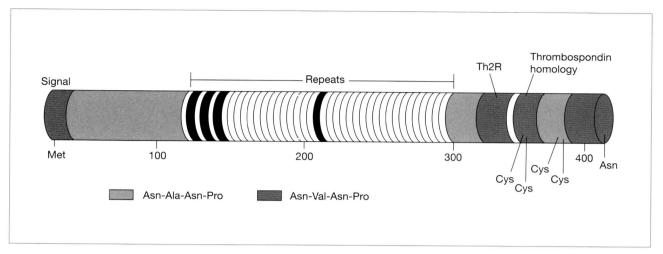

Figure 11 Circumsporate protein of malaria

vaccinia into which has been inserted the *Plasmodium falciparum* surface 25-kDa protein designated Pfs25. Attempts have been made to increase natural antibodies against circumsporozoite (CS) protein to prevent the prehepatoinvasive stage. The high mutability of *P. falciparum* makes prospects for an effective vaccine dim.

Plague vaccine *Yersinia pestis* microorganisms killed by heat or formalin are injected intramuscularly to induce immunity against plague. It is administered in three doses, 4 weeks or more apart. The duration of the immunity is approximately 6 months. A live attenuated vaccine, used mainly in Java, has also been found to induce protective immunity.

Typhus vaccination Protective immunization against typhus transmitted by lice or fleas and against Rocky mountain spotted fever is achieved by the administration of inactivated vaccines. Rickettsiae prepared in chick embryo yolk sacs or tissues are treated with formaldehyde to render them inactive. Rather than provide protective immunity that prevents the disease, these vaccines condition the host to experience a milder or less severe form of the disease than that which occurs in a non-vaccinated host.

Meningococcal vaccine is an immunizing preparation that contains bacterial polysaccharides from certain types of meningococci. Meningococcal polysaccharide vaccines A, C, Y and W135 are available for preventing diseases induced by those

serogroups. There is no vaccine for meningococcal serogroup B.

A **DNA vaccine** is an immunizing preparation comprising a bacterial plasmid containing a cDNA encoding a protein antigen. The mechanism apparently consists of professional antigen-presenting cells transfected *in vivo* by the plasmid, which then express immunogenic peptides that induce specific immune responses. The CpG nucleotides present in the plasmid DNA serve as powerful adjuvants. DNA vaccines may induce powerful cytotoxic T lymphocyte responses. This is an immunizing preparation prepared by genetic engineering in which the gene that encodes an antigen is inserted into a bacterial plasmid which is injected into the host. Once inside, it employs the nuclear machinery of the host cell to manufacture and express the antigen. In contrast to other vaccines, DNA vaccines may induce cellular as well as humoral immune responses.

Cytokines and chemokines

Leukocytes or other types of cells produce soluble proteins or glycoproteins termed cytokines that serve as chemical communicators from one cell to another. Cytokines are usually secreted, although some may be expressed on a cell membrane or maintained in reservoirs in the extracellular matrix. Cytokines combine with surface receptors on target cells that are linked to intracellular signal transduction and second messenger pathways. Their effects may be autocrine, acting on cells that produce them, or paracrine, acting on neighboring cells, and only rarely endocrine, acting on cells at distant sites.

Cytokines are immune system proteins that are biological response modifiers. They coordinate antibody and T cell immune system interactions, and amplify immune reactivity. Cytokines include monokines synthesized by macrophages and lymphokines produced by activated T lymphocytes and natural killer cells. Monokines include interleukin-1, tumor necrosis factor, α and β interferons and colony-stimulating factors. Lymphokines include interleukins-2–6, γ interferon, granulocyte macrophage colony-stimulating factor (GM-CSF) and lymphotoxin. Endothelial cells, fibroblasts and selected other cell types may also synthesize cytokines (Figure 12).

Lymphokine research can be traced to the 1960s when macrophage migration inhibitory factor was described. It is believed to be due to more than one cytokine in lymphocyte supernatants. Lymphotoxin was described in activated lymphocyte culture supernatants in the late 1960s, and lymphokines were recognized as cell-free soluble factors formed when sensitized lymphocytes respond to specific antigen. These substances were considered responsible for cell-mediated immune reactions. Interleukin-2 was described as T cell growth factor. Tumor necrosis factor (TNF) was the first monocyte/macrophage-derived cytokine or monokine to be recognized. Other cytokines derived from monocytes include lymphocyte activation factor (LAF), later named interleukin-1. It was found to be mitogenic for thymocytes. Whereas immunologists described lymphokines and monokines, virologists described interferons. Interferon is a factor formed by virus-infected cells that are able to induce resistance of cells to infection with homologous or heterologous viruses. Subsequently, interferon-γ, synthesized by T lymphocytes activated by mitogen, was found to be distinct from interferon-α and -β and to be formed by a variety of cell types. Colony stimulating factors (CSFs) were described as proteins capable of promoting proliferation and differentiation of hematopoietic cells. CSFs promote granulocyte or monocyte colony formation in semisolid media. Proteins that facilitate the growth of non-

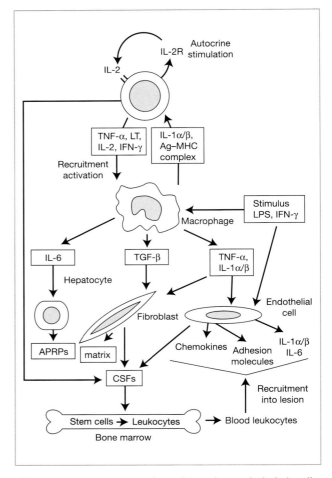

Figure 12 Generation of cytokines by endothelial cells, fibroblasts, T helper lymphocytes and monocyte/macrophages. TNF, tumor necrosis factor; IL, interleukin; LT, leukotriene; Ag, antigen; IFN, interferon; MHC, major histocompatibility complex; TGF, transforming growth factor; LPS, lipopolysaccharide; CSF, colony-stimulating factor; APRP, acute-phase reactant protein

hematopoietic cells are not usually included with the cytokines. Transforming growth factor-β has an important role in inflammation and immunoregulation as well as immunosuppressive actions on T cells.

Interferons (IFNs) constitute a group of immunoregulatory proteins synthesized by T lymphocytes, fibroblasts and other types of cells following stimulation with viruses, antigens, mitogens, double-stranded DNA or lectins. Interferons are classified as α and β, which have antiviral properties, and as γ, which is known as immune interferon. The α and β interferons share a common receptor, but γ has its own. Interferons have immunomodulatory functions. They enhance the ability of macrophages to destroy tumor cells, viruses and bacteria. Interferons α and β were formerly classified as type I interferons. They are acid-stable and synthesized mainly by leukocytes and fibroblasts. Interferon γ is acid-labile and is formed mainly by T lymphocytes stimulated by antigen or mitogen. This immune interferon has been termed type II interferon in the past. Whereas the ability of interferon to prevent infection of non-infected cells is species-specific, it is not virus-specific. Essentially, all viruses are subject to its inhibitory action. Interferons induce formation of a second inhibitory protein that prevents viral messenger RNA translation. In addition to γ interferon formation by T cells activated with mitogen, natural killer cells also secrete it. Interferons are not themselves viricidal.

Chemokines are a family of 8–10-kDa chemotactic cytokines that share structural homology. They are chemokinetic and chemotactic, stimulating leukocyte movement and directed movement. Two internal disulfide loops are present in chemokine molecules that may be subdivided according to the position of the two amino-terminal cysteine residues, i.e. adjacent (cys–cys) or separated by a single amino acid (cys–X–cys). Activated mononuclear phagocytes as well as fibroblasts, endothelium and megakaryocytes synthesize cys–X–cys chemokines, including interleukin-8, that act mainly on polymorphonuclear neutrophils as acute inflammatory mediators. Activated T lymphocytes synthesize cys–cys chemokines that act principally on mononuclear inflammatory cell subpopulations. Cys–X–cys and cys–cys chemokines combine with heparan sulfate proteoglycans on endothelial cell surfaces. They may activate chemokinesis of leukocytes that adhere to endothelium via adhesion molecules. Chemokine receptors are being characterized, and selected ones interact with more than one chemokine.

Immunodeficiencies: congenital and acquired

Immunodeficiencies are classified as either primary diseases with a genetic origin or those that are secondary to an underlying disorder. **X-linked (congenital) agammaglobulinemia** results from a failure of pre-B cells to differentiate into mature B cells. The defect in

Bruton's disease is in rearrangement of immunoglobulin heavy-chain genes. It occurs almost entirely in males, and is apparent after 6 months of age following disappearance of the passively transferred maternal immunoglobulins. Patients have recurrent sinopulmonary infections caused by *Haemophilus influenzae*, *Streptococcus pyogenes*, *Staphylococcus aureus* and *Streptococcus pneumoniae*. These patients have absent or decreased B cells and decreased serum levels of all immunoglobulin classes. The T-cell system and cell-mediated immunity appear to be normal.

Immunodeficiency disorders are conditions characterized by decreased immune function. They may be grouped into four principal categories based on recommendations from a committee of the World Health Organization. They include: antibody (B cell) deficiency, cellular (T cell) deficiency, combined T cell and B cell deficiencies and phagocyte dysfunction. The deficiency can be congenital or acquired. It can be secondary to an embryologic abnormality, an enzymatic defect or may be attributable to an unknown cause. Types of infections produced in the physical findings are characteristic of the type of immunodeficiency disease. Screening tests identify a number of these conditions, whereas others have an unknown etiology. Antimicrobial agents for the treatment of recurrent infections, immunotherapy, bone marrow transplantation, enzyme replacement and gene therapy are all modes of treatment.

Transient hypogammaglobulinemia of infancy is a temporary delay in the onset of antibody synthesis during the first 12 months or even 24 months of life. This leads to only a transient, physiologic immunodeficiency following catabolism of maternal antibodies passed to the infant across the placenta to the fetal circulation. Helper T cell function is impaired, yet B cell numbers are at physiologic levels.

X-linked agammaglobulinemia (Bruton's X-linked agammaglobulinemia) affects males who develop recurrent sinopulmonary or other pyogenic infections at 5–6 months of age after disappearance of maternal IgG. There is a defective B lymphocyte gene (chromosome Xq21.3–22). Whereas B cells and immunoglobulins are diminished, there is normal T cell function. Supportive therapy includes gammaglobulin injections and antibiotics. Repeated infections may lead to death in childhood. Their bone marrow contains pre-B cells with constant regions of immunoglobulin μ chains in the cytoplasm. There may be defective VH–D–JH (variable–diversity–joining) gene rearrangement.

btk is a protein tyrosine kinase encoded by the defective gene in X-linked agammaglobulinemia (XLA). B lymphocytes and polymorphonuclear neutrophils express the btk protein. In XLA (Bruton's disease) patients, only the B lymphocytes manifest the defect, and the maturation of B lymphocytes stops at the pre-B cell stage. There is rearrangement of heavy-chain genes but not of the light-chain genes. The btk protein might have a role in linking the pre-B cell receptor to nuclear changes that result in growth and differentiation of pre-B cells.

Selective immunoglobulin deficiency is an insufficient quantity of one of the three major immunoglobulins or a subclass of IgG or IgA. The most common is selective IgA deficiency followed by IgG3 and IgG2 deficiencies. Patients suffering from selective immunoglobulin deficiency may be either normal or manifest increased risk for bacterial infections.

DiGeorge syndrome is a T cell immunodeficiency in which there is failure of T cell development, but normal maturation of stem cells and B lymphocytes. This is attributable to failure in the development of the thymus, depriving the individual of the mechanism for T lymphocyte development. DiGeorge syndrome is a recessive genetic immunodeficiency characterized by failure of the thymic epithelium to develop. Maldevelopment of the thymus gland is associated with thymic hypoplasia. Anatomical structures derived from the third and fourth pharyngeal pouches during embryogenesis fail to develop. This leads to a defect in the function of both the thymus and parathyroid glands. DiGeorge syndrome is believed to be a consequence of intrauterine malfunction. It is not familial. Tetany and hypocalcemia, both characteristics of hypoparathyroidism, are observed in DiGeorge syndrome in addition to the defects in T cell immunity. Peripheral lymphoid tissues exhibit a deficiency of lymphocytes in thymic-dependent areas. By contrast, the B or bursa equivalent-dependent areas, such as lymphoid follicles, show normal numbers of B lymphocytes and plasma cells. Serum immunoglobulin levels are within normal limits, and there is a normal immune response following immunization with commonly employed immunogens. A defect in delayed-type hypersensitivity is demonstrated by the failure of affected patients to develop positive skin tests to commonly employed antigens such as candidin or streptokinase, and the inability to develop an allograft response. Defective cell-mediated immunity may increase susceptibility to opportunistic infections and render the individual vulnerable to a graft-versus-host reaction in blood transfusion recipients. There is also minimal or absent *in vitro* responsiveness to T cell antigens or mitogens. The most significant advance has been the identification of microdeletions on human chromosome 22q in most DiGeorge syndrome patients. Considerable success in treatment has been achieved with fetal thymic transplants and by the passive administration of thymic humoral factors.

Severe combined immunodeficiency syndrome (SCID) is a profound immunodeficiency characterized by functional impairment of both B and T lymphocyte limbs of the immune response. It is inherited as an X-linked or autosomal recessive disease. The thymus has only sparse lymphocytes and Hassal's corpuscles, or is bereft of them. Several congenital immunodeficiencies are characterized as SCID. There is T and B cell lymphopenia and decreased production of IL-2. There is an absence of delayed-type hypersensitivity, cellular immunity and normal antibody synthesis following immunogenic challenge. SCID is a disease of infancy with failure to thrive. Affected individuals frequently die during the first 2 years of life. Clinically, they may develop a measles-like rash, show hyperpigmentation and develop severe recurrent (especially pulmonary) infections. These subjects have heightened susceptibility to infectious disease agents such as *Pneumocystis carinii*, *Candida albicans* and others. Even attenuated microorganisms, such as those used for immunization, e.g. attenuated poliomyelitis viruses, may induce infection in SCID patients. Graft-versus-host disease is a problem in SCID patients receiving unirradiated blood transfusions. Maternal–fetal transfusions during gestation or at parturition, or blood transfusions at a later date, provide sufficient immunologically competent cells entering the SCID patient's circulation to induce graft-versus-host disease. SCID may be manifested in one of several forms. SCID is classified as a defect in adenosine deaminase (ADA) and purine nucleoside phosphorylase (PNP) enzymes and in a DNA-binding protein needed for human leukocyte antigen (HLA) gene expression. Treatment is by bone marrow transplantation or by gene therapy and enzyme reconstitution in those cases caused by a missing gene, such as adenosine deaminase deficiency.

Adenosine deaminase (ADA) deficiency is a form of severe combined immunodeficiency (SCID) in which affected individuals lack an enzyme, adenosine deaminase (ADA), which catalyzes the deamination of adenosine as well as deoxyadenosine to produce inosine and deoxyinosine, respectively. Cells of the thymus, spleen and lymph node, as well as red blood cells, contain free ADA enzyme. In contrast to the other forms of SCID, children with ADA deficiency possess Hassall's corpuscles in the thymus. The accumulation of deoxyribonucleotides in various tissues, especially thymic cells, is toxic and is believed to be a cause of immunodeficiency. As deoxyadenosine and deoxy-adenosine triphosphate (ATP) accumulate, the latter substance inhibits ribonucleotide reductase activity, which inhibits formation of the substrate needed for synthesis of DNA. These toxic substances are especially injurious to T lymphocytes. The auto-somal recessive ADA deficiency leads to death. Two-fifths of severe combined immunodeficiency cases are of this type. The patient's signs and symptoms reflect defective cellular immunity with oral candidiasis, persistent diarrhea, failure to thrive and other disorders, with death occurring prior to 2 years of age. T lymphocytes are significantly diminished. There is eosinophilia and elevated serum and urine adenosine and deoxyadenosine levels. As bone marrow transplantation is relatively ineffective, gene therapy is the treatment of choice.

Immunodeficiency with thrombocytopenia and eczema (Wiskott–Aldrich syndrome) is an X-linked recessive disease characterized by thrombocytopenia, eczema and susceptibility to recurrent infections, sometimes leading to early death. The life span of young boys is diminished as a consequence of extensive infection, hemorrhage and sometimes malignant disease of the lymphoreticular system. Infectious agents affecting these individuals include the Gram-negative and Gram-positive bacteria, fungi and viruses. The thymus is normal morphologically, but there is a variable decline in cellular immunity, which is thymus dependent. The lymph node architecture may be altered as paracortical areas become depleted of cells with progression of the disease. IgM levels in serum are low, but IgA and IgG may be increased.

Isohemagglutinins are usually undetectable in the serum. Patients may respond normally to protein antigens, but show defective responsiveness to polysaccharide antigens. There is decreased immune responsiveness to lipopolysaccharides from enteric bacteria and B blood group substances.

Phagocyte disorders are conditions characterized by recurrent bacterial infections that can involve the skin, respiratory tract and lymph nodes. Evaluation of phagocytosis should include tests of motility, chemotaxis, adhesion, intracellular killing (respiratory burst), enzyme testing and examination of the peripheral blood smear. Phagocyte disorders include the following conditions: chronic granulomatous disease; myeloperoxidase deficiency; Job syndrome (hyperimmunoglobulin E syndrome); Chediak–Higashi syndrome; leukocyte adhesion deficiency; together with less common disorders.

Phagocytic cell function deficiencies Patients with this group of disorders frequently show an increased susceptibility to bacterial infections, but are generally able successfully to combat infections by viruses and protozoa. Phagocytic dysfunction can be considered as either extrinsic or intrinsic defects. Extrinsic factors include diminished opsonins that result from deficiencies in antibodies and complement, immunosuppressive drugs or agents that reduce phagocytic cell numbers, corticosteroids that alter phagocytic cell function and autoantibodies against neutrophil antigens that diminish the number of polymorphonuclear cells (PMNs) in the blood circulation. Complement deficiencies or inadequate complement components may interfere with neutrophil chemotaxis to account for other extrinsic defects. By contrast, intrinsic defects affect the ability of phagocytic cells to kill bacteria. This is related to deficiencies of certain metabolic enzymes associated with the intracellular digestion of bacterial cells. Among the disorders are chronic granulomatous disease, myeloperoxidase deficiency and defective glucose-6-phosphate-dehydrogenase.

Chemotactic disorders are conditions attributable to abnormalities of the complex molecular and cellular interactions involved in mobilizing an appropriate phagocytic cell response to injuries or inflammation. This can involve defects in either the humoral or cellular components of chemotaxis that usually lead to recurrent infections. The process begins with the generation of chemoattractants. Among these chemoattractants that act *in vivo* are the anaphylatoxins (C3a, C4a and C5a), leukotriene B_4 (LTB$_4$), interleukin-8 (IL-8), granulocyte macrophage colony-stimulating factor (GM-CSF) and platelet-activating factors. Once exposed to chemoattractant, circulating neutrophils embark upon a four-stage mechanism of emigration through the endothelial layer to a site of tissue injury where phagocytosis takes place. The four stages include:

(1) Rolling or initial margination by the selectins (L-, P-, E-);

(2) Stopping on the endothelium by CD18 integrins and intercellular adhesion molecular (ICAM)-1;

(3) Neutrophil–neutrophil adhesion by CD11b/CD18;

(4) Transendothelial migration by CD11b/CD18, CD11a/CD18, ICAM-1.

Chemotactic defects can be either acquired or inherited.

Complement deficiency conditions are rare. In healthy Japanese blood donors, only one in 100 000 persons had no C5, C6, C7 and C8. No C9 was contained in three of 1000 individuals. Most individuals with missing complement components do not manifest clinical symptoms. Additional pathways provide complement-dependent functions that are necessary to preserve life. If C3, factor I or any segment of the alternative pathway is missing, the condition may be life-threatening, with markedly decreased opsonization in phagocytosis. C3 is depleted when factor I is absent. C5, C6, C7 or C8 deficiencies are linked with infections, mainly meningococcal or gonococcal, which usually succumb to complement's bactericidal action. Deficiencies in classical complement pathway activation are often associated with connective tissue or immune complex diseases. Systemic lupus erythematosus may be associated with C1qrs, C2 or C4 deficiencies. Hereditary angioedema (HAE) patients have a deficiency of C1 inactivator. A number of experimental animals with specific complement deficiencies have been described, such as C6 deficiency in rabbits and C5 deficiency in mice. Acquired complement deficiencies may be caused either by accelerated complement consumption in immune complex diseases with a type III mechanism or by diminished formation of complement proteins as in acute necrosis of the liver.

Secondary immunodeficiency is an immunodeficiency that is not due to a failure or intrinsic defect in the T and B lymphocytes of the immune system. It is a consequence of some other disease process, and may be either transient or permanent. The transient variety may disappear following adequate treatment, whereas the more permanent type persists. Secondary immunodeficiencies are commonly produced by many effects. For example, those that appear in patients with neoplasms may result from effects of the tumor. Secondary immunodeficiencies may cause an individual to become susceptible to microorganisms that would otherwise cause no problem. They may occur following immunoglobulin or T lymphocyte loss, the administration of drugs, infections, cancer, effects of ionizing radiation on immune system cells and other causes.

Acquired immune deficiency syndrome (AIDS)

Acquired immune deficiency describes a decrease in the immune response to immunogenic (antigenic) challenge as a consequence of numerous diseases or conditions that include acquired immune deficiency syndrome (AIDS), chemotherapy, immunosuppressive drugs such as corticosteroids, psychological depression, burns, non-steroidal anti-inflammatory drugs, radiation, Alzheimer's disease, celiac disease, sarcoidosis, lymphoproliferative disease, Waldenström's macroglobulinemia, multiple myeloma, aplastic anemia, sickle cell disease, malnutrition, aging, neoplasia, diabetes mellitus and numerous other conditions.

Acquired immune deficiency syndrome (AIDS) is a retroviral disease marked by profound immunosuppression that leads to opportunistic infections, secondary neoplasms and neurologic manifestations. It is caused by the human immunodeficiency virus HIV-1, the causative agent for most cases worldwide, with a few in western Africa attributable to HIV-2. Principal transmission routes include sexual contact, parenteral inoculation and passage of the virus from infected mothers to their newborns. Although originally recognized in homosexual or bisexual men in the United States, it is increasingly a heterosexual disease. It appears to have originated in Africa, where it is a heterosexual disease and has been reported from more than 193 countries. The CD4 molecule on T lymphocytes serves as a high-affinity receptor for HIV. HIVgp120 must also bind to other cell surface molecules termed coreceptors for cell entry. They include CCR5 and CXCR4 receptors for β chemokines and α chemokines. Some HIV strains are macrophage-tropic, whereas others are T cell-tropic. Early in the disease, HIV colonizes the lymphoid organs. The striking decrease in $CD4^+$ T cells is a hallmark of AIDS that accounts for the immunodeficiency late in the course of HIV infection, but qualitative defects in T lymphocytes can be discovered in HIV-infected persons who are asymptomatic. Infection of macrophages and monocytes is very important, and the dendritic cells in lymphoid tissues are the principal sites of HIV infection and persistence. In addition to the lymphoid system, the nervous system is the major target of HIV infection. It is widely accepted that HIV is carried to the brain by infected monocytes. The microglia in the brain are the principal cell type infected in that tissue. The natural history of HIV infection is divided into three phases that include: an early acute phase, a middle chronic phase and a final crisis phase. Viremia, measured as HIV-1 RNA, is the best marker of HIV disease progression, and it is valuable clinically in the management of HIV-infected patients. Clinically, HIV infection can range from a mild acute illness to a severe disease. The adult AIDS patient may present with fever, weight loss, diarrhea, generalized

lymphadenopathy, multiple infections, neurologic disease and in some cases secondary neoplasms. Opportunistic infections account for 80% of deaths in AIDS patients. Prominent among these is pneumonia caused by *Pneumocystis carinii* as well as other common pathogens. AIDS patients also have a high incidence of certain tumors, especially Kaposi sarcoma, non-Hodgkin's lymphoma and cervical cancer in women. No effective vaccine has yet been developed.

AIDS serology Three to 6 weeks after infection with HIV-1 there are high levels of HIV p24 antigen in the plasma. One week to 3 months following infection there is an HIV-specific immune response resulting in the formation of antibodies against HIV envelope protein gp120 and HIV core protein p24. HIV-specific cytotoxic T lymphocytes are also formed. The result of this adaptive immune response is a dramatic decline in viremia and a clinically asymptomatic phase lasting from 2 to 12 years. As $CD4^+$ T cell numbers decrease, the patient becomes clinically symptomatic. HIV-specific antibodies and cytotoxic T lymphocytes decline, and p24 antigen increases.

AIDS belt refers to the geographic area across central Africa that describes a region where multiple cases of heterosexual AIDS, related to sexual promiscuity, were reported. Nations in this belt include Burundi, Central African Republic, Kenya, the Congo, Malawi, Rwanda, Tanzania, Uganda and Zambia.

Human immunodeficiency virus (HIV) (Figures 13–15) is the retrovirus that induces acquired immune

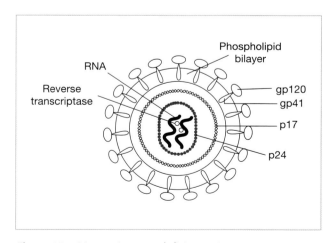

Figure 13   Human immunodeficiency virus (HIV)-1 structure

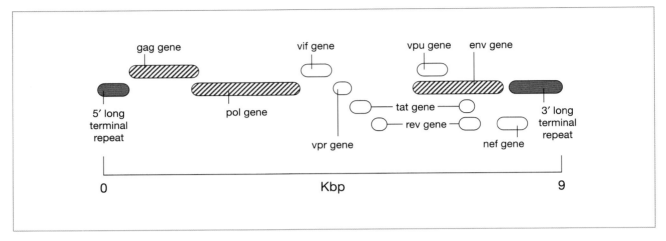

Figure 14 Human immunodeficiency virus (HIV)-1 genes

deficiency syndrome (AIDS) and associated disorders. It was isolated in early 1983 by Luc Montagnier, F. Barre-Sinoussi and J.C. Chermann from a culture of activated T lymphocytes derived from a lymph node biopsy of a homosexual patient with lymphadenopathy. Thus, Montagnier is credited with the original isolation. Another investigator, Robert Gallo of the US National Institutes of Health successfully propagated the virus in cell culture and developed critically needed diagnostic tests. Both groups have made major contributions to AIDS biology. It infects CD4$^+$ T lymphocytes, mononuclear phagocytes carrying CD4 molecules on their surface, follicular dendritic cells and Langerhans cells. It produces profound immunodeficiency affecting both humoral and cell-mediated immunity. There is a progressive decrease in CD4$^+$ helper/inducer T lymphocytes until they are finally depleted in many patients. There may be polyclonal activation of B lymphocytes with elevated synthesis of immunoglobulins. The immune response to the virus is not protective and does not improve the patient's condition. The virus is composed of an envelope glycoprotein (gp160) which is its principal antigen. It has a gp120 external segment and a gp41 transmembrane segment. CD4 molecules on CD4$^+$ lymphocytes and macrophages serve as receptors for gp120 of HIV. It has an inner core that contains RNA and is encircled by a lipid envelope. It contains structural genes designated *env*, *gag* and *pol* that encode the envelope protein, core protein and reverse transcriptase, respectively. HIV also possesses at least six additional genes, i.e. *tat*, that regulate HIV replication. It can increase production of viral protein several 1000-fold.

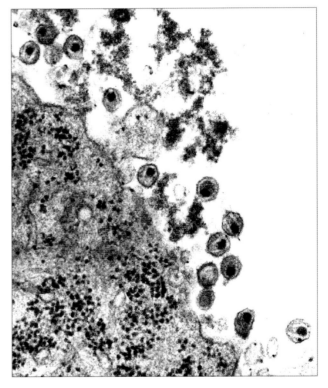

Figure 15 Human immunodeficiency virus (HIV): electron micrograph

rev encodes proteins that block transcription of regulatory genes. *vif* (*sor*) is the virus infectivity gene whose product increases viral infectivity and may promote cell-to-cell transmission. *nef* is a negative regulatory factor that encodes a product that blocks replication of the virus. *vpr* (viral protein R) and *vpu* (viral protein U) genes have also been described. No successful vaccine has yet been developed, although several types are under investigation.

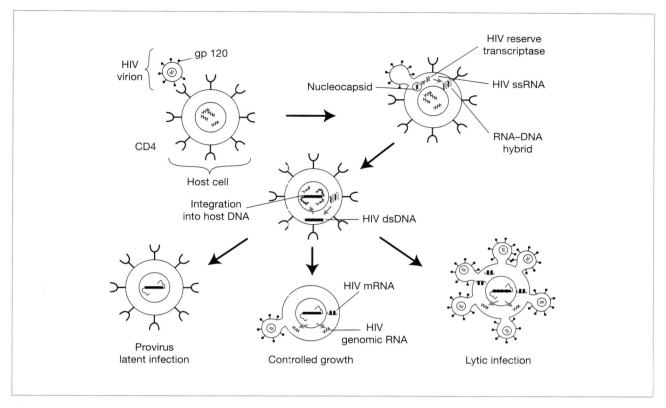

Figure 16   Human immunodeficiency virus (HIV) infection

HIV infection (Figure 16) The recognition of infection by the human immunodeficiency virus (HIV) is through seroconversion. Following conversion to positive reactivity in an antibody screening test, a Western blot analysis is performed to confirm the result of positive testing for HIV. HIV mainly affects the immune system and the brain. It affects primarily the CD4$^+$ lymphocytes which are necessary to initiate an immune response by interaction with antigen-presenting cells. This also deprives other cells of the immune system from receiving a supply of interleukin-2 through CD4$^+$ lymphocyte stimulation, leading to a progressive decline in immune system function. HIV transmission is by either sexual contact, through blood products or horizontally from mother to young.

HIV-1 genes include the *gag* gene which encodes the structural core proteins p17, p24, p15 and p55 precursor. *pol* encodes a protease that cleaves *gag* precursors. It also encodes reverse transcriptase that produces proviral DNA from RNA and encodes an integrase that is necessary for proviral insertion. *env* encodes gp160 precursor, gp120 and gp41 in mature

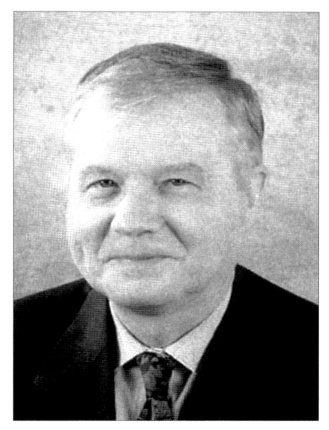

Figure 17   Luc Montagnier, Institut Pasteur, Paris

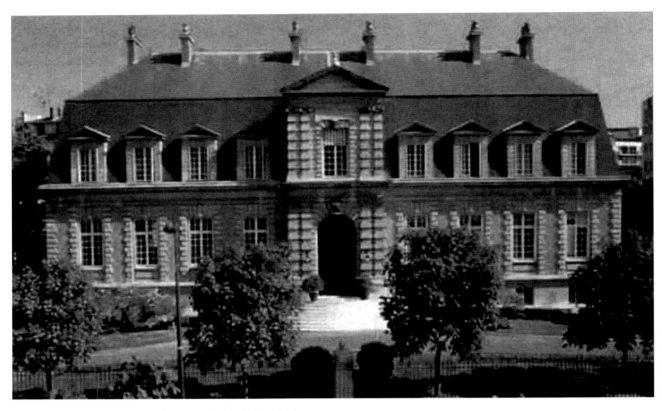

Figure 18   Institut Pasteur administration building, Paris

proteins. gp120 binds CD4 molecules, and gp41 is needed for fusion of the virus with the cell. *vpr*'s function is unknown. *vif* encodes a 23-kDa product that is necessary for infection of cells by free virus and is not needed for infection from cell to cell. *tat* encodes a p14 product that binds to viral long-terminal repeat (LTR) sequence and activates viral gene transcription. *rev* encodes a 20-kDa protein product that is needed for post-transcriptional expression of *gag* and *env* genes. *nef* encodes a 27-kDa protein that inhibits HIV transcription and slows viral replication. *vpu* encodes a 16-kDa protein product that may be required for assembly and packaging of new virus particles.

HIV-2 is an abbreviation for human immunodeficiency virus-2. Its clinical course resembles that of AIDS produced by HIV-1, but it is confined principally to western Africa and is transmitted principally through heterosexual promiscuity.

AIDS treatment   Two classes of antiviral drugs are used to treat HIV infection and AIDS. Nucleotide analogs inhibit reverse transcriptase activity. They include azidothymidine (AZT), dideoxyinosine and dideoxycytidine. They may diminish plasma HIV RNA levels for considerable periods, but often fail to stop disease progression because of the development of mutated forms of reverse transcriptase that resist these drugs. Viral protease inhibitors are now used to block the processing of precursor proteins into mature viral capsid and core proteins. Currently, a triple-drug therapy consisting of protease inhibitors together with two separate reverse transcriptase inhibitors is used to reduce plasma viral RNA to very low levels in patients treated for more than 1 year.

Further reading

Parish HJ. *A History of Immunization*. Edinburgh: E and S Livingstone, 1965

Parish HJ. *Victory with Vaccines*. Edinburgh: E and S Livingstone, 1968

Baxby D. *Jenner's Smallpox Vaccine*. London: Heinemann Educational Books, 1981

Plotkin SA, Orenstein WA. *Vaccines*. Philadelphia: WB Saunders Co, 1999

CHAPTER 13

Immunological methods

ASSAYS OF ANTIGENS AND ANTIBODIES

Just as the eclectic science of immunology intersects essentially all of the basic biological sciences, it makes use of many biochemical techniques such as chromatography and protein fractionation. It also employs the newer methods of molecular genetics such as gene sequencing and related techniques. Advances in technology have armed the immunologist with the powerful tools of polymerase chain reaction (PCR) technology, immunophenotyping by flow cytometry, hybridomas and monoclonal antibodies, DNA typing, enzyme-linked immunosorbent assay (ELISA) and radiolabeling of immune system molecules. In addition, the time-honored methods of precipitation, agglutination, complement fixation and related techniques have long been used by the immunologist. Since its inception, immunologic science has not only maintained a unique nomenclature but also special techniques that have elucidated some of nature's most jealously guarded secrets through scientific investigation. Inbred mice, of known genetic constitution, and more recently, transgenic animals including knockout mice, offer new avenues for elucidating some of immunology's most perplexing conundrums. Great tomes are currently available that describe the myriad immunological techniques now available.

Although Charrin and Roger observed that immune serum could produce clumping of bacteria in suspension[1], Durham in 1896 discovered bacterial agglutination by immune serum and applied the method as a diagnostic tool[2]. Widal applied the principle discovered by von Grüber (Chapter 2, Figure 27) and Durham

(Chapter 2, Figure 26) that the blood serum of typhoid patients would agglutinate typhoid bacilli to develop a clinically useful test for typhoid fever in which blood sera of patients were tested against known bacteria in an agglutination assay[3]. Kraus introduced the precipitin test the following year[4]. He discovered precipitation in a mixture of immune serum and culture filtrates of *Vibrio cholerae*. Both of these methods found immediate widespread use in diagnostic bacteriology. When Landsteiner (Chapter 2, Figure 39) described the human blood groups in 1900, he found natural isohemagglutinins in the serum[5]. The next year (1901), Bordet and Gengou discovered the complement fixation test and applied it to measure antigen–antibody reactions[6]. The complement fixation test found widespread use in the diagnosis of infectious diseases. When used to diagnose syphilis, the test became known as the Wassermann reaction[7]. After the demonstration by Denys and Leclef in 1895 that immunization has an enhancing effect upon phagocytosis[8], Wright and Douglas (1903) discovered antibodies in the blood, called opsonins, that attached to bacteria or other particles and assisted their phagocytosis[9]. This constituted the basis of an opsonocytophagic index that correlated the ability of patient leukocytes to phagocytize bacteria *in vitro* with the patient's level of immunity against the infectious disease agent. Although these studies had limited significance, they did yield some valuable information concerning opsonins in immunity.

Agglutination, precipitation and complement fixation were the tool of serology, the study of antigen–antibody interactions *in vitro*. Dean and Webb (1928) developed an optimal proportions procedure for the quantitation of precipitating antibodies[10]. In the 1930s, Heidelberger (Chapter 3, Figure 15) and Kendall developed precise methods for the quantitation of antibody, and they discovered and characterized nonprecipitating antibodies, which were functionally univalent or incomplete[11]. Pappenheimer and Robinson in the 1930s described a variant of precipitation called flocculation, which was observed in studies on horse antisera against bacterial toxins and later in the human reaction to thyroglobulin[12]. In 1934, Marrack (Chapter 3, Figures 9–12) proposed a lattice theory of secondary aggregates of antigen and antibody in his monograph on *The Chemistry of Antigens and Antibodies*[13]. A significant breakthrough in methodology came in 1937 when Tiselius proposed the electrophoretic method of separating serum proteins and the assignment of antibody activity to the globulin fraction[14]. In 1929, Kabat and Tiselius demonstrated by electrophoresis and ultracentrifugation that 19S antibody is found early and 7S antibody late in the immune response[15].

August von Wassermann (1866–1925), German physician who, with Neisser and Bruck, described the first serological test for syphilisis, i.e. the Wassermann reaction. *Handbuch der Pathogenen Mikroorganismen* (with Kolle), 1903.

Gaston Ramon (1886–1963), French immunologist who perfected the flocculation assay for diphtheria toxin.

Bela Schick (1877–1967), Austro-Hungarian pediatrician whose work with von Pirquet resulted in the discovery and description of serum sickness. He developed the test for diphtheria that bears his name. *Die Serumkrankheit* (with Pirquet), 1905.

Michael Heidelberger and associates in 1933 reported the use of colored materials in quantitative studies of the precipitation reaction[16]. They attached a salt of benzidine to egg albumin through a diazo linkage. Spectrophotometric methods were employed in the studies. Marrack (1934) showed that dyes could be introduced into antibody molecules without altering their immunological specificity[17]. In 1941, Coons (Figure 1a) and associates at Harvard Medical School first labeled antibody molecules with fluorescent dyes[18]. Coons' group later developed an improved optical filter system, a procedure for the preparation of isocyanate

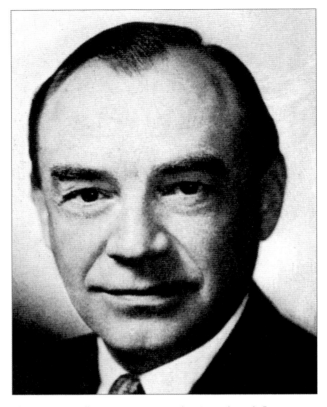

Figure 1a Albert H. Coons, who introduced fluorescent antibody methods

and a technique for the conjugation of antibody globulin with fluorescence dye[19]. Tissue sections or smears of material containing antigen were covered with specific antibody labeled with a fluorescent compound, and observed in ultraviolet light for fluorescence (Figure 1b). Although non-fluorescent dyes were first employed, they were inferior to the fluorescence variety because of the greater ease of detecting a minute amount of light against a dark background compared with detecting a small amount of color in a bright microscopic field. This fluorescent antibody method found wide application in diagnostic medicine as well as in research.

Albert Hewett Coons (1912–78), American immunologist and bacteriologist who was an early leader in immunohistochemistry with the development of fluorescent antibodies. Coons, a Professor at Harvard, received the Lasker medal in 1959, the Ehrlich Prize in 1961 and the Behring Prize in 1966.

The antiglobulin technique described in 1908 by Moreschi (Chapter 10, Figure 26) was rediscovered and perfected in 1945 by Coombs[20] (Chapter 9, Figure 4).

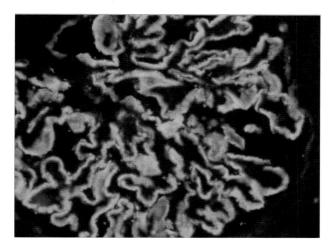

Figure 1b The fluorescence antibody method showing immune deposits in glomerulonephritis

This has been a useful tool in the detection of incomplete (i.e. more correctly termed non-agglutinating) antibodies, such as those found in certain types of autoimmune hemolytic anemia and hemolytic disease of the newborn. It detects antibodies attached to cell surfaces that are unable to bridge the gap between cells to produce agglutination in saline. The use of a medium that reduces the zeta potential surrounding cells and the use of rabbit antihuman immunoglobulin permitted Coombs to develop the test.

Jules Freund (1890–1960), Hungarian physician who later worked in the USA. He made many contributions to immunology, including work on antibody formation, studies on allergic encephalomyelitis and the development of Freund's adjuvant. He received the Lasker Award in 1959.

Jacques Oudin (1908–86), French immunologist who was director of analytical immunology at the Institut Pasteur, Paris. His accomplishments include discovery of idiotypy and the agar single diffusion method antigen–antibody assay.

Orjan Thomas Gunnersson Ouchterlony (1914–), Swedish bacteriologist who developed the antibody detection test that bears his name. Two-dimensional double diffusion with subsequent precipitation patterns is the basis of the assay. *Handbook of Immunodiffusion and Immunoelectrophoresis*, 1968.

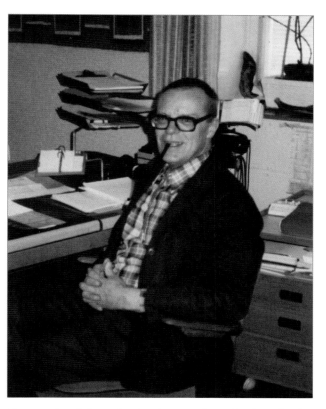

Figure 2 Orjan Ouchterlony, who developed the precipitation in gel technique by diffusion in two dimensions

In 1946, Oudin discovered that bands of precipitation occurred in tubes containing antiserum and antigen incorporated into agar[21]. This represented diffusion in a single dimension. The technique was expanded by Ouchterlony[22] (Figures 2 and 3) and independently by Elek[23] who used agar in Petri plates to allow antigen and antibody to diffuse from wells cut in the agar in two dimensions. With this technique, relative similarities or differences in antigens reacting with a common antiserum could be detected. Laser nephelometry proved beneficial in quantifying the precipitin reaction.

In 1953, Grabar (Figure 4) and Williams developed the immunoelectrophoresis technique in which a serum sample or other antigen preparation was electrophoresed to separate its components prior to interaction with antibody to produce precipitation lines in gel[24]. This method proved that certain immunoglobulin classes were lacking in the sera of hypogammaglobulinemia patients. This valuable technique found broad applications in both clinical diagnosis and research.

Pierre Grabar (1898–1986), French-educated immunologist, born in Kiev, who served as chef de

Figure 3   Precipitation in gel using the Ouchterlony technique

service at the Institut Pasteur and as director of the National Center for Scientific Research, Paris. He is best known for his work with Williams in the development of immunoelectrophoresis. He studied antigen–antibody interactions and developed the 'carrier' theory of antibody function. He was instrumental in reviving European immunology in the era after World War II.

Singer first developed methods for the detection and localization of antigen or antigen–antibody complexes by electron microscopy. He conjugated ferritin to antibody molecules, rendering them highly electron scattering, thus permitting their detection as a row of gray points along a cell membrane where antigens were located[25].

Rosalyn Sussman Yalow (1921–) (Figure 5), American investigator who shared the 1977 Nobel Prize with Guillemin and Schally for her endocrinology research and perfection of the radioimmunoassay (RIA) technique[26]. With Berson, Yalow made an important discovery of the role that antibodies play in insulin-resistant diabetes. Her technique provided a test to estimate nanogram or picogram quantities of various types of hormones and biologically active molecules, thereby advancing basic and clinical research. RIA revolutionized the treatment of hormonal disorders. It made possible the diagnosis of medical conditions associated with minute changes in hormones and launched the new field of neuroendocrinology.

The immunoperoxidase technique was introduced in the 1970s for immunohistopathologic evaluation of cells and tissues that formerly relied on fluorescence antibody staining[27]. This technique offered several advantages that include high sensitivity, the use of conventional light microscopy rather than special fluorescence microscopy, the detection of antigenic markers on cells fixed in paraffin sections for many years, and permanent sections which obviate the need for photographs required for immunofluorescence. This technique found wide application in diagnostic pathology.

Without the significant advances in the techniques of biochemistry made in the past 30 years, the great strides made in immunological research would not have been possible. Highly sophisticated hybridoma

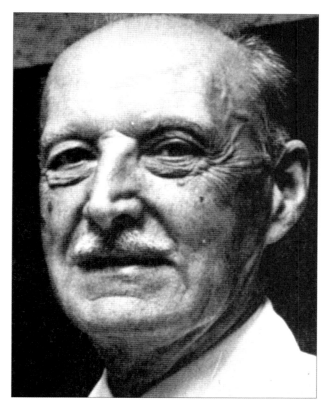

Figure 4 Pierre Grabar, who, with Williams, developed the immunoelectrophoresis technique

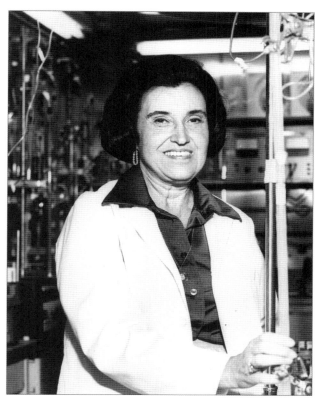

Figure 5 Rosalyn Yalow, Nobel Laureate in Medicine or Physiology for her perfection of the radioimmunoassay

technology and monoclonal antibodies, DNA sequencing, flow cytometry, chromatographic and ultracentrifugal techniques, amino acid analysis and synthesis, X-ray diffraction studies, immunoenzymology, recombinant DNA technology and advances in genetic engineering account for the windfall of progress in immunological research.

Techniques for the study of cell-mediated immunity are mentioned elsewhere in this book. Following the demonstration that ficoll-hypaque could be used to isolate lymphocytes as well as neutrophils, techniques were employed to separate T and B cells from each other[28]. The affinity of B cells for nylon wool permitted their separation from T cells, which pass through as the B cells adhere. This was later replaced by magnetic beads. Different subpopulations of macrophages have also been separated by ultracentrifugal methods. Flow cytometry has largely replaced more primitive methods for T cell subset analysis and B and T cell sorting. This method permits the rapid and accurate separation of cells with different antigenic markers and functional capabilities into distinct populations for further studies. The enzyme linked immunosorbent (ELISA) assay replaced many of the radioisotypic immunoassays of serum antibodies developed in the modern era.

Monoclonal antibody (MAb) (Figure 6), is an antibody synthesized by a single clone of B lymphocytes or plasma cells. The first to be observed were produced by malignant plasma cells in patients with multiple myeloma and associated gammopathies. The identical copies of the antibody molecules produced contain only one class of heavy chain and one type of light chain. Köhler and Milstein in the mid-1970s developed B lymphocyte hybridomas by fusing an antibody-producing B lymphocyte with a mutant myeloma cell that was not secreting antibody. The B lymphocyte product provided the specificity, whereas the myeloma cell conferred immortality on the hybridoma clone.

Today, MAbs are produced in large quantities against a plethora of antigens for use in diagnosis and sometimes in treatment. MAbs are homogeneous and are widely employed in immunoassays, single antigen identification in mixtures, delineation of cell surface molecules and assay of hormones and drugs in serum, among many other uses. Since the response to some

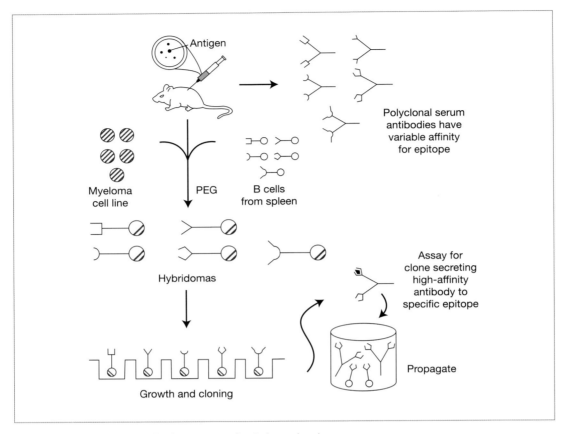

Figure 6 Monoclonal antibodies. PEG, polyethylene glycol

immunogens is inadequate in mice, monoclonal antibodies have also been generated using rabbit cells. Monoclonal antibodies have been radioactively labeled and used to detect tumor metastases; to differentiate subtypes of tumors, with monoclonal antibodies against membrane antigens or intermediate filaments; to identify microbes in body fluids; and for circulating hormone assays. MAbs may be used to direct immunotoxins or radioisotopes to tumor targets with potential for tumor therapy.

A **B lymphocyte hybridoma** is a hybrid cell produced by the fusion of a splenic antibody-secreting cell immunized against that particular antigen with a mutant myeloma cell from the same species that no longer secretes its own protein product (Figure 7). Polyethylene glycol is used to effect cell fusion. Antibody-synthesizing cells do not secrete hypoxanthine guanine phosphoribosyl transferase (HGPRT), an enzyme needed for DNA nucleotide synthesis, but do provide the ability to produce a specific monoclonal antibody. The mutant myeloma cell line confers

immortality upon the hybridoma. If the nucleotide synthesis pathway is inhibited, the myeloma cells become HGPRT-dependent. The antibody-synthesizing cells provide the HGPRT and the mutant myeloma cell enables endless reproduction. Once isolated through use of a selective medium such as hypoxanthine aminopterin thymidine (HAT), hybridoma cell lines can be maintained for relatively long periods. Hybridomas produce specific monoclonal antibodies that may be collected in great quantities for use in diagnosis and selected types of therapy.

Georges J. F. Köhler (1946–) (Figure 8), German immunologist who shared the Nobel Prize in Medicine or Physiology in 1984 with César Milstein for their work on the production of monoclonal antibodies by hybridizing mutant myeloma cells with antibody-producing B cells (hybridoma technique). Monoclonal antibodies have broad applications in both basic and clinical research as well as in diagnostic assays.

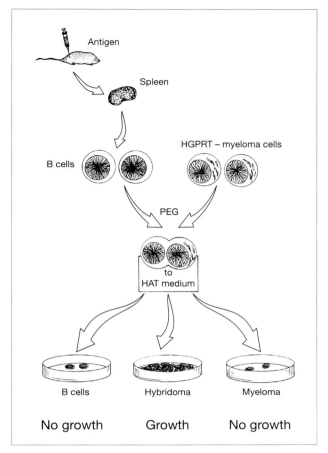

Figure 7   B lymphocyte hybridoma. HGPRT, hypoxanthine guanine phosphoribosyl transferase; HAT, hypoxanthine aminopterin thymidine

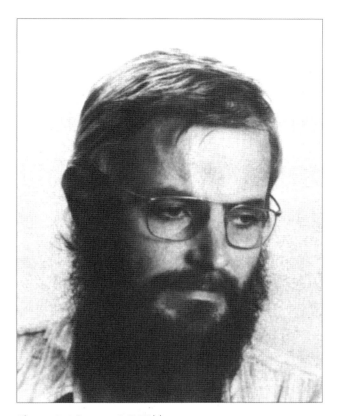

Figure 8   Georges J. F. Köhler

Köhler was born in Munich and educated at the University of Freiburg, Germany, where he received a diploma in biology in 1971 and a PhD in 1974. His research for the doctorate was conducted at the Institute for Immunology in nearby Basel. Visiting the Basel Institute in 1973 to present a seminar, Milstein invited Köhler to join him at Cambridge as a postdoctoral fellow in 1974. Köhler accepted, and later returned to Basel in 1976 as a Member of the Institute. The pivotal advance made by Köhler and Milstein had neither been planned nor was it an accident. Michael Potter, in 1962, had devised technology to produce myelomas in mice, and described their maintenance. Milstein and Cotton had already used rat and mouse myelomas to investigate whether or not different chromosomes encode variable and constant regions of immunoglobulins. Their results revealed that both variable and constant regions were always of one species, even though heavy and light chain hybrids did occur.

Köhler began his postdoctoral fellowship in Milstein's laboratory at Cambridge University in 1974. His dissertation research had shown that 1000 different murine immunoglobulins were able to react with a single epitope. He embarked upon a project with Milstein on antibody gene mutations.

Encountering difficulties with the research, Köhler sought ways to synthesize myeloma antibodies of known specificity. He conceived the idea of producing hybridomas at the end of 1974, while lying in bed halfway between wakefulness and sleep. On learning his concept the next morning, Milstein encouraged Köhler to proceed. Initial failures were traced to the use of toxic reagents, but eventually the experiments succeeded. They fused antibody-forming spleen cells with mutant myeloma cells to create hybridomas, to study the genetic basis of antibody diversity. The mutant myeloma cells conferred immortality on the fused cell line, whereas the spleen cells conferred antibody specificity. Thus, the hybrid cell or hybridoma cell line was endowed with the ability for long-term survival in culture, producing an unlimited quantity of monoclonal antibodies. The success of the technique depended upon a selective method to recover only fused cells. Therefore, they employed a mutant myeloma cell line that was deficient in the enzyme hypoxanthine phosphoribosyltransferase. Cells deficient in this enzyme would perish in a medium containing hypoxanthine, aminopterine and thymidine (HAT). However, hybrid cells would survive and could be isolated, since the antibody-synthesizing cell incorporated into the hybridoma would furnish the enzyme. Thus, the immortal hybridoma clone would produce abundant quantities of monoclonal antibodies with specificity for a specific antigenic determinant. Milstein wrote the report and received most of the initial honors and credit. Yet both were awarded the Nobel Prize in Medicine for 1984, together with N. K. Jerne. Monoclonal antibodies have broad applications in both basic science and clinical research. They have been developed against a multitude of antigens, including tissue markers that are of critical importance in surgical pathologic diagnosis of tumors, to cite but one example. The thousands of articles and dozens of monographs on monoclonal antibodies published in the last quarter century reflect their widespread use and significance.

Further reading

Köhler GF, Milstein C. Continuous cultures of fused cells secreting antibody of predefined specificity. *Nature (London)* 1975;256:495–7

Milstein C. Monoclonal antibodies from hybrid myelomas: theoretical aspects and some general comments. In McMichael AJ, Fabre JW, eds. *Monoclonal Antibodies in Clinical Medicine.* London: Academic Press, 1982:3–13

Clark WR. *The Experimental Foundations of Modern Immunology.* New York: John Wiley & Sons, 1991

LeBlanc PA. Monoclonal antibodies: novel to Nobel. In Cruse JM, Lewis RE, eds. *The Year in Immunology 1984–85.* Basel: Karger, 1985:136–42

César Milstein (1927–) (Figure 9), an Argentinian molecular biologist who, with Georges Köhler, perfected the technique of monoclonal antibody production from hybridomas, for which they received

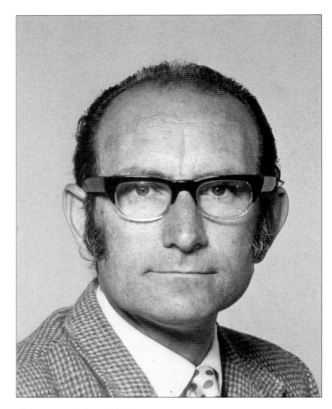

Figure 9 César Milstein

the Nobel Prize in Medicine or Physiology (1984) which was shared with Niels K. Jerne. This technology revolutionized immunological research.

César Milstein was born on October 8, 1927 in Bahia Blanca, Argentina. He attended the Collegio Nacional, Bahia Blanca, from 1939 to 1944, earning his Bachiller degree. He matriculated at the University of Buenos Aires in 1945 and graduated in 1952. He continued studies for the doctorate, which he received in 1957, and continued as a staff member in the Institute of Microbiology until 1963. During a leave of absence, Milstein worked in the Department of Biochemistry at Cambridge University in England, receiving a second doctorate there in 1960. Returning to Cambridge in 1963, he joined the staff of the Medical Research Council Laboratory of Molecular Biology as a Member, later directing its Protein Chemistry Division together with F. Sanger. Milstein and associates established the complete sequence of the light-chain portion of an immunoglobulin molecule. He determined the nucleotide sequence of a large segment of the light-chain messenger RNA discovering that there is only one type of RNA for both domains within that chain. The separate domains of light and heavy chains are designated constant and variable.

Milstein reasoned that the constant domain genes may be separate in the germ line but that they must come together in antibody-synthesizing cells. Milstein and Köhler proceeded to develop a method for preparing monoclonal antibodies from hybridomas in 1975, for which they subsequently shared the Nobel Prize in Medicine or Physiology. They fused mutant myeloma cells, which contributed immortality, with spleen cells, which produced antibodies against a designated antigen, contributing specificity to produce a hybridoma (hybrid cells) that could be cultured perpetually, producing antibodies against any antigen used to immunize the spleen cells. By selecting clones, Milstein and Köhler developed cell lines that produced monoclonal antibodies of a single antigen-bonding specificity. This revolutionary technique permitted the development of permanent cultures from a single clone that could be maintained indefinitely, providing an unlimited amount of specific monoclonal antibody. The technique developed with mouse cells was later extended to perfect human hybridomas, and could even be used to synthesize purified monoclonal antibodies against impure antigens.

The **immunoperoxidase method** (Figure 10) was introduced by Nakene and Pierce in 1966 who proposed that enzymes be used in the place of fluorochromes as labels for antibodies. Horseradish peroxidase (HRP) is the enzyme label most widely employed. The immunoperoxidase technique permits the demonstration of antigens in various types of cells and fixed tissues. This method has certain advantages that include:

(1) The use of conventional light microscopy;

(2) The stained preparations may be kept permanently;

(3) The method may be adapted for use with electron microscopy of tissues;

(4) Counterstains may be employed.

The disadvantages include:

(1) The demonstration of relatively minute positively staining areas is limited by the light microscope's resolution;

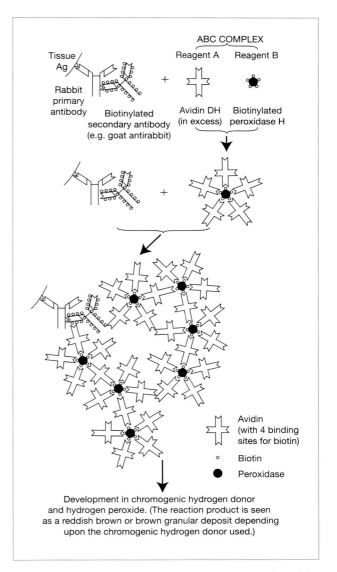

Figure 10 The immunoperoxidase method introduced by Nakene and Pierce

(2) Endogenous peroxidase may not have been completely eliminated from the tissue under investigation;

(3) Diffusion of products resulting from the enzyme reaction away from the area where antigen is localized.

The PAP (peroxidase–antiperoxidase) technique (Figure 11) is a method for immunoperoxidase staining of tissue to identify antigens with antibodies. This method employs unlabeled antibodies and a PAP reagent. The same PAP complex may be used for dozens of different unlabeled antibody specificities. If the primary antibody against the antigen being sought

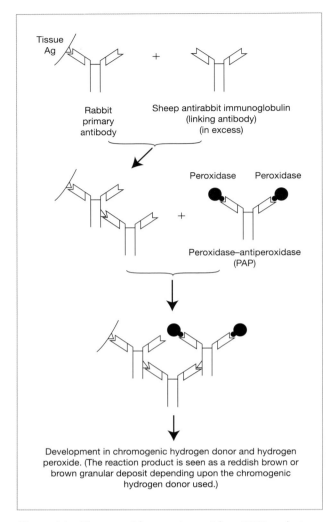

Development in chromogenic hydrogen donor and hydrogen peroxide. (The reaction product is seen as a reddish brown or brown granular deposit depending upon the chromogenic hydrogen donor used.)

Figure 11   The peroxidase–antiperoxidase (PAP) technique

is made in the rabbit, then tissue sections treated with this reagent are exposed to sheep antirabbit immunoglobulin followed by the PAP complex. For human primary antibody, an additional step must link the human antibody into the rabbit sandwich technique. Paraffin-embedded tissue sections are first treated with xylene, and after deparaffinization, they are exposed to hydrogen peroxide to destroy the endogenous peroxidase. Sections are next incubated with normal sheep serum to suppress non-specific binding of immunoglobulin to tissue collagen. Primary rabbit antibody against the antigen to be identified combined with the tissue section. Unbound primary antibody is removed by rinsing the sections which are then covered with sheep antibody against rabbit immunoglobulin. This linking antibody will combine with any primary rabbit antibody in the

tissue. It is added in excess, which results in one of the antigen-binding sites remaining free. After washing, the PAP is placed on the section, and the rabbit antibody part of this complex will be bound to the free antigen-binding site of the linking antibody. The unbound PAP complex is then washed away by rinsing. A substrate of hydrogen peroxide and AEC is placed on the tissue section leading to formation of a visible color reaction product that can be seen by light microscopy. Peroxidase is localized only at sites where the PAP is bound via linking antibody and primary antibody to antigen molecules, permitting the antigen to be identified as an area of reddish-brown pigment. Tissues may be counterstained with hematoxylin.

The **enzyme-linked immunosorbent assay (ELISA)** (Figure 12) is an immunoassay that employs an enzyme linked to either anti-immunoglobulin or antibody specific for antigen and detects either antibody or antigen. This method is based on the sandwich or double-layer technique, in which an enzyme rather than a fluorochrome is used as the label. In this method, antibody is attached to the surface of plastic tubes, wells, or beads to which the antigen-containing test sample is added. If antibody is being sought in the test sample, then antigen should be attached to the plastic surface. Following antigen–antibody interaction, the enzyme–anti-imunoglobulin conjugate is added. The ELISA test is read by incubating the reactants with an appropriate substrate to yield a colored product that is measured in a spectrophotometer. Alkaline phosphatase and horseradish peroxidase are enzymes that are often employed. ELISA methods have replaced many radioimmunoassays because of their lower cost, safety, speed and technical simplicity.

The **polymerase chain reaction (PCR)** is a method to amplify minute quantities of genetic information into large amounts of material that can be analyzed. In the 1980s, Kary Mullis, working at Cetus Corporation, conceived of a way to start and stop a polymerase's action at specific points along a single strand of DNA. He understood that by harnessing this type of molecular reproduction technology, the target DNA could be amplified exponentially. Once Cetus scientists developed PCR to perform in a reliable manner, it became useful. They had a powerful technique to generate unlimited quantities of precise genetic material in a

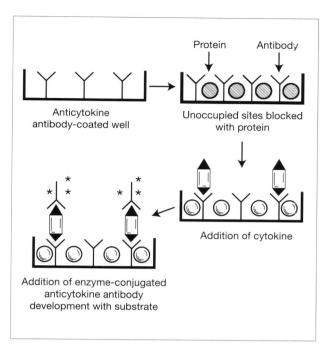

Protein   Antibody

Anticytokine
antibody-coated well

Unoccupied sites blocked
with protein

Addition of cytokine

Addition of enzyme-conjugated
anticytokine antibody
development with substrate

Figure 12   The enzyme-linked immunosorbent assay (ELISA)

brief time period. The first article on PCR was published in *Science* in 1985. With increased applications, innovations and variations in technique, there has been a virtual explosion in molecular biological information generated by this methodology. PCR is one of the most significant biotech discoveries ever made and Kary Mullis was awarded the Nobel Prize in Chemistry in 1993 for inventing the technique.

Further reading

Robinson P. *Making PCR, A Story of Biotechnology*. Chicago, IL: University of Chicago Press, 1996

PCR (Figure 13) is a technique to amplify a small DNA segment beginning with as little as 1 μg. The segment of double-stranded DNA is placed between two oligonucleotide primers through many cycles of amplification. Amplification takes place in a thermal cycler, with one step occurring at a high temperature in the presence of DNA polymerase that is able to withstand the high temperature. Within a few hours, the original DNA segment is transformed into millions of copies. PCR methodology has been used for multiple purposes, including detection of human immunodeficiency virus 1 (HIV-1), the prenatal diagnosis of

sickle cell anemia, and gene rearrangements in lymphoproliferative disorders, among numerous other applications. The technique is used principally to prepare enough DNA for analysis by available DNA methods and is used widely in DNA diagnostic work. PCR has a 99.99% sensitivity.

Coulter, in 1959, developed an instrument that electronically counted and sized cells flowing in a conductive fluid with one cell at a time passing a measuring point. This represented the first flow analyzer. In 1965, Kamentsky and colleagues constructed a two-parameter flow cytometer capable of measuring absorption and block-scattered illumination of unstained cells. This enabled the determination of cell nucleic acid content and size. Thus, Kamentsky's apparatus constituted the first multiparameter flow cytometer. Also in 1965, Fulwyler perfected the first cell sorter. That same year, Sweet employed an electrostatic deflection ink-jet method which permitted cell sorting at a rate of 1000 cells/s. Based on the real volume differences of cells, Van Dilla and associates (1967) prepared purified (> 95%) human granulocyte and lymphocyte suspensions. The subsequent perfection of monoclonal antibodies, labeled with various fluorochromes, and inexpensive powerful computers enabled flow cytometry to become a routine procedure. This was a welcome successor to the previously used cell-by-cell analysis by microscope-based static cytometry which had been widely employed in diagnosis. Flow cytometry came into widespread use in the diagnosis and management of various diseases, especially hematopathology, as further refinements permitted the measurement of as many as five parameters on 20 000 cells in a second (Macey, 1994).

Further reading

Coulter WH. High speed automatic blood cell counter and cell analyzer. *Proc Natl Elec Conf* 1956;12:1034–5

Kamentsky LA, Melamed MR, Derman H. Spectrophotometer: new instrument for ultrarapid cell analysis. *Science* 1965;150:630–1

Fulwyler MJ. Electronic separation of biological cells by volume. *Science* 1965;36:131–2

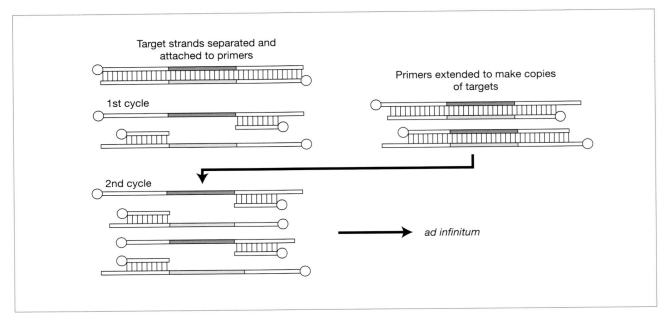

Figure 13   The polymerase chain reaction (PCR)

Van Dilla MA, Fulwyler MJ, Boone IV. Volume distribution and separation of normal human leukocytes. *Proc Soc Exp Biol Med* 1967;125:367–70

Macey MG, ed. *Flow Cytometry, Clinical Applications*. Oxford: Blackwell Scientific Publications, 1994

Flow cytometry (Figures 14 and 15) is an analytical technique to phenotype cell populations that requires a special apparatus, termed a flow cytometer, that can detect fluorescence on individual cells in suspension and thereby ascertain the number of cells that express the molecule binding a fluorescent probe. Cell suspensions are incubated with fluorescent-labeled monoclonal antibodies or other probes and the quantity of probe bound by each cell in the population is assayed by passing the cells one at a time through a spectrofluorometer with a laser-generated incident beam. Sample cells flow single file past a narrowly focused excitation light beam that is used to probe the cell properties of interest. As the cells pass the focused excitation lightbeam, each cell scatters light and may emit fluorescent light, depending on whether or not it is labeled with a fluorochrome or is autofluorescent. Scattered light is measured in both the forward and perpendicular directions relative to the incident beam.The fluorescent emissions of the cell are measured in the perpendicular directions by a photosensitive detector. Measurements of light scatter and fluorescent emission intensities are used to characterize each cell as it is processed. Flow cytometry is a fast, accurate way to measure multiple characteristics of a single cell simultaneously. These objective measurements are made one cell at a time, at routine rates of 500–4000 particles per second in a moving fluid stream. A flow cytometer measures relative size (FSC), relative granularity or internal complexity (SSC), and relative fluorescence. Three-color flow cytometry is used to analyze blood cells by size, cytoplasmic granularity, and surface markers labeled with different fluorochromes. Flow cytometry serves as the basis for numerous very different, highly specialized assays. It is a multifactorial analysis technique and provides the capability for performing many of these assays simultaneously.

Further reading

Milstein C. Monoclonal antibodies from hybrid myelomas: theoretical aspects and some general comments. In *Monoclonal Antibodies in Clinical Medicine*. McMichael AJ and Febre JW, eds. London: Academic Press, 1982:3–13

Köhler GF, Milstein C. Continuous cultures of fused cells secreting antibody of predefined specificity. *Nature (London)* 1975;256:495–7

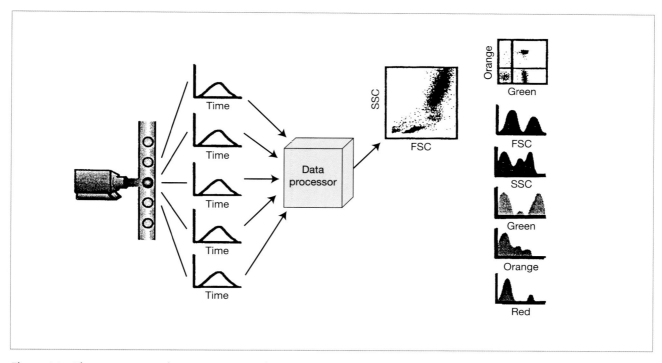

Figure 14 Flow cytometry. Flow cytometry is a fast, accurate way to measure multiple characteristics of a single cell simultaneously. These objective measurements are made one cell at a time, at routine rates of 500 to 5000 particles per second in a moving fluid stream. A flow cytometer measures relative size (FSC), relative granularity or internal complexity (SSC), and relative fluorescence. Use of three-color flow cytometry to analyze blood cells by size, cytoplasmic granularity, and surface markers labeled with different fluorochromes. With recent advances in technology, five-color flow cytometry is readily available

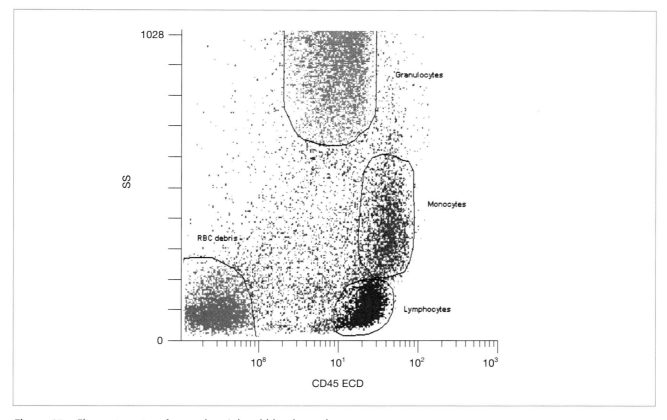

Figure 15 Flow cytometry of normal peripheral blood sample

Clark WR. *The Experimental Foundations of Modern Immunology*. New York: John Wiley & Sons, 1991

LeBlanc PA. Monoclonal antibodies: novel to Nobel. In Cruse JM, Lewis RE, eds. *The Year in Immunology 1984–85*. Basel: Karger, 1985:136-42

The foregoing brief descriptions of immunological and molecular methods are merely representative of a virtual explosion of technological advances. These developments have greatly accelerated and intensified both basic and clinical immunological research that is proceeding at an unprecedented pace.

For a more complete and detailed account, the reader is referred to the following sources.

Further reading

Rose NR, Hamilton RG, Detrick B. *Manual of Clinical Laboratory Immunology*, 6th edn. Washington, DC: ASM Press, 2002

Lefkovits I. *Immunology Methods Manual*. Vol. 1–4. San Diego, CA: Academic Press, 1997

REFERENCES

1. Charrin A, Roger J. Note sur le developpment des microbes pathogens dans le serum des animaux vaccines. *C R Soc Biol* 1889;41:667–99

2. von Grüber M, Durham HE. Eine neue Methode zur racshen Erkennung des Cholervibrio und des Typhusbacillus. *Münch Med Wschr* 1896;43:285–6

3. Widal GFI, Sicard A. Recherches de la reaction agglutinante dans le sang et le serum desséches des typhiques et dans le serosité des vesicatoires. *Bull Mem Soc Med Hop (Paris)* 1896;13:681–2

4. Kraus R. Ueber Specifische Reaktionen in keimfreien Filtraten aus Cholera, Typhus und Pestbouillonculturen, erzeugt durch homologes Serum. *Wien Klin Wschr* 1897;10:736–8

5. Landsteiner K. Zur Kenntniss der antifermentativen, lytischen und agglutinierenden Wirkungen des Blutserums und der Lymphe. *Zentralbl Bakteriol* 1900;27:357–62

6. Bordet J, Gengou O. Sur l'existence de substance sensibilisatrices dans la plupart des serums antimicrobiens. *Ann Inst Pasteur* 1901;15:289–302

7. Wasserman A, Neisser A, Bruck C. Eine serodiagnostische Reaktion bei Syphilis. *Deutche Med Wschr* 1902;32:745–6

8. Denys J, Leclef J. Sur le mechanisme de l'immunité chez le lapin vaccine contre le streptocoque pyogene. *Cellule* 1895;11:175–221

9. Wright A, Douglas SR. An experimental investigation of the blood fluids in connection with phagocytosis. *Proc R Soc (London)* 1903–04; 72: 357–70, 73:128–42

10. Dean HR, Webb RA. The determination of the rate of antibody (precipitin) production in rabbit's blood by the method of 'optimal proportions'. *J Pathol Bacteriol* 1928;31:89–99

11. Heidelberger M, Kendall FE. A quantitative theory of the precipitin reaction. *J Exp Med* 1935;62:697–720

12. Pappenheimer AM Jr, Robinson ESJ. Quantitative study of Ramon diphtheria flocculation reaction. *J Immunol* 1937;32:291–300

13. Marrack JR. *The Chemistry of Antigens and Antibodies*. Medical Research Council. Special report series, 194. London: HMSO, 1934

14. Tiselius A. Electrophoresis of serum globulin. *J Biochem* 1937;31:313–17; Electrophoresis of purified antibody preparations. *J Exp Med* 1937;65:641–6

15. Tiselius AWK, Kabat E. An electrophoretic study of immune sera and purified antibody preparations. *J Exp Med* 1929;69:119–31

16. Heidelberger M, Kendall FE, Soo Hoo CM. Quantitative studies on precipitin reaction. Antibody production in rabbits injected with azoprotein. *J Exp Med* 1933;58:132–52

17. Marrack J. Derived antigens as means of studying relation of specific combination to chemical structure. *Proc R Soc Med (London)* 1934;27:1063–5

18. Coons AH, Creech HH, Jones RN. Immunological properties of an antibody containing a fluorescent group. *Proc Soc Exp Biol Med* 1941;47:200–2

19. Coons AH, Kaplan MH. Localization of antigen in tissue cells. II. Improvements in a method for the detection of antigen by means of fluorescent antibodies. *J Exp Med* 1950;91:1–13

20. Coombs RRA, Race RR, Mourant AE. Detection of weak and 'incomplete' Rh agglutinins: a new test. *Lancet* 1945;2:15–16

21. Oudin J. Methode d'analyse immunochemique par precipitation specifique en milieu gelifie. *C R Acad Sci* 1946;222:115

22. Ouchterlony O. *In vitro* methods for testing the toxin-producing capacity of diphtheria bacteria. 8th Scandanavian Pathological Congress, 1947. *Acta Path Microbiol Scand* 1948;25:186

23. Elek SD. The recognition of toxicogenic bacterial strains *in vitro*. *Br Med J* 1948;1:493

24. Grabar P, Williams CA. Methode permettante l'etude conjugée des propriétés electrophoretiques et immuno-chemiques d'un mélange de proteines. *Biochim Biophys Acta* 1953;10:193–4

25. Singer SJ. Preparation of an electron-dense antibody conjugate. *Nature (London)* 1959;183:1523

26. Yalow RS. Radioimmunoassay. *Ann Rev Biophys Bioeng* 1980;9:327–345

27. Nakane PK, Pierce CB Jr. Enzyme-labeled antibodies for the light and electron microscope localization of tissue antigens. *J Cell Biol* 1967;33:307–18

28. Macqueen JM, Tardif G, eds. *Tissue Typing Reference Manual*. Richmond, VA: Southeastern Organ Procurement Foundation (SEOPF), 1987

CHAPTER 14

Immunological societies

THE FOUNDING OF THE AMERICAN ASSOCIATION OF IMMUNOLOGISTS[1]

The ferment in immunological research in European laboratories in the early 1900s attracted American and Canadian physicians to Germany, France and England, where they became acquainted with late-breaking scientific discoveries. In addition to Ehrlich, von

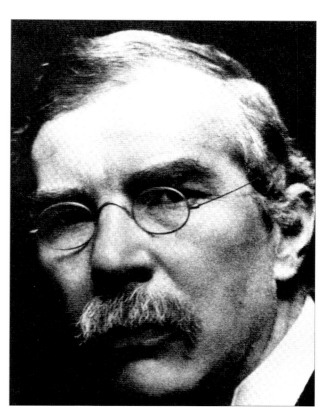

Figure 1 Sir Almroth E. Wright MD, FRS, founder and teacher of the principles of vaccine therapy. From the Cruse Collection, University of Wisconsin, Middleton Library

Behring, Koch and Mechnikov on the continent, Sir Almroth E. Wright, Director of the Inoculation Department of St Mary's Hospital, London, was a favorite mentor (Figure 1). In his Praed Street Laboratories, Sir Almroth taught his students the 'new immunotherapy' that employed preventive vaccines and mass inoculation (Figure 2). As von Behring proved the therapeutic efficacy of diphtheria antitoxin, Wright, in 1898–1900, established the efficacy and feasibility of typhoid vaccine and the practicability of mass inoculation of British forces in the South African War and in India.

In 1903, Wright and a colleague, Stewart R. Douglas, discovered antibodies in the blood, termed opsonins, that attach to bacteria or other particles and facilitate their phagocytosis. They developed an opsonocytophagic index that correlated the ability of a patient's leukocytes to phagocytize bacteria *in vitro* with the level of immunity against an infectious disease agent. Leonard Colebrook joined Wright and Douglas in 1907. Recognizing that it would take many years to gain sufficient fundamental knowledge to understand immune processes, Wright predicted that 'the physician of the future will be an immunisator'.

Among the North American disciples attracted to Wright's laboratory were Drs Martin J. Synnott (Figure 3) of Montclair, NJ; Gerald Bertram Webb (Figure 4) of Colorado Springs, CO; F. J. Clemenger of Ashville, NC; R. Matson of Portland; Benjamin H. Matthews of Denver, CO; and F. M. Pottenger of Monrovia, CA. On returning to the United States following studies on immunity at the Praed Street Laboratory, Synnott suggested that the American and Canadian students of Wright form a 'society of vaccine therapists'. Dr Gerald

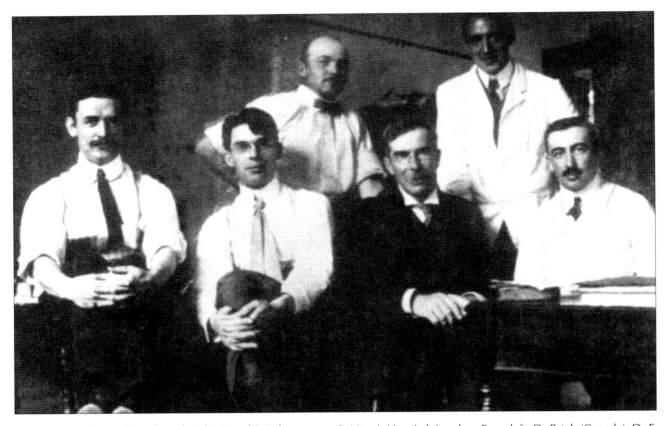

Figure 2 Students of Sir Almroth in his Praed St Laboratory at St Mary's Hospital, London. From left: Dr Patch (Canada), Dr F. M. Pottenger (Monrovia, CA), Dr O. H. Brown (Wisconsin), Sir Almroth, Dr G. B. Webb (Colorado Springs, CO), Dr Alymer May (Africa). Courtesy of Mrs Marka Webb Stewart

Bertram Webb, who had also been a pupil of Wright's, expressed the belief that laboratory researchers should be included together with therapists to form an inter-disciplinary society with a philosophy sufficiently flexible to accommodate changes in direction as immuno-logical knowledge increased. He believed that the proposed objective of the society and the criteria and qualifications for membership were too narrowly focused and too restricted. Dr Webb suggested that physicians who had studied under other founders of immunology besides Sir Almroth, including Metchnikoff, von Behring, Ehrlich and Koch should also be invited to membership.

Dr Victor Clarence Vaughan (Figure 5), of Ann Arbor, MI, champion of laboratory researchers inter-ested in the biochemistry of serology and vaccine therapy, expressed the view that progress in medicine was not possible without advances in physical, chemical and biological sciences. Webb's wise counsel prevailed, and his suggestion was adopted by the few 'charter members' at a National Tuberculosis Association

Meeting in May, 1913, in Washington, DC. The society was not chartered formally until June 1913, at a meeting of the American Medical Association in Minneapolis. Drs Webb, Synnott and A. Parker Hitchens and appar-ently the 52 enrolled charter members met on June 19 and founded the American Association of Immunologists (AAI), the name proposed by Dr Gerald B. Webb. Other officers included Drs George W. Ross as vice-president, Martin J. Synnott as secretary and Willard J. Stone as treasurer.

The council, which comprised Dr A. Parker Hitchens (Figure 6) as Chairman, Drs Oscar Berghausen, Campbell Laidlaw, Henry L. Ulrich and J. E. Robinson, was charged with governance of the Association. The elected officers served as *ex officio* members. The council and officers proposed three principal objectives for the Association, which were subsequently adopted by the charter members. The first annual meeting was held on June 22, 1914, in Hotel Chelsea in Atlantic City, NJ. During this meeting, Dr A. Parker Hitchens presented a draft of the Association's

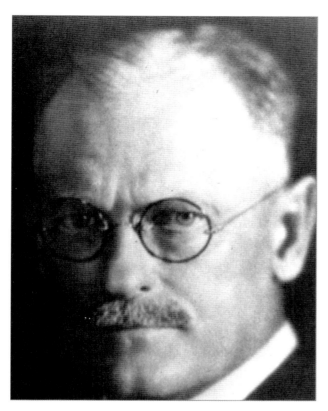

Figure 3   Martin J. Synnott MD, who in 1912, had the idea for the formation of a 'Society of Vaccine Therapists'. Courtesy of the New York Academy of Medicine Library

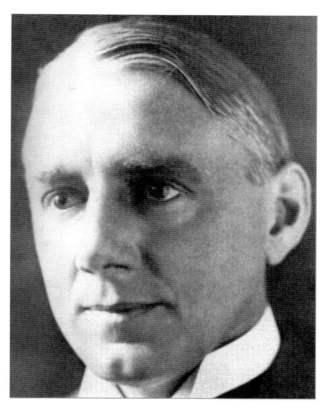

Figure 4   Gerald Bertram Webb, MD, who coined the name 'The American Association of Immunologists', and served two terms as the Association's first president. Courtesy of Mrs Marka Webb Stewart

constitution and by-laws, which was adopted unanimously. The constitution and by-laws were subsequently enacted on 6 April 1917. Seven applicants were elected to charter membership. Sir Almroth Wright and Captain S. R. Douglas were elected to honorary membership. Sir Alexander Fleming, Dr Leonard Colebrook and Dr John Freeman were named corresponding members. The first scientific meeting of the Association consisted of three sessions. Dr Webb's Presidential Address was on 'History of Immunity'.

In principle, the 1917 constitution and by-laws still serve as the basis for governance of the Association. They were modified or expanded in 1936 to make past presidents honorary members of the council. Later the membership, rather than the council, elected new members. The Association, by vote of council, accepted membership in the Federation of American Societies for Experimental Biology (FASEB) on April 1, 1942. At that time the council also voted unanimously to include the Editor-in-Chief and four associate editors of the *Journal of Immunology* as *ex officio* members of the AAI

Council. Although traditionally officers had served only 1 year, during World War II Dr J. J. Bronfenbrenner served as president from 1942 until 1946, when Dr Michael Heidelberger was elected to succeed him. He sought changes in the governance policies of the Association. In 1947 the constitution and by-laws were revised and were formally adopted in 1950.

The changes applied to the classes of membership, i.e. active, emeritus and honorary, together with specific qualifications for active, criteria for transfer to emeritus and the professional achievements associated with honorary membership. Active and honorary members, nominated by the council, were to be elected by the membership-at-large. Besides the officers, four councilors, one elected each year, with 4-year terms of service, would be elected. The council would consist of the four elected officers and five councilors, one of whom would be the Editor-in-Chief of the *Journal of Immunology*. Past presidents would be invited to attend council meetings but would not vote. It was not until 1965 that a central office for Association affairs was

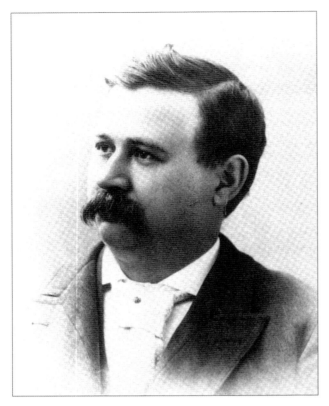

Figure 5 Victor Clarence Vaughan MD, championed the cause of the laboratory researcher as vital to the interdisciplinary goals of the Association. Courtesy of the University of Michigan Library

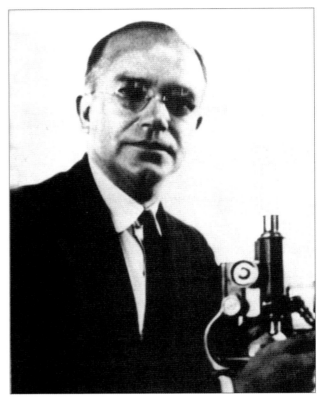

Figure 6 A. Parker Hitchens MD, first chairman of the American Association of Immunologists (AAI) council, 'father' of the Association's constitution and by-laws and the force behind an Association journal. Courtesy of the New York Academy of Medicine Library

established in Beaumont House at FASEB headquarters in Bethesda, MD.

Twelve qualified members per year were accepted between 1914 and 1938, resulting in a total of 275 active members. Only 28 new members were added between 1939 and 1945 because of World War II. Approximately 35 new active members were added each year from 1946 through 1963, resulting in 626 new members on the Association's 50th anniversary. In 1972, specific criteria for membership eligibility were established. These were modified in 1975, 1977 and 1978. Trainee members were first admitted in 1983. Other categories of membership included honorary, emeritus and sustaining associate (corporate) members.

At the time of the Association's 75th anniversary meeting in 1988, membership had risen to 5142, and by 1998, the Association's 85th anniversary, total membership was 5774. The Association was invited to meet with FASEB first in 1939, and became a Corporate Member Society in 1942. Until 1948, the secretary of the Association was responsible for preparing and

programming the annual scientific sessions. Thereafter, the council enlisted the assistance of two members to assist the secretary in program activities to improve the quality of sessions at the annual meeting. By 1958, FASEB had begun to hold intersociety symposia involving all member societies.

Symposia were included in the annual meeting for the first time in 1948. Members were permitted to submit abstracts of 10-min volunteered papers to be presented at the annual meeting as the highlight of the program. By 1967, the program committee suggested that distinguished foreign, as well as non-member, immunologists be invited to participate in symposia. Poster presentations were begun in 1975 and represented a major departure from the volunteered oral presentations. Since that time, posters have gained considerable popularity over oral presentations, which, nevertheless, provided valuable experience for younger investigators. By 1986, poster presentations developed into poster workshop/discussion groups led by senior investigators. The number of mini-symposia was increased in 1979, and volunteered papers were integrated into them.

The time allotted for the presentation of brief papers was increased to 15 min. Slide sessions were eliminated, and all abstracts not chosen for mini-symposia were programmed into poster sessions, which constitute more than three-quarters of volunteered papers. The format of mini-symposia and poster sessions has been modified in various ways during the past 20 years. The Association has also met apart from the traditional FASEB annual meeting, combining efforts with other FASEB societies or immunology groups with related interests.

THE AAI ESTABLISHES AN OFFICIAL JOURNAL

In 1915, Dr A. Parker Hitchens announced to the AAI council, on which he had served as Chairman, that a movement was afoot outside of the AAI to launch a *Journal of Immunity* with Dr Arthur F. Coca of New York City as editor (Chapter 6, Figure 3). To avoid working at cross-purposes, the AAI council authorized Dr Hitchens to contact Dr Coca and the New York Society of Serology and Hematology, which Coca served as President, concerning the establishment of the journal. Representatives of the two organizations met in 1915, together with a representative of Williams and Wilkins Company, to work out details for founding the *Journal of Immunology*.

Dr Coca was chosen unanimously to become Managing Editor, supported by an editorial board selected by a committee comprising two members from each of the two societies, with the Managing Editor serving *ex officio*. It was decided that the journal would publish scientific research articles on immunity, serology and bacterial therapy. It would appear bimonthly with each volume consisting of six numbers and containing from 500 to 525 total pages. By 1930 the Association's financial position improved and the journal showed a profit for the first time. In 1940 the council decided to make the publication international by inviting Latin-American immunologists to serve on the editorial board. They appointed Dr A. Sordelli of Buenos Aires and Dr M. Ruiz Castaneda of Mexico City as the first two non-US immunologists to serve on the board. After 30 years of service, Dr Arthur F. Coca resigned as Managing Editor, and was succeeded by Dr Geoffrey Edsall, who brought considerable fiscal

responsibility to the journal and worked with the council to arrange for the publisher to credit the Association with journal pages saved per year. Dr John Y. Sugg succeeded him in 1954. By 1963, the total pages published increased to 1400 as the quality improved with the acceptance of meritorious articles representing the forefront of immunologic research. Two thousand pages were published in 1964. This number more than doubled to 4650 by 1978, and in 1986, 9400 published pages were printed. Financial arrangements with the publisher continued to improve in favor of the Association.

With the proliferation of immunological research, the journal developed subsections of Immunochemistry, Cellular Immunology, Immunopathology, Immunogenetics, and Microbial and Viral Immunology, each with its own subeditor. In 1968, Dr Harry Rose succeeded Dr Sugg. In 1971, Dr Joseph D. Feldman became the fifth Editor-in-Chief. He proposed a new format for an 8 1/2′×11′ page size that would diminish the cost of published papers. This was implemented in 1975, and students were offered the journal at reduced rates. The Association was given copyright to the *Journal of Immunology* in 1972, which strengthened its role in working with the publisher to regulate journal income and to set the ratio for net income distribution. Subsequently, in 1982, the editorial board arranged for a cost-plus arrangement with the publisher. The council established a journal reserve fund in 1983, and charged the editorial board with reorganization of scientific and business management functions. Editorial matters were transferred to the AAI Central Office at FASEB headquarters in Bethesda, and scientific functions were separated from financial responsibilities. In 1984, the editorial board became the publications committee, which gave it stature as a standing committee of the Association. In 1985, the journal began publication twice monthly. The publications committee became responsible to the council for the quality of the *Journal of Immunology*. With the transfer of the journal's editorial office from San Diego to Bethesda in early 1987, Dr Ethan M. Shevach succeeded Dr Joseph D. Feldman as Editor-in-Chief with scientific responsibility for the journal, and Dr Joseph Saunders, Executive Officer, became Managing Editor. Subsequent Chief Editors included Drs Peter Lipsky and Frank Fitch. In the intervening decade, the *Journal of Immunology* continued to increase in size and prestige, publishing scholarly articles not only from Americans, but from the international community as well.

THE AAI SUPPORTS IMMUNOLOGY EDUCATION

The Association has played a vital role in immunology education, sponsoring an advanced course which was first authorized by the council in 1964 at the suggestion of the AAI secretary/treasurer, Dr Sheldon Dray. It began as a summer course, with 2–3 weeks of intensive training at the professional level. Its purpose was to facilitate dissemination of immunological information to individuals, who were themselves teachers and would pass on this knowledge to their students. The first course was held in the summer of 1966 at Lake Forest College in Illinois. It was designed for university instructors and investigators desiring to improve their knowledge of basic immunology. In succeeding years, both PhDs and MDs enrolled. In 1976, the council adopted the recommendation of an expert committee that two courses be organized each year at different locations on the east and west coasts. One would be on basic immunology and the other on clinical immunology. By 1981, the annual course became self-sustaining, and in 1982, the council and the Education Committee elevated the course level to include topics in advanced basic and clinical immunology. The Education Committee selected course instructors who taught the faculty members, PhD and MD postdoctoral fellows, graduate students and industrial staff scientists, who registered. In 1984, the course was moved to Lindenwood College, St Charles, MO, under the capable leadership of Drs Carl W. Pearce and Judith A. Kapp. In 1980, the Education Committee recommended that a course be established for high-school science teachers. Subsequently, the council approved a grant to develop an instructional monograph on advances in immunology for use by high-school and college biology teachers and students.

THE AAI ADDRESSES CLINICAL IMMUNOLOGY

In 1973, the council established an *ad hoc* committee on hospital-based clinical immunology that was designed to address problems and increase the standards of diagnostic immunology. In 1976, the AAI council established a Committee on Clinical Immunology and Immunopathology. Whereas the council decided against

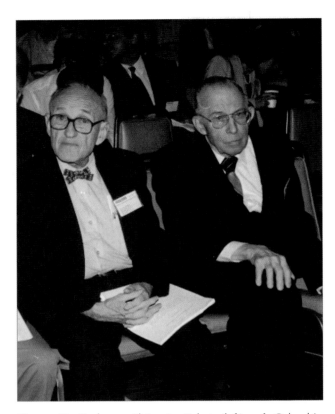

Figure 7 Professor Elvin A. Kabat (left), of Columbia University and Professor Merrill W. Chase (right) of the Rockefeller University, at the 75th annual meeting of the American Association of Immunologists in Las Vegas, NV, 1988

involvement in certification activities, it consented to cooperate with groups engaged in certification to ensure fair and sound procedures. In 1979, the council determined that AAI representation on the certification boards of the American Academy of Microbiology, the American Board of Pathology and the American Board of Allergy and Immunology would be desirable. The council appointed representatives recommended by the Clinical Immunology and Immunopathology Committee.

In 1983, clinical diagnostic laboratory immunologists formed a new international society named the Clinical Immunology Society (CIS). The AAI council consented to support and co-sponsor a meeting of the CIS in the fall of 1986. Earlier that year, representatives of the CIS met with the AAI council to define further the affiliation and interaction between the two organizations. The AAI council recognized the CIS as an autonomous society formally affiliated with the AAI, and designated the CIS to serve as its clinical regent. The AAI council determined that the affiliation would include exchange of council/board members on each organization's council to

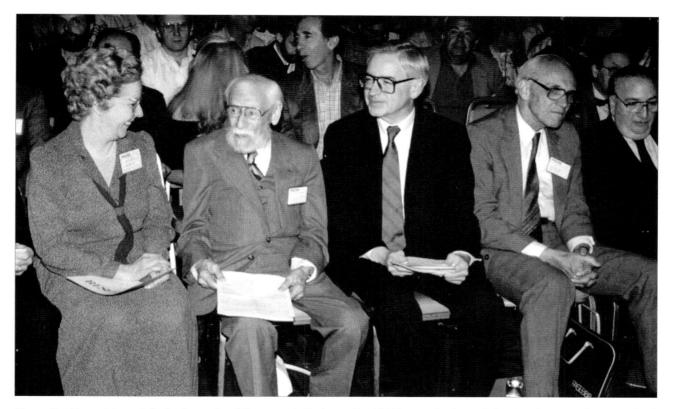

Figure 8 From right to left: Professor Baruj Benacerraf; Professor David Talmage; Professor Julius M. Cruse; Professor Michael Heidelberger; Mrs D. C. Schreffler; (Professor Donald Schreffler, AAI President, not shown) at the symposium honoring Professor Michael Heidelberger on his 100th birthday at the 75th annual meeting of the American Association of Immunologists in Las Vegas, NV, 1988

facilitate future meetings and other activities of mutual interest. At further meetings, representatives from the two groups identified areas of mutual interest and planned future interactions. The two societies decided to hold joint meetings and to exchange not only representatives to society councils but also selected committees, such as those for programs and publications. They decided that an *ad hoc* committee comprising representatives from each society would meet annually to facilitate future interactions between the AAI and the CIS.

Dr Bernhard Cinader of the Canadian Immunology Society approached the council in 1967 with a proposal to establish an International Congress of Immunology that would be held quadrennially. The following year, the council established an *ad hoc* steering committee that led to formation of the International Union of Immunological Societies (IUIS), which met first in 1969 in Bruges, Belgium. It was then decided that the first Congress would be held in Washington, DC in August 1971. Since that time, International Congresses of Immunology have been held around the world, most recently in Montreal in 2004.

On its 75th anniversary, the AAI honored Professor Michael Heidelberger, of Columbia University, on his 100th birthday. Among the distinguished members present were Professor Elvin Kabat, Heidelberger's first PhD graduate in immunochemistry, and Professor Merrill W. Chase, long-term associate of Karl Landsteiner at the Rockefeller Institute for Medical Research (Figure 7).

Awaiting commencement of the celebratory proceeding were Professor Baruj Benacerraf, Professor David W. Talmage, Professor Julius M. Cruse, who introduced Professor Heidelberger, Dr Heidelberger, Mrs D. Schreffler and Professor D. Schreffler, AAI President (Figure 8).

Following the founding of the American Association of Immunologists, national immunological societies were established in many other countries. The International Union of Immunological Societies (IUIS) was established in 1969 by representatives from ten societies meeting in Bruges, Belgium to facilitate communication and cooperation among immunologists of all nations. The IUIS is an umbrella organization for many of the regional and national societies of immunology throughout the world. The objectives of IUIS are: to organize international cooperation in immunology and to promote communication among the various branches of immunology and allied subjects; to encourage, within each scientifically independent territory, cooperation among the societies that represent the interests of immunology; and to contribute to the advancement of immunology in all its aspects.

There are currently 54 member societies of the IUIS. International Congresses of Immunology are held every 3 years under the auspices of the IUIS. The IUIS also contributes to the staging of regular congresses and conferences by each of the four Regional Federations and to various educational activities in immunology.

REFERENCE

1. Saunders JF, Cruse JM, Cohen SG, Lewis RE Jr. The AAI, 1913 to 1988 in the first century of immunology. *J Immunol* 1988;141: 537–54

CHAPTER 15

Landmarks in the history of immunology

1798   Vaccination

Edward Jenner published *Inquiry...* on vaccination

1830–50   Modern microscopes

1839   Francois Magendie, *Lectures on the Blood*, described secondary injection of egg albumin causing death, first description of anaphylaxis

1835–36   Bassi described pathogenic microorganism of silkworm

1840   F. G. J. Henle's essay on miasms and contagions, etiological relation of bacteria to disease

1850   Anthrax in sheep blood

1858   Fermentation due to microbe

Natural selection

1860   H. H. Salter, *On Asthma*, 'best work in 19th century', G. M.

1864   Spontaneous generation disproved

1865   J. A. Willemin, tuberculosis inoculable in rabbits

1867   Aseptic surgery

1870   T. Klebs, observed bacteria in wounds

1871   DNA in trout sperm

1876   Robert Koch, description of anthrax

Anthrax transmitted from culture

1878   Koch's masterpiece on the etiology of traumatic infections, the role of bacteria in infection and the specificity of infection

1879–81   Attenuated vaccine

1880   Pasteur's first paper on attenuation of infective organisms, studying fowl cholera; followed by work on anthrax, rabies and swine erysipelas

1883   Phagocytic theory

1884   Elie Metchnikoff described phagocytosis, studied the phenomenon in starfish larvae and *Daphnia*

1885   Paul Ehrlich's book on the need of the organism for oxygen, first reference to his side-chain theory, *Das Sauerstoff-Bedurfniss des Organismus*

1886   D. E. Salmon and Theobald Smith found that dead virus could produce immunity against the living virus

Louis Pasteur described method of preventing rabies

1887   F. B. Loffler, a first history of bacteriology, incomplete

1888   George Nuttall, demonstration of the bactericidal power of the blood of certain animals

Emile Roux and A. E. J. Yersin found that a bacterium-free filtrate of the diphtheria bacillus culture contained the exotoxin

Killed vaccines

First antigen and antibody

1889 Hans Buchner demonstrated that the bactericidal power of defibrinated serum was in cell-free serum and was lost on heating the serum to 55 °C for 1 h

A. Charrin and J. Roger observed clumping of bacterial suspension by immune serum

1890 Emil von Behring and Shibasaburo Kitasato published papers describing the use of antitoxins against diphtheria and tetanus in therapy, passive transfer of immunity

Koch announced the preparation of 'tuberculin' prematurely at the 10th International Congress of Medicine in Berlin

Hypersensitivity

Antitoxins

1891 Ehrlich studied the plant toxins ricin and abrin and raised antibodies to them

1892 Filterability of virus

Complement

Richard Pfeiffer recorded the occurrence of bacteriolysis in cholera vibrio incubated with specific antibody and fresh guinea pig serum, the 'Pfeiffer' phenomenon first demonstrated *in vivo*

1895 Jules Bordet described properties of the sera of immunized animals. He found both a heat-stable and a heat-labile component, antibody and alexine (complement: Ehrlich)

J. Denys and J. Leclef: immunization greatly increased phagocytosis

Precipitins

1896 Max von Grüber and Henry Durham discovered agglutination of the typhoid bacillus, by the serum of typhoid patient

Fernand Widal used the same reaction in reverse, testing sera of patients against

known bacteria to identify typhoid, the Grüber–Widal test

1897 Ehrlich developed a method for standardizing the antitoxin used in treatment of diphtheria, one of the founding discoveries of immunochemistry

R. Kraus showed that bacterial culture filtrate could produce an antibody which formed precipitate when added to the filtrate used for injection. The precipitin reaction could be demonstrated with a variety of protein and complex polysaccharides

1898 Bordet published paper on bacterial hemolysis, bringing it to the attention of many investigators

Side-chain theory

Intracellular growth of virus

1900 Karl Landsteiner mentioned the agglutination of red blood cells of healthy human blood from another individual, perhaps due to inborn differences, in a footnote

Blood groups

P. Ehrlich and J. Morgenroth studied blood of six goats, finding that there are clumping reactions between some, not published until 1901, the 'horror autotoxicus' theory

1901 J. Bordet and O. Gengou developed the complement fixation test, basis of many laboratory tests

Emil von Behring awarded Nobel Prize in Medicine for diphtheria, tetanus antitoxin sera

Max Neisser and R. Lubowski demonstrated complement deviation

Complement fixation

Yellow fever transmission

1902 Jan Danysz studied the 'Danysz phenomenon', different results from mixing antitoxin–toxin in equal parts or the antitoxin added in two doses, resulting in continued toxicity

August von Wassermann: studies on hemolysin, cytotoxin and precipitin

Paul Portier and Charles Richet described anaphylaxis in dogs using Portugese man-of-war and anemone poisons

P. T. Uhlenhuth: tissue-specific antigens, recognition of bird egg albumin

Anaphylaxis

1903 Nicholas Arthus studied local necrotic lesion resulting from a local antigen–antibody reaction in an immunized animal, the 'Arthus reaction' (type III hypersensitivity)

Opsonins

Allergy

1904 Almroth E. Wright and Stewart R. Douglas studied opsonization reactions (coined from *opsono*: I prepare food for). A bridge between the cellular and humoral theories

George Nuttall's *Blood Immunity and Blood Relationships* published. Precipitin reactions used to demonstrate blood relationships amongst various animals

F. Obermayer and C. P. Pick described altered protein antigens, first hapten study

Fred Neufeld: bacteriotropins named and described

Svante Arrhenius delivered a series of lectures in Berkeley, later to be published in the book *Immunochemistry*, term coined by him

1905 Clemens von Pirquet and Bela Schick published text on serum sickness of children receiving serum therapy. Pirquet coined 'allergy' to indicate an altered reactivity of the body, *ergcia* reactivity and *allos* altered

Robert Koch: Nobel Prize, for investigations in tuberculosis

1906 Wassermann developed the test for syphilis which bears his name

Richard Otto, the 'Theobald Smith phenomenon' described: anaphylactic death of guinea pigs

1907 A. Besredka and E. Steinhardt gave term 'anti-anaphylaxis' to the desensitization of animals sensitized to an antigen

1908 Paul Ehrlich, Elie Metchnikoff: Nobel Prize, for work on immunity

1909 Inbred mice

1910 John Auer and Paul Lewis; S. J. Meltzer identified the physiological reaction in anaphylaxis, recognized that asthma was a phenomenon of anaphylaxis

L. Hirzfeld and E. von Dungern: blood groups were genetically determined

Sir Henry Dale isolated histamine from ergot, demonstrated allergic contraction of muscle

William H. Schultz developed Shultz–Dale test for anaphylaxis

1911 John Freeman, Leonard Noon, treated hay fever with injection of pollen extract

Tumor viruses

1912 Alexis Carrell: Nobel Prize, for organ grafting

Charles Richet: Nobel Prize, for work on anaphylaxis

Viruses cultured

1913 Ludvig Hektoen proved that X-rays suppressed the antibody response

American Association of Immunologists founded

1914 Frederick Twort announced the transmissible lyis of bacteria by viruses, first mention of bacteriophage

1915 G. Sanarelli observed what was later called 'Shwartzman reaction'

Bacterophage discovered

1916 Landsteiner began study on haptens, carriers and antibody specificity

1919 Jules Bordet: Nobel Prize, for theories of immunity, complement

1920 Felix D'Herelle wrote *Le Bacteriophage*, filterable substance capable of bacteriolysis

Albert Calmette and Camile Guérin used BCG vaccine in experimental vaccination of newborns, later in mass vaccinations to control tuberculosis

1921 Carl W. Prausnitz and Heinz Küstner studied reagin; allergy to fish was passively transmitted, Prausnitz–Küstner test

Bacterial lysogeny

1922 Alexander Fleming described lysozyme

Michael Heildelberger and O. T. Avery: studies of antibody binding using capsular polysaccharides of pneumococci

Clarence Little established that the homograft reaction was due to genetic differences between donor and recipient

Sir Thomas Lewis wrote on the role of a histamine-like substance in the anaphylaxis complex

Carl S. Williamson of the Mayo Clinic described the pathology of transplant rejection

Hans Zinsser identified immediate and delayed hypersensitivity

1924 Besredka, local immunity, oral immunizations

BCG vaccine

1928 Gregory Shwartzman: local skin reactivity to *B. typhosus* filtrate, the Shwartzman phenomenon

1929 L. Dienes and E. W. Schoenheit wrote on delayed hypersensitivity to simple protein antigens injected into tubercles, forerunner of the adjuvant

Alexander Fleming, penicillin described

William Taliaferro's monograph on immunity to parasitic infections

1930 Friedrich Breinl and Felix Haurowitz: the template theory of antibody formation

Direct template theory

1931 Thomsen's description of the panagglutination reaction named for him in human erythrocytes

Virus culture on embryo

Virus size measured

1933 Landsteiner's 1st edition of *The Specificity of Serological Reactions*

1934 John Marrack proposed the 'lattice' theory of antibody–antigen secondary aggregates of antibody–antigen

1935 Tobacco mosaic virus crystalized

Viral interference

1935–36 Michael Heidelberger and Forrest E. Kendall isolated pure antibodies, performed quantitative precipitin reactions

P. D. McMaster and S. S. Hudack: antibody produced by cells of lymph nodes

1936 Gorer identified the first histocompatibility antigens

MHC antigens

Specificity of serologic reactions

Viral nucleoproteins

1935–39 Peter Gorer detected antigenic differences in mouse erythrocytes using immune sera

1938 Arne Tiselius and Elvin Kabat demonstrated that antibodies were gammaglobulins in Sweden using analytical ultracentrifuge; 19S antibody found early, 7S late in immune response

1939 Philip Levine and R. E. Stetson studied hemolytic disease of newborn, case of Mary Seno

γ-globulins

1940 Karl Landsteiner and Alexander Wiener: Rh antigens

Linus Pauling proposed a theory of antibody formation, the template idea again, the necessity of stereophysical complementarity of reaction

Variable folding theory

1941 George Hirst discovered virus hemagglutination. Also independently discovered by McClelland and Hare

F. M. Burnet, Freeman, Jackson and Lush proposed an early theory of antibody formation

1942 Jules Freund: Freund's complete adjuvant which enhanced antibody response to antigen and directed response to development of delayed hypersensitivity

A. H. Coons and H. H. Creech used fluorescein labeling, immunofluorescence as a tool for research

Lloyd D. Felton observed immunological tolerance in mice injected with minute amounts of polysaccharides

Karl Landsteiner and Merrill Chase demonstrated cellular transfer of sensitivity in guinea pigs

Immunofluorescence

Delayed-type hypersensitivity transferred with cells

Bacterial transformation with DNA

1944 Peter Medawar proved that the mechanism of tissue transplant rejection was immunological

Acquired immunological tolerance

1945 R. R. A. Coombs, R. R. Race and A. E. Mourant developed the antiglobulin test for incomplete Rh antibody

Ray Owen, Wisconsin, bovine twins were chimeras

T. N. Harris, E. Grimm, E. Mertens, W. E. Ehrich, the role of the lymphocyte in antibody formation

Cattle chimeras

Recombination in phage

1946 Jacques Oudin: precipitin reaction in gels

1948 Orjan Ouchterlony and Stephen Elek independently: double diffusion of antigen and antibody in gels

Antibodies in plasma cells

1949 Astrid Fagraeus, thesis on the correlation of antibody formation with the plasma cell series

Elvin Kabat, W. T. J. Morgan and others worked out the structure of ABO blood group antigens

Burnet and Frank Fenner introduced the 'self-marker' hypothesis in *The Production of Antibodies*

P. S. Hench and others at Mayo found that adrenocorticotropic hormone inhibited allergic reaction

Adaptive enzyme theory

Polio virus in culture

1950 A. H. Coons and Melvin H. Kaplan on the fluorescent antibody technique

1951 Max Theiler: Nobel Prize, development of yellow fever vaccine

1952 Ogdon Bruton described agammaglobinemia in humans

James R. Riley and Geoffrey B. West found histamine in mast cells

Transduction in phage

Infective agent was DNA

1953 Pierre Grabar and C. S. Williams: immunoelectrophoretic analysis

P. Medawar, R. E. Billingham and L. Brent on 'actively acquired tolerance' of foreign cells, proof for Burnet and Fenner's theory of antibody production

L. Pillemer, and others, properdin and its role in immune phenomena

John F. Enders, F. C. Robbins, T.H. Weller: poliomyelitis virus grown in tissue cultures, Nobel Prize

Chimeric tolerance

The double helix

1955 Rodney Porter: splitting IgG into Fab and Fc fragments

Niels K. Jerne developed the natural selection theory of antibody production

1956 Ernest Witebsky and Noel Rose: induction of autoimmune thyroiditis in animals

Discovery of human immunodeficiencies

1957 Roitt and Doniach, *et al.*, autoantibodies in thyroid disease, Hashimoto's thyroiditis

B. Glick, T. S. Chang and R. G. Jaap discussed the bursa of Fabricius in antibody production, 'B cells'

Alick Isaacs and Jean Lindenmann, discovery of interferon

L. D. McLean, S. Zak, R. Varco and R. Good: the role of the thymus in antibody production

Hugh Fudenberg and H. G. Kunkel: macroglobulins with antibody activity, cold agglutinins, rheumatoid factor

Daniel Bovet, Nobel Prize for antihistamine research

Cell selection theories

Interferon

1958 Jean Dausset, Rapaport: histocompatibility antigens on leukocytes

R. S. Farr: quantitative measure of primary interaction between bovine serum albumin and antibody

George Snell: the histocompatibility antigens of the mouse

Solomon Berson and Rosalyn Yalow: radioimmunoassay

1959 Burnet's clonal selection theory of antibody production

Gerald Edelman, Alfred Nisonoff and Rodney Porter studied the structure of antibody molecule using pepsin, papain

J. L. Gowans, lymphocyte recirculation

1960 Nowell, lymphocyte transformation (phytohemagglutinin)

Sir F. Macfarlane Burnet, Peter B. Medawar, Nobel Prize for work on acquired immunological tolerance

Messenger RNA

1961 J. F. A. P. Miller, Robert Good: thymus dependence of immune responses

1964 A. E. Reif and J. M. V. Allen, the AKR thymic antigen and its distribution in leukemia and nervous tissues, the theta antigen

1966 T and B cells

Genetic code completed

Spleen cell cultures

1966–67 H. N. Claman, Davies A, N. A. Mitchison: T–B cell cooperation

1967 Kimishige Ishizaka and T. Ishizaka: IgE as reaginic antibody

Johansson and Bennich study an atypical myeloma globulin, E myeloma

1968 Immune response genes linked to MHC

1970 Site-specific restriction enzymes

Reverse transcriptase

1971 Richard K. Gershon and Kazumnari Kondo: T cell suppression

1972 Rodney R. Porter, Gerald M. Edelman: Nobel Prize for immunoglobulin structure

Recombined DNA

1973 Niels Jerne: network theory of immune regulation

Recombined DNA replicated

Recombinant DNA

1974 T cell restriction

1975 H. Cantor and E. A. Boyse: T-cell subclasses distinguished by their Ly antigens, cell cooperation in the cell-mediated lympholysis reaction

Georges Köhler and César Milstein: monoclonal antibodies from hybridomas

R. M. Zinkernagel and P. C. Doherty: the altered self-concept dual recognition by T cells

Monoclonal antibodies

1977 Rosalyn S. Yalow: Nobel Prize for radio-immunoassay

1978 Immune response gene rearrangement

1980 Jean Dausset, Baruj Benacerraf, George Snell: Nobel Prize for immunogenetics research, MHC

W. Szmuness: hepatitis vaccine clinical trials

Henry Kaplan, Lennart Olsson: human hybridomas

Transgenic mice

1983 T cell receptors

1984 Human immunodeficiency virus (HIV-1) discovered to be the etiologic agent of acquired immune deficiency syndrome (AIDS) by Luc Montagnier, F. Barre–Sinoussi and J. C. Chermann, Institut Pasteur, Paris

T cell receptor genes

1987 Pamela Bjorkman and associates determined the structure of the human class I histocompatibility antigen and its antigen binding and T cell recognition regions

Susumu Tonegawa received the Nobel Prize in Medicine or Physiology for his demonstration of how antibody diversity is generated

1996 Peter Doherty and Rolf Zinkernagel received the Nobel Prize in Medicine or Physiology for their demonstration of MHC restriction of cytotoxic T-cell recognition of viral antigens on infected cells

What better way to end our discussion of milestones in the history of immunology than to use them as a window to the future, fulfilling our hopes and aspirations for successfully combating devastating microbial and neoplastic diseases not with toxic chemotherapeutic agents, but with substances manufactured within the animal body, devised by nature to aid our survival.

Suggested further reading

HISTORY OF IMMUNOLOGY

Bäumler E. *Paul Ehrlich Scientist for Life.* (Transl. Grant Edwards). New York: Holmes & Meier, 1984

Bibel DJ. *Milestones in Immunology: a Historical Exploration.* Madison, WI: Science Tech Publishers, 1988

Brent L. *A History of Transplantation Immunology.* San Diego, CA: Academic Press, 1997

Brock TD. *Robert Koch: a Life in Medicine and Bacteriology.* Madison, WI: Science Tech Publishers, 1988

Bulloch W. *The History of Bacteriology.* University of London Heath Clark Lectures, 1936. London: Oxford University Press, 1960 (1938)

Cunningham A, Williams P, eds. *The Laboratory Revolution in Medicine.* Cambridge: Cambridge University Press, 1992

Dubos RJ. *Louis Pasteur: Free Lance of Science.* Boston, MA: Little, Brown & Co, 1950

Ford WW. *Bacteriology.* (Clio Medica). New York: Paul B. Hoeber, Inc. Medical Book Department of Harper & Brothers, 1939

Foster WD. *A History of Medical Bacteriology and Immunology.* London: William Heinemann Medical Books Ltd, 1970

Mazumdar PMH. *Immunology 1930–1980: Essays on the History of Immunology.* Toronto: Wall & Thompson, 1989

Mazumdar PMH. *Species and Specificity: an Interpretation of the History of Immunology.* Cambridge: Cambridge University Press, 1995

Parish HJ. *A History of Immunization.* Edinburgh: E&S Livingstone Ltd, 1965

Parish HJ. *Victory with Vaccines.* Edinburgh: E&S Livingstone Ltd, 1968

Silverstein AM. *A History of Immunology.* San Diego, CA: Academic Press, 1989

Silverstein AM. *Paul Ehrlich's Receptor Immunology: the Magnificent Obsession.* With Introduction by Sir Gustav Nossal. San Diego, CA: Academic Press, 2002

Szentivanyi A, Friedman H, eds. *The Immunologic Revolution: Facts and Witness.* Boca Raton, FL: CRC Press, 1994

Talmage DW. A century of progress: beyond molecular immunology. *J Immunol* 1988;141:S5–16

Tauber AI, Chernyak L. *Metchnikoff and the Origins of Immunology: from Metaphor to Theory.* New York: Oxford University Press, 1991

Terasaki PI, ed. *History of HLA: Ten Recollections.* Los Angeles, CA: UCLA Tissue Typing Laboratory, 1990

Terasaki PI, ed. *History of Transplantation. Thirty-Five Recollections.* Los Angeles, CA: UCLA Tissue Typing Laboratory, 1991

CONTEMPORARY IMMUNOLOGY

Abbas A, Lichtman AH. *Cellular and Molecular Immunology.* Philadelphia: Saunders (Elsevier), 2000

Cruse JM, Lewis RE. *Illustrated Dictionary of Immunology,* 2nd edn. Boca Raton, FL: CRC Press, 2003

Cruse JM, Lewis RE. *Atlas of Immunology.* 2nd edn. Boca Raton, FL: CRC Press, 2004

Cruse JM, Lewis RE, Wang H. *Immunology Guidebook.* London: Academic Press, Elsevier, 2004

Janeway C, Travers P, Walport M, Shlomchik MJ. *Immunobiology,* 6th edn. New York: Garland Science, 2005

Goldsby RA, Kindt TJ, Osborne BA. *Kuby Immunology,* 4th edn. New York: Freeman Publishing, 2000

Lahita RG, ed. *Textbook of the Autoimmune Diseases.* Philadelphia, PA: Lippincott Williams & Wilkins, 2000

Parham P. *The Immune System.* New York: Garland, 2000

Paul WE. *Fundamental Immunology,* 5th edn. Philadelphia, PA: Lippincott Williams & Wilkins, 2003

Roitt IM. *Essential Immunology,* 9th edn. Oxford: Blackwell Science, 1997

Rose NR, Mackay IR, eds. *The Autoimmune Diseases,* 3rd edn. San Diego, CA: Academic Press, 1998

Epilogue

Michael Heidelberger (1888–1991), longest lived founder and eyewitness to the history of immunology in the 20th century.

Like a good parent, Michael Heidelberger nurtured immunochemistry from infancy through adolescence to adulthood. Master investigator and *mensch*, he trained a spate of highly gifted investigators including Elvin Kabat, Manfred Mayer and a host of others who have passed on his knowledge and expertise from generation to generation.

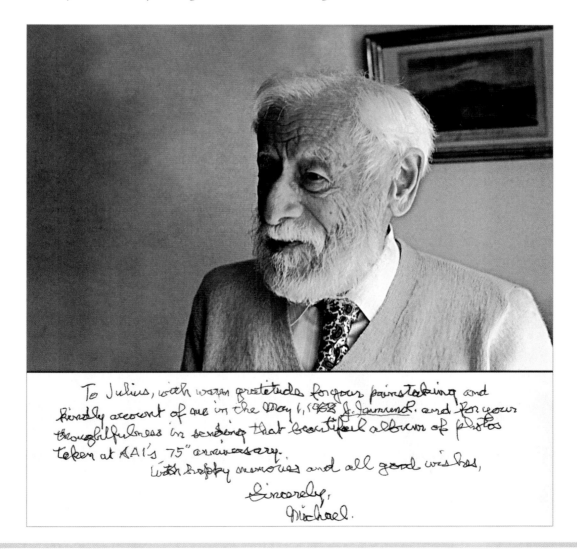

To Julius, with warm gratitude for your painstaking and kindly account of me in the May 1, 1968 J. Immunol. and for your thoughtfulness in sending that beautiful album of photos taken at AAI's 75" anniversary.
With happy memories and all good wishes,
Sincerely,
Michael.

Heidelberger's passing represented the end of the beginning for immunology – for he was the last of the founders, following Jules Bordet's death in 1961, who witnessed a century of spectacular advances in immunologic research. With the publication of his final investigative work in the 1990s, Michael contributed novel and innovative original scientific research articles to the literature in every decade of the 20th century! This final triumph of his magnificent career is unmatched in the annals of science. Michael's accomplishments in research are legion and well chronicled[1–7] and are not for further discussion here.

Michael's lifetime achievements in immunochemistry are a testament to the universality of science. His international outreach for the cause of science and humanity and quest for world peace command our respect not only for his professional skill and contributions to science but for an exceptional and exemplary life – *a hymn to the universe.*

When a new student performs his first experiment in immunology, he will be there. When a young investigator forges a new pathway in research, he will be there. When a senior scientist makes a breakthrough discovery that changes the course of medical science, Michael will be there – for it was his genius that illuminated and molded the facts, one by one, into the modern science that is immunology. When future generations ask, let it be said that we have stood on the shoulders of giants. What better use of a life than to spend it for something that outlasts its.

Lebe wohl, Michael … with our eternal thanks.

REFERENCES

1. Heidelberger M. A 'pure' organic chemist's downward path. *Annu Rev Microbiol* 1977;31:1

2. Heidelberger M. A 'pure' organic chemist's downward path; Chapter 2 – the years at P. and S. *Annu Rev Biochem* 1979;48:1

3. Kabat E. Michael Heidelberger as a carbohydrate chemist. *Carbohydrate Res* 1975;40:1

4. Cruse JM. A centenary tribute: Michael Heidelberger and the metamorphosis of immunologic science. *J Immunol* 1988;140:2861–3

5. Cruse JM. Introduction of Professor Michael Heidelberger. *J Immunol* 1988;141:52

6. Kabat EA. Michael Heidelberger – active at 100. *FASEB J* 1988;2:2233–4

7. Heidelberger M. *Lectures in Immunochemistry*. New York: Academic Press, 1956

8. Cruse JM. Michael Heidelberger (1888–1991): transition from life to legend. *Immunol Res* 1992;11:1–2

Credits for illustrations

ABOUT THE CRUSE COLLECTIONS

The Julius M. Cruse Collection in Immunology and Medicine at the Middleton Health Sciences Library, University of Wisconsin, Madison, was donated by Dr Julius M. Cruse in 1980.

The Julius M. Cruse Collection in the History of Immunology was donated to Rowland Medical Library, University of Mississippi Medical Center, Jackson, Mississippi in 2003.

CHAPTER 1

1. Courtesy of New York Academy of Medicine
2. Cruse Collection
3. Courtesy of National Library of Medicine
4. Cruse Collection
5. Courtesy of the Jenner Museum, The Chantry, Berkeley, Gloucestershire
6. Courtesy of the Jenner Museum, The Chantry, Berkeley, Gloucestershire
7. Cruse Collection
8. Courtesy of World Book Encyclopedia
9. Cruse Collection
10. Cruse Collection
11. Courtesy of the Wellcome Library, London
12. Courtesy of the Mary Evans Picture Library
13. Courtesy of the National Library of Medicine
14. Cruse Collection
15. Cruse Collection

16. Courtesy of the Harvey Cushing/John Hay Whitney Library, Yale University, New Haven, CT
17. Cruse Collection
18. Authors' Collection
19. Courtesy of the Wellcome Library, London
20. Courtesy World Health Organization
21. Courtesy World Health Organization
22. Courtesy World Health Organization
23. Photo courtesy of Dr Jason Weisfeld

CHAPTER 2

1. Cruse Collection
2. Cruse Collection
3. Cruse Collection
4. Courtesy of the Institut Pasteur, Paris
5. Cruse Collection
6. From the British magazine *Punch*
7. Cruse Collection
8. Parish H. J. *History of Immunization*. (plate 16) E&S Livingstone Ltd., Edinburgh and London, 1965. With permission of Elsevier Publishers
9. Cruse Collection
10. Cruse Collection
11. Cruse Collection
12. Cruse Collection
13. Cruse Collection
14. Cruse Collection
15. Cruse Collection
16. Cruse Collection

17. Cruse Collection
18. Cruse Collection
19. Courtesy of the Institut Pasteur, Paris
20. Cruse Collection
21. Cruse Collection
22. Cruse Collection
23. Cruse Collection
24. Parish H. J. *History of Immunization*. (plate 11) E&S Livingstone Ltd., Edinburgh and London, 1965. With permission of Elsevier Publishers
25. Cruse Collection
26. Cruse Collection
27. Cruse Collection
28. Marquardt M. *Paul Ehrlich als Mensch und Arbeiter*, 1924
29. Cruse Collection
30. Cruse Collection
31. Proceedings of the Royal Society, London, 1900. The Croonian lecture
32. Proceedings of the Royal Society, London, 1900. The Croonian lecture
33. Cruse Collection
34. Authors' Collection
35. Marquardt M. *Paul Ehrlich als Mensch und Arbeiter*, 1924
36. Marquardt M. *Paul Ehrlich als Mensch und Arbeiter*, 1924
37. Marquardt M. *Paul Ehrlich als Mensch und Arbeiter*, 1924
38. Marquardt M. *Paul Ehrlich als Mensch und Arbeiter*, 1924
39. Courtesy of George Mackenzie Collection, American Philosophical Society, Philadelphia, PA
40. Cruse Collection
41. Cruse Collection
42. Cruse Collection, courtesy of Dr M. W. Chase
43. Felix Haurowitz, an early proponent of the instructive theory of antibody formation
44. Courtesy of The Linus Pauling Institute
45. Cruse Collection
46. Cruse Collection
47. Cruse Collection
48. Cruse Collection
49. Cruse Collection
50. Cruse Collection
51. Cruse Collection
52. Cruse Collection
53. Courtesy of Dr D. W. Talmage
54. Cruse Collection

55. Courtesy of Sir Gustav Nossal
56. Courtesy of Sir Gustav Nossal
57. Cruse Collection
58. Courtesy of Dr Susumu Tonegawa
59. Authors' Collection
60. Authors' Collection
61. Authors' Collection
62. Courtesy of Dr Leroy Hood
63. Authors' Collection
64. Parish H. J. *History of Immunization*. (plate 18) E&S Livingstone Ltd., Edinburgh and London, 1965. With permission of Elsevier Publishers
65. Cruse Collection
66. Courtesy of the Wright-Fleming Institute, Imperial College, London

CHAPTER 3

1. Cruse Collection
2. Cruse Collection
3. Courtesy of George Mackenzie Collection, American Philosophical Society, Philadelphia, PA
4. Cruse Collection
5. Courtesy Dover Publications
6. Cruse Collection
7. Cruse Collection
8. Cruse Collection
9. Cruse Collection
10. Cruse Collection
11. Cruse Collection
12. Cruse Collection
13. Cruse Collection
14. Cruse Collection
15. Courtesy of the National Library of Medicine
16. Cruse Collection
17. Cruse Collection
18. Cruse Collection
19. Cruse Collection
20. *Ann Rev Immunol* – Annual Reviews Inc., Palo Alto, CA
21. Cruse Collection
22. Courtesy of the National Library of Medicine
23. Authors' Collection
24. Courtesy of Dr Gerald Edelman
25. Courtesy of Dr Gerald Edelman
26. Cruse Collection

27. *Nature,* Courtesy of Macmillan Magazines, London
28. Authors' Collection
29. Authors' Collection
30. Authors' Collection
31. Authors' Collection
32. Authors' Collection
33. Authors' Collection
34. Authors' Collection
35. Authors' Collection
36. Authors' Collection
37. Authors' Collection
38. Authors' Collection
39. Authors' Collection
40. Authors' Collection
41. Authors' Collection
42. Authors' Collection
43. Authors' Collection
44. Authors' Collection
45. Authors' Collection
46. Authors' Collection
47. Authors' Collection
48. Authors' Collection
49. Authors' Collection
50. Authors' Collection
51. Courtesy *Immunologic Research,* Humana Press, Totowa, NJ
52. Courtesy *Immunologic Research,* Humana Press, Totowa, NJ
53. Authors' Collection
54. Authors' Collection
55. Authors' Collection

CHAPTER 4

1. Cruse Collection
2. Cruse Collection
3. Cruse Collection
4. Cruse Collection
5. Cruse Collection
6. Authors' Collection
7. Cruse Collection
8. Cruse Collection
9. Authors' Collection
10. Authors' Collection
11. Authors' Collection
12. Authors' Collection

13. Authors' Collection
14. Cruse Collection
15. Authors' Collection
16. Cruse Collection
17. Cruse Collection
18. Authors' Collection
19. Authors' Collection

CHAPTER 5

1. Courtesy National Library of Medicine
2. Cruse Collection
3. Cruse Collection
4. Cruse Collection
5. Cruse Collection
6. Cruse Collection
7. Cruse Collection
8. Cruse Collection
9. Cruse Collection
10. Cruse Collection
11. Cruse Collection
12. Cruse Collection
13. Cruse Collection
14. Authors' Collection
15. Authors' Collection
16. Authors' Collection
17. Courtesy of Dr Zoltan Ovary
18. Authors' Collection
19. Cruse Collection

CHAPTER 6

1. Cruse Collection
2. Courtesy of Johns Hopkins Press
3. Cruse Collection
4. Cruse Collection
5. Cruse Collection
6. Cruse Collection
7. Courtesy of the National Library of Medicine
8. Authors' Collection
9. Authors' Collection
10. Courtesy of Mt Sinai Medical Center, New York, NY
11. Cruse Collection

12. Authors' Collection
13. Cruse Collection
14. Cruse Collection
15. With permission from Elsevier
16. Authors' Collection
17. *Immunology*. A Scope Publication. The UpJohn Co., 1985
18. Authors' Collection
19. Authors' Collection
20. Authors' Collection
21. Authors' Collection
22. Authors' Collection
23. Cruse Collection
24. Authors' Collection
25. Authors' Collection
26. Authors' Collection

CHAPTER 7

1. Cruse Collection
2. Parish H. J. *History of Immunization*. E&S Livingstone Ltd., Edinburgh and London, 1965. With permission of Elsevier
3. Courtesy National Library of Medicine
4. Courtesy National Library of Medicine
5. Authors' Collection
6. Authors' Collection
7. *Immunology*. A Scope Publication. The Upjohn Co., 1985
8. Authors' Collection
9. Authors' Collection
10. *Immunology*. A Scope Publication. The Upjohn Co., 1985
11 Courtesy of Dr John R. David

CHAPTER 8

1a. Cruse Collection
1b. *Acta Scandinavica Hematologica*
1c. Cruse Collection
1d. Cruse Collection
1e. Cruse Collection
2. Cruse Collection
3. Courtesy of Dr Robert A. Good
4. Courtesy of Dr Robert A. Good

5. Cruse Collection
6. Courtesy National Library of Medicine
7. Courtesy of Prof. Nicole Suciu-Foca, Columbia University, New York, NY
8. Cruse Collection
9. Cruse Collection
10. Cruse Collection
11. Cruse Collection
12. Cruse Collection
13. Authors' Collection
14. Authors' Collection
15. Authors' Collection
16. Authors' Collection
17. Authors' Collection
18. Authors' Collection
19. Authors' Collection
20. Authors' Collection
21. Authors' Collection
22. Authors' Collection
23. Authors' Collection
24. Authors' Collection
25. Authors' Collection
26. Authors' Collection
27. Authors' Collection
28. Authors' Collection
29. Authors' Collection
30. Authors' Collection
31. Authors' Collection
32. Authors' Collection
33. Authors' Collection
34. Authors' Collection
35. Authors' Collection

CHAPTER 9

1. Marquardt M. *Paul Ehrlich als Mensch und Arbeiter*. Stuttgart, 1924
2. Cruse Collection
3. Cruse Collection
4. Cruse Collection
5. Cruse Collection
6. Cruse Collection
7. Cruse Collection
8. Cruse Collection
9. Cruse Collection
10. Courtesy of INOVA Diagnostics and Mrs Carol Peebles, San Diego, CA, USA

CHAPTER 10

1. Courtesy of the National Library of Medicine
2. Cruse Collection
3. Cruse Collection
4. Cruse Collection
5. Cruse Collection
6. Cruse Collection
7. Cruse Collection
8. Cruse Collection
9. Authors' Collection
10. Authors' Collection
11. Authors' Collection
12. Authors' Collection
13. Authors' Collection
14. Cruse Collection
15. Cruse Collection
16. Cruse Collection
17. Courtesy of Simon and Schuster Publishers
18. Authors' Collection
19. Authors' Collection
20. Authors' Collection
21. Cruse Collection
22. Authors' Collection
23. Authors' Collection
24. Courtesy of Simon and Schuster Publishers
25. Cruse Collection
26. Courtesy of the Wellcome Trust Library, London

CHAPTER 11

1. Burgos Cathedral Museum, Burgos, Spain
2. From a 15th century miniature ascribed to Andrea or Francesco Mantegna
3. Courtesy of The Royal College of Surgeons of England, London
4. Gaspare Tagliacozzi, *Du Curtorum Chirurgia Per Institonem*. 1597
5. Putti's Donation of the Instituto Ortopedico Rizzoli, Bologna
6. Cruse Collection
7. Cruse Collection
8. Courtesy of the National Library of Medicine
9. Cruse Collection
10. Cruse Collection, Courtesy of Dr Rupert Billingham

11. Cruse Collection
12. Cruse Collection
13. Cruse Collection
14. Cruse Collection
15. Cruse Collection
16. Cruse Collection
17. Cruse Collection
18. Courtesy of UCLA Tissue Typing Laboratory
19. Courtesy of Dana Farber Cancer Institute, Boston, MA
20. Cruse Collection
21. Courtesy of UCLA Tissue Typing Laboratory
22. Courtesy of Dr Paul Terasaki
23. Courtesy of UCLA Tissue Typing Laboratory
24. Courtesy Jerry Berndt
25. Courtesy of Dr Rolf Zinkernagel
26. Authors' Collection
27. Authors' Collection
28. Authors' Collection
29. Authors' Collection
30. Authors' Collection
31. Authors' Collection
32. Authors' Collection
33. Authors' Collection
34. Authors' Collection
35. Authors' Collection
36. Authors' Collection
37. Authors' Collection
38. Authors' Collection
39. Authors' Collection
40. Authors' Collection
41. Authors' Collection
42. Authors' Collection
43. Authors' Collection
44. Authors' Collection
45. Authors' Collection
46. Authors' Collection
47. Authors' Collection
48. Authors' Collection

CHAPTER 12

1. Courtesy of Johns Hopkins University Press
2. Cruse Collection
3. Cruse Collection
4. Cruse Collection
5. Cruse Collection

6. Cruse Collection
7. Cruse Collection
8. Cruse Collection
9. Authors' Collection
10. Authors' Collection
11. Authors' Collection
12. Authors' Collection
13. Authors' Collection
14. Authors' Collection
15. Authors' Collection
16. Authors' Collection
17. Courtesy of the Institut Pasteur
18. Courtesy of the Institut Pasteur

10. Cruse Collection
11. Cruse Collection
12. Cruse Collection
13. Cruse Collection
14. Cruse Collection
15. Cruse Collection

CHAPTER 14

1. Cruse Collection
2. Courtesy of Mrs Marka Webb Stewart
3. Courtesy of New York Academy of Medicine
4. Courtesy of Mrs Marka Webb Stewart
5. Courtesy of the Bentley Historical Library, University of Michigan
6. Courtesy of New York Academy of Medicine
7. Authors' Collection
8. Authors' Collection

CHAPTER 13

1a. Cruse Collection
1b. Cruse Collection
2. Cruse Collection
3. Cruse Collection
4. Cruse Collection
5. Cruse Collection
6. Cruse Collection
7. Cruse Collection
8. Cruse Collection
9. Cruse Collection

EPILOGUE

Photograph of Michael Heidelberger, inscribed to Julius Cruse

Index

Abzyme 90
Ackroyd, J.F. 183
acquired immune deficiency syndrome (AIDS) 273–274, 284–288
  AIDS belt 285
  serology 285
  treatment 288
Adams, R.D. 192
Addison's disease 190
adenosine deaminase (ADA) deficiency 283
adoptive immunity 259
adoptive immunization 259
adoptive immunotherapy 175
affinity 89, 90
  functional 89
  maturation 89
AIDS *see* acquired immune deficiency syndrome (AIDS)
alexine 93–94
allelic exclusion 43–44
allergen 130
allergic contact dermatitis 146–147
allergic reaction 128–129
allergic rhinitis 129
allergoids 130
allergy 121, 128
  atopic 129
  autoallergy 197, 198
  bacterial allergy 142
  drug allergy 130
  food allergy 129
  house dust allergy 129
  infection allergy 142
  see also hypersensitivity
alloantibodies 84
  tumor transplantation and 229–232
allogeneic 260
allograft 258
  fetus allograft 257–258
allotope 84
allotype 83–84
altered self 199
Am allotypic marker 84

amboceptor 71
American Association of Immunologists (AAI) 305–309
  Committee on Clinical Immunology 310–311
  Journal of Immunology 309
  role in education 310
Amos, Bernard 213–215, 236
anaphylactic shock 116
anaphylactoid reaction 118
anaphylaxis 114–119
  active 117
  aggregate 118
  cutaneous 118–119
  generalized 117
  local 117
  passive 117
  passive cutaneous anaphylaxis (PCA) 119
    reverse (RPCA) 119
  systemic 117
  see also hypersensitivity
anaphylatoxins 118
Anderson, J.R. 188
anergy 145, 146, 244
  clonal anergy 37, 244
  lymphocyte anergy 244
anthrax 18
antiantibody 73
antibodies 70
  affinity 89, 90
  anti-D antibody 219–220
  anti-idiotypic antibody 91
  anti-immunoglobulin antibody 73
  antiglobulin antibodies 220
  as globulins 51–55
  assays 289–293
    see also specific methods
  autoantibodies 196–197
    cytokine autoantibodies 199
    natural autoantibodies 199–200
    pathologic autoantibodies 200
  blocking antibody 91
  catalytic antibodies 73
  chimeric antibodies 74

complement-fixing antibody 96
cross-reacting antibody 72
cytotoxic antibody 73
cytotrophic antibody 73
designer antibody 90
detection of 71
Donath–Landsteiner antibody 221
formation of see antibody formation
heteroconjugate antibodies 173
heterophile antibody 70
humanized antibody 75
immune antibody 219
isoantibody 258
monoclonal antibodies (MAb) 39, 70, 293–294
natural antibodies 218
non-precipitating antibodies 73
polyclonal antibodies 87
screening 254–255
skin-fixing antibody 73
skin-sensitizing antibody 114
specificity 71
synthesis see antibody formation
titer 71, 72
univalent antibody 72
see also immunoglobulins
antibody formation 72, 232
    instructive theory 39–40
    recombinatorial germ line theory 40, 232
    selection theory 31, 35–39, 40, 69, 179, 232
        clonal selection 36–38, 44, 45, 69, 179, 232
    self-marker hypothesis 39
    side-chain theory 26–30, 39, 50
    template theories 31–34, 39, 51, 232
    see also immunoglobulins
antibody screening 254–255
antibody-binding site 71
antibody-dependent cell-mediated cytotoxicity (ADCC)
    133, 134, 163–164, 172, 173
antigen–antibody interaction 44–45, 49–51
antigen-binding site 72
antigenic deletion 172
antigenic determinant 60, 61, 62, 66
    hidden determinant 65
antigenic diversion 172
antigenic gain 172
antigenic modulation 172
antigenic reversion 172
antigenic transformation 172
antigenicity 65
antigens 60–64
    assays 289–293
        see also specific methods
    autoantigens 196
    blood group antigens 218
        O antigen 219
        P antigen 221
        rhesus antigen 219
    carbohydrate antigens 64
    cross-reacting antigens 64
    Dander antigen 114

definition 61
    embryonic antigens 171
    fetal antigens 171
    Forssman antigen 69
    heterophile antigen 69
    histocompatibility 250
        human leukocyte antigens (HLA) 213–215, 234,
            238, 251–254
        minor 250
    indirect presentation 262
    oncofetal antigens 170–171
    platelet antigens 221–222
    private antigen 69, 256
    prostate-specific antigen (PSA) 169–170
    public (supratypic) antigen 69, 256
    sequestered 200
    superantigen 61
    synthetic antigens 61–64
    T cell-dependent (TD) antigens 64, 68
    T cell-independent (TI) antigens 64, 69
    tumor antigens 169
    tumor-associated antigens 169
        carcinoma-associated antigens 171
        melanoma-associated antigens 171–172
antiglobulin antibodies 220
    direct antiglobulin test 220
    indirect antiglobulin test 220
antiserum 71
antithymocyte globulin (ATG) 249
antitoxin 71
    assay 72
    diphtheria 22–24, 26, 126–127
    tetanus 275
    unit 72
antivenom 72
arachidonic acid (AA) 116
Arrhenius, Svante 44, 49, 50
Arthus, Nicolas Maurice 122, 123, 126
Arthus reaction 122, 123, 135–136
    passive 136
asthma 130
atopy 121, 129
attenuation 274
autoallergy 197, 198
autograft 259–260
autoimmune diseases 200
    animal models 201
    see also specific diseases
autoimmune hemolytic anemia 181–183
autoimmune thyroiditis 188–189
autoimmunity 177–181, 193, 196
    chronology of developments 194–195
    drug-induced 199
    liver disease and 191–192
    neurologic disorders 192–193
    sex hormones and 200
    skin reactions 193
autosensitization 198
Avery, Oswald T. 51, 54–55
avidity 88–89

hypothesis 89
azoprotein 68

B cell receptor 162
B cells 153, 162, 180
   tolerance 243
B lymphocyte hybridoma 87, 294, 295
bacillus Calmette–Guérin (BCG) vaccine 169, 269, 276
Bacon, P.A. 192
bacteriology 15–16
Baehr, G. 183
Bartholin, Thomas 2
basophils 167
Bassi, Agnostino 15
Benacerraf, Baruj 181, 186, 235–236, 311
Bendixen, G. 192
Bennett, J.C. 41, 232
Besredka, Alexandre 80, 111, 112, 119–120
Beutner, Ernst 179, 189, 193
Billingham, Rupert E. 139, 230–231
biological response modifiers (BRMs) 174
Blizzard, R.M. 190
blood groups 210–213, 218
   ABO system 210–211, 218
   Lewis system 221
   MNS system 211–212, 221
   rhesus (Rh) system 212–213, 214, 219
blood transfusions 207–208, 222, 238
   platelet transfusion 222
   transfusion reactions 222
   universal donor 222
   universal recipient 222
Bloom, Barry R. 139
Blundell, James 208, 209
bone marrow transplantation 259, 273
   allogeneic 260
   autologous (ABMT) 260
Bordet, Jules Jean Baptiste Vincent 1, 22, 24, 25, 45,
   94–96, 98, 289
Bovet, Daniel 120
Boyden, S. 179
Boyle, Robert 208
Boylston, Zabdiel 3
Boyse, E.A. 155
Brambell, F.W.R. 88
Brambell receptor 88
Breinl, F. 31
Brester–Cohn theory 240
Bronfenbrenner, J.J. 307
Brown–Pearce sarcoma 169
Bruton's X-linked agammaglobulinemia 281–282
Buchner, Hans 1, 18, 93, 94
bullous diseases 193
Burkitt's lymphoma 169
Burnet, Frank Macfarlane 1, 32–37, 168, 178, 179–180,
   191, 232
bursa of Fabricius 149, 162, 180
Buschard, K. 190

Calmette, Albert 138, 270

cancer 168–169
Cantell, Kari 273
Cantor, H. 155
carcinoembryonic antigen (CEA) 169
carcinoma-associated antigens 171
Carrel, Alexis 227–228
carrier 66
   specificity 67
carrier effect 67
Casey, A.E. 169
Catherine the Great, of Russia 4
cell-mediated immunity (CMI) 139–140, 149–157,
   179–181
cell-mediated lympholysis (CML) 155
Charrin, A. 289
Chase, Merrill W. 31, 139, 149, 211
Chauffard, M.A. 181
chemokines 281
chemotactic disorders 284
Chinitz, A. 181
Chorzelski, T.P. 193
chromosome 6 250, 251
Cinader, Bernhard 311
Claman, Henry N. 153, 154, 155–156, 180
clonal anergy 37, 244
clonal balance 244
clonal deletion 240–241
clonal ignorance 242–243
clonal selection theory 36–38, 44, 45, 69, 179, 232
   forbidden clone 36–37, 44, 178, 180
Coca, Arthur Fernandez 121, 122–123, 309
Cochrane, C.G. 128, 183
Cohn, Ferdinand 15
Colebrook, Leonard 305
Coley, William 168
collagen disease 183
complement deficiency conditions 284
complement deviation 97
complement fixation 95, 96–97
   assay 96, 289
complement system 55, 93–107
   activation unit 102
   alternative pathway 98, 101–103, 104–105, 106–107
   C1 complex 101, 102, 104
   classical pathway 98, 99, 101–102, 106–107
   complement multimer 102
   doughnut structure 102
   lectin pathway 105, 107
   membrane attack complex (MAC) 99–100, 102–104
   proteins 9
   recognition unit 102
   type II hypersensitivity 130–131
complementarity-determining region (CDR) 74
Condamine, Charles La 4
conjugate 66–67
constant domain 74
constant region 74
contact hypersensitivity 146
contact sensitivity 146–147
Cooke, Robert Anderson 121, 126

Coombs' antiglobulin test 215, 220
Coombs, Robin R.A. 122, 127–128, 182, 183, 184, 214, 291
Coons, Albert Hewett 149, 290
cowpox 4–10
cross-match testing 255
Cruse, Julius M. 311
cyclooxygenase pathway 116
cyclophilin 247
cyclosporine 245–246, 247
cytokine autoantibodies 199
cytokines 279–281

Dacie, J.V. 182–183
Dale, Henry Hallett 111, 112
Dameshek, William 181, 182
Dander antigen 114
Danysz, Jan 44–45
Danysz phenomenon 45
Dausset, Jean Baptiste Gabriel 234
David, John R. 139
Davies, A.J. 180
Dean, H.R. 186–187, 289
delayed-type hypersensitivity (DHT) *see* hypersensitivity
dendritic cells 165–166
Denis, Jean 208
Denys, J. 289
desensitization 117
determinant spreading 193–196
diazo salt 68
diazotization 68
DiGeorge syndrome 273, 282
Dimsdale, Thomas 4, 8
dinitrochlorobenzene (DNCB) 65, 66
dinitrofluorobenzene (DNFB) 67
2,4-dinitrophenyl (DNP) 65
diphtheria 22–24
    antitoxin 22–24, 26, 126–127
Dixon, Frank James 127, 128, 183, 186
DNA vaccine 279
doctrine of original antigenic sin 68, 87
Doherty, Peter 156, 157, 238, 239
Donath, J. 178
Donath–Landsteiner antibody 221
Doniach, Deborah 184, 190
donor 258–259
Douglas, Stewart R. 45, 289, 305, 307
Dray, Sheldon 310
Dreyer, W.J. 41, 232
drug allergy 130
drug-induced autoimmunity 199
DTaP vaccine 275
Durham, Herbert 25, 289

Ecker, E.E. 98
Edelman, Gerald Maurice 1, 56–58, 60, 187
Edsall, Geoffrey 309
Ehrlich, Paul vii–viii, 1, 25–30, 49, 94, 98, 177–178, 208, 269
eicosanoids 118

Eisen, Herman Nathaniel 60
electrophoresis 290
Elek, S.D. 291
Enders, John F. 270, 271
engraftment 261
enzyme-linked immunosorbent assay (ELISA) 298
eosinophils 167
epitopes 60, 61, 65
    definition 65
    immunodominant epitope 65
    tumor-specific 172
Epstein, W. 187
euglobulin 71

Fab fragments 56, 57, 70, 75, 81–82
Fab' fragments 82–83
Fabc fragment 82
Facb fragment 83
factor P see properdin
Fagraeus–Wallbom, Astrid Elsa 149, 155, 180
Fambrough, D.M. 193
Fb fragment 83
Fc fragments 56, 57, 70, 75, 81, 82
Fc' fragment 82
pFc' fragment 81
Fc receptor 91
Fd fragment 82
Fd' fragment 83
Feldman, Joseph D. 309
Fenner, F. 32–33, 35, 178, 179, 232
Ferrata, A. 97–98
fetus allograft 257–258
Fiessinger, N. 191
Finn, Ronald 212–213, 216
FK506 247, 248
FKBP (FK-binding proteins) 247
flocculation 290
flow cytometry 255–256, 300, 301
fluorescence antibody method 290–291
Foley, E.J. 169
food allergy 129
Forssman substance 69
Fracastoro, Girolamo 15
Fraenkel, Carl 22
framework regions (FRs) 91
Franklin, E.C. 187
Freund, Jules 178, 291
Fudenberg, Hugh 56, 182, 187
Fv fragment 83
Fv region 82

Gell, P.G.H. 122, 127–128, 183
Gengou, O. 289
Gershon, Richard K. 153, 155, 157, 186
Glick, Bruce 149, 152, 155, 180
globulins 70
    antithymocyte globulin (ATG) 249
    Rhesus immune globulin 220
    γ-globulin 71
    see also immunoglobulins

Gm allotype 82, 84
Gold, Phil 169
Gomagk, Gerhard 269
Good, Robert Alan 149–153, 156, 180, 193, 273
Goodpasture, Ernest W. 133
Goodpasture's antigen 133–134
Goodpasture's syndrome 131–133, 134
Gorer, Peter Alfred 229–230, 233
Gowans, J.L. 153, 154, 156, 180
Grabar, Pierre 179, 291–292, 293
graft rejection 179, 230–232, 261, 262–266
    first-set rejection 262
    second-set rejection 262
    see also transplantation
graft-versus-host reaction (GVHR) 139, 266
Green, I. 180
Green, N.M.J. 58
Gross, L. 183
Guérin, C. 138

H substance 218–219
Haemophilus influenzae type b vaccine (HB) 278
Haldane, J.B.S. 229
haplotype 92, 255
    extended 253
haptens 49–51, 60–61, 65–66
    carriers 66
        specificity 67
    hapten inhibition test 67–68
    hapten–carrier conjugate 66
        hapten conjugate response 67
Hargreaves, M.D. 183
Harris, T.N. 153, 180
Hasek, Milan 153, 154, 155
Hata, Sachahiro 26, 28
Haurowitz, Felix 31, 32
hay fever 129
heart–lung transplantation 256
heat inactivation 97
heavy chains 75, 76, 77
Heidelberger, Michael 51, 54, 58–59, 97, 98, 289–290,
    311, 321–322
Hektoen, L. 188
Hellström, Ingegerd 169
Hellström, Karl 169
Helmont, J.B. von 15
hemagglutination test 219
hemagglutinin 219
hematopoietic chimerism 261
hematopoietic stem cell (HSC) transplants 260–261
hemolytic disease of the newborn (HDN) 213, 216,
    220–221
Henle, Jacob 15
hepatitis vaccine 277–278
Heremans, J.F. 80
Hewson, William 153
hidden determinant 65
Hilleman, Maurice 272
hinge region 74
Hirszfeld, Ludwik 210, 212

histocompatibility 232–238, 249–250
    testing 250
histocompatibility antigen 250
    minor 250
histocompatibility locus 250
    minor 250
hives 116
HLA see human leukocyte antigens (HLA)
homograft 258
homology region 75–76
Hong, Richard 273
Hood, Leroy 43
'horror autotoxicus' 178, 179, 197–198
horse serum sensitivity 129–130
hot spots 72, 74
house dust allergy 129
Huang, S.W. 190
human immunodeficiency virus (HIV) 273–274,
    285–288
    HIV infection 287
    HIV-1 genes 287–288
    HIV-2 288
    see also acquired immune deficiency syndrome (AIDS)
human leukocyte antigens (HLA) 213–215, 234, 238,
    251–254
    disease association 253–254
    extended haplotype 253
    HLA non-classical class I genes 253
    HLA-A 252
    HLA-B 252
    HLA-C 252
    HLA-D region 251
        HLA-DP subregion 252
        HLA-DQ subregion 252
        HLA-DR subregion 252
    HLA-DM 252–253
    HLA-DR antigen specificities 252
    HLA-G 253
    HLA-H 253
    linkage disequilibrium 253
    splits 256
    tissue typing 254
humoral immunity 71
humoral–cellular immunity controversy 45, 93
Hunter, John 225, 226
Hutchinson, R. 188
hybridoma 39, 157, 181
    B lymphocyte hybridoma 87, 294, 295
hyperimmunization 274
hypersensitivity 113, 127–128
    delayed (type IV) 16, 127, 138–139, 140–142, 143
        contact sensitivity 146–147
        demonstration of 139
        infection hypersensitivity 142
        Jones–Mote reaction 147
        patch test 147
        poison ivy hypersensitivity 147
        tuberculin hypersensitivity 144
    immediate 114, 127
        prick test 116

scratch test 116–117
    type I (anaphylaxis) 114–119
    type II (antibody-mediated) 130–134
    type III (immune complex-mediated) 122, 124, 128,
      134–135
  pollen hypersensitivity 130
  see also allergy
hypervariable regions 77–78

idiopathic hypoparathyroidism 190
idiotype 84–85
  network theory 85–86, 181
immune complexes 122, 124, 128, 134–135, 183
  tissue injury and 183
immunization 10, 18, 269–272
  adoptive 259
  anthrax 18
  diphtheria 22.24
  hepatitis 277–278
  hyperimmunization 274
  influenza 272, 276, 278
  malaria 272, 278–279
  measles 270, 275, 277
  meningococcus 279
  mumps 272, 275, 277
  passive 90–91
  plague 279
  polio 270, 275, 276
  rabies 18, 270, 276
  rubella 272, 275, 277
  smallpox 2–11, 272
  tuberculosis 144–146, 276–277
  typhoid 276
  typhus 279
  yellow fever 270, 276
immunochemistry 49–50
  immunodeficiencies 273, 281–285
  secondary immunodeficiency 284
  with thrombocytopenia and eczema 283
  see also specific disorders
immunofluorescent staining of C4d 262, 263
immunogenetics 228
immunogenicity 65
immunogens 60–61, 64
  see also antigens
immunoglobulin genes 43
  allelic exclusion 43–44
  junctional diversity 44
  rearrangement 39–43, 44, 69–70
  recombination activating genes (RAG-1/RAG-2) 44
immunoglobulin superfamily 70
immunoglobulins 70, 75
  classes of 58, 70, 75, 78
    class switching 80, 91, 153, 180
    IgA 80
    IgD 80
    IgE 80, 111–117
    IgG 79, 187–188
    IgM 79–80
    subclasses 78–79

constant region 74
diversity 39–44, 69–70
domains 76, 77
  constant domain 74
  fold 76–77
fragments 81–83
framework regions (FRs) 91
function 76
heavy chains 75, 76, 77
hinge region 74
homology region 75–76
hypervariable regions 77–78
J chain 78
light chains 75, 76, 77, 78
maternal 87
papain digestion 55–56, 57, 81
pepsin digestion 58–59, 80–81
selective immunoglobulin deficiency 282
structure 28, 38, 56–58, 75, 77
variable region 91
see also antibodies; antibody formation
immunohematology 207–215
immunologic facilitation 174
immunologic paralysis 245
immunological enhancement 168–169, 174, 257
immunological escape 174
immunological ignorance 244–245
immunological inertia 239
immunological unresponsiveness 239
  Sulzberger–Chase phenomenon 244
immunologically privileged sites 256–257
immunology
  origins 1–2
  subspecialties 1
immunoperoxidase method 297
immunophilins 246
immunoregulation 239
immunoselection 174
immunosuppression 245
immunosuppressive agents 245
immunosurveillance 173
immunotherapy 174
  adoptive immunotherapy 175
immunotoxin 174–175, 260
indirect antigen presentation 262
infection, germ theories 15
influenza vaccine 272, 276
inoculation, smallpox 2–4
  see also immunization
insulin-dependent (type I) diabetes mellitus (IDDM)
  189–190
insulitis 189
interferon (IFN) 272–273, 280–281
interleukin (IL) 140
International Congress of Immunology 311, 312
International Union of Immunological Societies (IUIS)
  311–312
Irvine, J. 184, 191
Irwin, M.R. 228, 229
Isaacs, Alick 272, 273

Ishizaka, Kimishige 111, 113
Ishizaka, Terako 111, 113
islet cell transplantation 259
isoantibody 258
isogeneic 258
isograft 258
isologous 258
isotype 83
    switching 86–87

J chain 78
Jenner, Edward 4–7, 140, 269
Jensen, C.D. 228
Jerne, Niels Kaj 34–36, 85, 153–155, 179, 181, 186, 232
Johnson, S.D. 192
Jones–Mote reaction 147
Jordan, R.E. 193
Joske, R.A. 191
Journal of Immunology 309

K (killer) cells 164
Kabat, Elvin Abraham 51, 55–56, 59, 192, 290, 310
Kaplan, Henry 157
Kaplan, Martin 270
Kaposi, M.K. 183
Kay, M.M.B. 179
Kendall, F.E. 51, 289–290
King, W.E. 191
Kirkpatrick, James 4
Kissmeyer-Nielsen, F. 236–238
Kitasato, Shibasaburo 22, 24
Klemperer, P. 183
Koch phenomenon 142, 143
Koch, Robert 1, 15–16, 22, 138
Köhler, Georges J.F. 39, 157, 181, 294–296
Kondo, K. 153
Koprowski, Hilary 270
Kraus, R. 289
Krugman, Saul 272
Kunkel, Henry George 56, 58, 184, 186, 187
Küstner, H. 122

Landsteiner, Karl 1, 30–31, 37–38, 49–51, 139, 149, 178, 181, 208–212, 215–217, 289
Laquer, L. 193
Lawrence, Henry Sherwood 139
Leclef, J. 289
Leder, P. 43, 181
Lederberg, Joshua 38, 39
Lepow, Irwin 103, 105
Lerman, J. 188
leukotrienes 116, 118
Levine, Philip 211, 212, 213, 217
Lewis, M.R. 139
light chains 75, 76, 77, 78
Lindenmann, Jean 272
Lindstrom, J. 193
linkage disequilibrium 253
lipoxygenase pathway 116
Little, C.C. 228–229

liver disease 191–192
Loeb, L. 228
Lower, Richard 208
lupoid hepatitis 191
lymphocytes 139, 156, 157
    anergy 244
    designer lymphocytes 172
    recirculation 153
    tumor-infiltrating lymphocytes 175
    see also B cells; T cells
lymphokine-activated killer (LAK) cells 175
lymphokines 139, 280
lysins 74

McDevitt, H.O. 181
Mackay, Ian R. 180, 191
Maclaren, N.K. 190
macrophage migration test 146
macrophages 164–165
Madsen, Thorvald 44, 45
Magendie, François 15, 109
magic bullet 175
major histocompatibility complex (MHC) 215, 233
Makinodan, T. 179
malaria vaccines 272, 278–279
Marrack, John Richardson 51, 53, 60, 290
mast cells 167–168
Mather, Cotton 3–4
Mayer, Manfred 55, 98, 99
measles vaccine 270, 275, 277
Medawar, Peter Brian 1, 33, 179, 230, 231
Meister, Joseph 18
melanoma antigen-1 gene (MAGE-1) 171
melanoma-associated antigens (MAAs) 171–172
membrane attack complex (MAC) 99–100, 102–104
meningococcal vaccine 279
Merklin, G.A. 209
Metchnikoff, Elie 1, 18–21, 93, 137–138, 178
Meyer, K. 185
Miescher, Peter 184, 185
migration inhibition factor (MIF) 139, 146
    assay 139, 145, 146
Milgrom, Felix 187, 189, 190
Miller, J. 192
Miller, J.F.A.P. 149–153, 156, 180, 193
Miller, K.B. 184
Milstein, César 39, 157, 181, 296–297
Mitchison, N.A. 180, 181, 186, 231–232
Mithridates, King of Pontus 2
molecular (DNA) typing 255
Mollison, P.L. 182
monoclonal antibodies (MAb) 39, 70, 293–294
monocytes 165
mononuclear phagocyte system 166
Montagnier, Luc 273, 287
Montagu, Lady Mary Wortley 3
Moreschi, Carlo Alberto 215, 217, 290–291
Morgan, I.M. 192
Morgenroth, Julius 177–178, 208
Morton, J.A. 182, 191

Mudd, S. 31
Müller-Eberhard, Hans J. 98, 105
mumps vaccine 272, 275, 277
Muromonab OKT3 249, 262
Murray, Joseph E. 238
myasthenia gravis 193
mycophenolate mofetil 248–249

natural killer (NK) cells 163–164, 173
Neisser-Wechsberg phenomenon 97
Nelmes, Sarah 4–7
Nerup, J. 190
network theory 85–86, 155, 181
neurologic disorders 192–193
neutrophils 166–167
Nisonoff, Alfred 56–58
non-secretor 219
Nossal, Gustav Joseph Victor 37, 38, 180
Nuttall, George 18, 19, 93

O antigen 219
Obermayer, F. 30, 49
OKT3 249, 262
Olsson, Lennart 157
opsonins 45
opsonization 131
organ bank 259
organ brokerage 259
original antigenic sin 68, 87
Osler, W. 183
Oswald, A. 188
Ouchterlony, Oerjan Thomas Gunnersson 291
Oudin, Jacques 291
Ovary, Dr Zoltan 119
Owen, Ray David 230–231

P antigen 221
pancreatic transplantation 259
PAP (peroxidase–antiperoxidase) technique 297–298
papain 81
Pappenheimer, A.M., Jr 290
paratope 72
Parker Hitchens, A. 306–307, 308, 309
passive cutaneous anaphylaxis (PCA) 119
     reverse (RPCA) 119
passive transfer 113–114
Pasteur, Louis 1, 16–18, 178, 269, 270
patch test 147
Patrick, J. 193
Pauling, Linus 31, 32, 51
Payne, Rose 234–235
pemphigus vulgaris 193
pentadecacatechol 147
pernicious anemia 190–191
Pfeiffer phenomenon 24
Pfeiffer, Richard 24, 25, 93–94
phagocyte disorders 283
phagocytic cell function deficiencies 283–284
phenotype 255
phytohemagglutinin (PHA) 139

Pick, E.P. 30, 49
Pickles, M.M. 182
Pike, B.L. 37, 180
Pillemer, Louis 98, 101, 102
plague vaccine 279
plasma 218
plasma cell 149–151, 162–163, 180
platelet antigens 221–222
platelet transfusion 222
poison ivy hypersensitivity 147
polio vaccine 270, 275, 276
pollen hypersensitivity 130
polyimmunoglobulin receptor 91
polymerase chain reaction (PCR) 298–299, 300
polymorphonuclear leukocytes (PMNs) 166
polysaccharide antigens 64
polyvalent pneumococcal vaccine 275–276
Porter, Rodney Robert 1, 55–56, 60
Portier, Paul Jules 109–111, 113
postvaccinal encephalomyelitis 10
Prausnitz-Giles, Carl 122, 123, 126
Prausnitz–Küstner (PK) reaction 129, 130
precipitation 289–290, 292
precipitin 72, 289
Prehn, R.T. 169
Pressman, David 51, 53
prick test 116
Procopius 2
properdin 98, 102, 104
properdin system 104
prostate-specific antigen (PSA) 169–170
Putnam, Frank 56
Pylarini, Jacob 3

rabies 18
     vaccination 18, 270, 276
Race, Robert 213, 217
Ramon, Gaston 290
rapamycin 247–248
reagins 76, 111, 121–122
recombination activating genes (RAG-1/RAG-2) 44
rejection 262, 263
     see also graft rejection
Rhazes 2
rhesus (Rh) blood group system 212–213, 214, 219
     rhesus immune globulin 220
     rhesus incompatibility 220
rheumatoid arthritis 185–188
rheumatoid factor 187–188
Rich, A.R. 139
Richet, Charles Robert 109–111, 113
Rivers, T.M. 192
Robbins, F.C. 270
Robinson, E.S.J. 290
Roger, J. 289
Roitt, Ivan 184, 189
Rose, Harry 309
Rose, Noel Richard 185–186, 187, 188, 189
Roux, Emile 18, 19
rubella vaccine 272, 275, 277

Sabin, Albert 270, 272
Salk, Jonas 270, 271
Salk vaccine 276
Salmon, David E. 18
Salvarsan 26, 29, 269
Sanger, Ruth 213, 217
Saunders, Joseph 309
Scheel, Paul 208
Schick, Bela 127, 290
Schlepper 67
Schultz–Dale test 111
Schwartz, M. 191
Schwartz, S.O. 181, 184
scratch test 116–117
Scripps Clinic and Research Foundation 128
secretor 219
selective immunoglobulin deficiency 282
self-tolerance 178, 240, 241
    see also autoimmunity
sensitization 113, 231–232
    autosensitization 198
sequence specific priming (SSP) 255
serum sickness 127–128, 135, 183
severe combined immunodeficiency (SCID) 273,
        282–283
sex hormones, autoimmunity and 200
Shevach, Ethan M. 309
Shulhof, K. 188
Shulman, Sidney 189
Shwartzman, Gregory 122, 125, 126, 168
Shwartzman reaction 122, 125–126, 136, 168
Simonsen, M. 139
Singer, S.J. 292
Sirolimus 248
Sjögren's syndrome 188
skin grafting 225–227, 259
    split thickness graft 259
    take 261
    see also transplantation
Sloane, Sir Hans 3, 4
smallpox 2–13
    eradication 10–12
    inoculation 2–4
    vaccination 4–11, 272
Smith, H.R. 179
Smith, Theobald 18, 19
Snell, George Davis 169, 232–233
Soborg, M. 192
'specific soluble substance' 64
Steinberg, Alfred D. 179, 184, 185
Sturli, A. 208–210
Sugg, John Y. 309
Sulzberger–Chase phenomenon 244
superantigen 61
Sutton, Robert 4
Swentker, F.F. 192
switch 86–87
syngeneic 258
syngraft 258

Synnott, Martin J. 305, 307
syphilis
    treatment 26, 29
    Wassermann test for 25, 94, 97, 178, 289
systemic lupus erythematosus 183–184
Szmuness, Wolf 272

T cell receptor (TCR) 157, 160, 161
    $\gamma\delta$ T cell receptor 160–162
    types of 160
T cells 153, 158–159, 180–181
    $\alpha\beta$ T cells 160
    autoreactive T cells 199
    cytotoxic T cells 159, 172
    development 157–158
    helper T cells 159, 181
    suppressor T cells 153, 159–160, 181
    $\gamma\delta$ T cells 160
    tolerance 243
tacrolimus 247
Tagliacozzi, Gaspare 225–227
Talal, Norman 184, 185
Talmage, David Wilson 34, 36, 37, 179, 311
Tan, E.M. 184
Taylor, K.B. 191
Terasaki, Paul 236, 237
tetanus antitoxin 275
Theiler, Max 270, 271, 272
Theofilopoulos, Argyrios. N. 184, 185
Thomas, E. Donnall 238, 273
Thomas, Lewis 168
Thucydides of Athens 1–2
thymus 153, 180
thyroglobulin 188–189
Timoni, Emmanuele 2
Tiselius, Arne 55, 59–60, 290
titer 72
    antibody 71, 72
tolerance 63, 239–240
    acquired tolerance 241, 242
    adoptive tolerance 240
    B cell tolerance 243–244
    central tolerance 242
    control tolerance 242
    high-dose tolerance 241
    high-zone tolerance 241
    immunologic tolerance 240
    infectious tolerance 245
    low-dose tolerance 241
    peripheral tolerance 242
    self-tolerance 178, 240, 241
    T cell tolerance 243
tolerogen 240
Tomasi, Thomas B., Jr 80
Tonegawa, Susumu 41–43, 181, 232
toxins 64
    anaphylatoxins 118
    immunotoxin 174–175, 260
toxoid 275
transfer factor 139

transient hypogammaglobulinemia of infancy 281
transplantation 225–227, 238–239, 249
   bone marrow transplantation 259, 273
      allogeneic 260
      autologous (ABMT) 260
   graft rejection 179, 230–232, 261, 262–266
      first-set rejection 262
      second-set rejection 262
   graft-versus-host reaction (GVHR) 139, 266
   heart–lung transplantation 256
   hematopoietic stem cell (HSC) transplants 260–261
   islet cell transplantation 259
   pancreatic transplantation 259
   skin grafting 225–227, 259
   tumor allografts 228–232
triple response of Lewis 114
tuberculin 144
   hypersensitivity 144
   reaction 140–142, 144
   test 144
tuberculin-type reaction 144
tuberculosis 16
   immunization 144–146, 276–277
Tudhope, G.R. 191
tumor allografts 228–232
tumor immunity 168–175
tumor rejection antigen 172
tumor-associated antigens 169, 170
   carcinoma-associated antigens 171
   melanoma-associated antigens 171–172
tumor-infiltrating lymphocytes 175
tumor-specific antigens (TSAs) 172, 173
tumor-specific determinants 172
tumor-specific transplantation antigens (TSTAs) 172
typhoid fever
   Grüber–Widal test for 25
   vaccine 276
typhus vaccination 279

ultracentrifugation 290
unitarian hypothesis 86
urushiols 147

vaccination 10, 18, 269–272, 274
   see also immunization
vaccines 274
   conjugate vaccine 278
   DNA vaccine 279
   killed vaccine 274
   live vaccine 274
      attenuated 274–275
   see also immunization; specific vaccines
vaccinia 10

   generalized 10
   progressive 10
Valentine, R.C. 56, 58
van Rood, J.J. 236, 237
variable region 91
   framework regions (FRs) 91
variolation 2–4
vasoactive amines 116
Vaughan, Victor Clarence 306, 308
Villemin 15
Vincent, C. 181
Voisin, G. 178
Voltaire 4
von Behring, Emil Adolph 1, 22–24
von Descastello, Alfred 208–210
von Dungern, Emil 210, 212
von Grüber, Max 25, 289
von Pirquet, Clemens Freiherr 121, 122, 126, 127
von Wassermann, August 25, 94, 290

Waaler, E. 185
Waksman, B.H. 192
Waldenström, Jan Gosta 58
Walker, J.G. 192
Wassermann reaction 25, 94, 97, 178, 289
Waterhouse, Benjamin 7
Webb, Gerald Bertram 305–306, 307
Webb, R.A. 289
Weigert, C. 193
Weller, T.H. 270, 272
Wells, Harry Gideon 51, 52
Wheal and flare reaction 129
Whittingham, S. 191
Widal, Fernand 25, 181, 289
Wiener, Alexander 211, 212
Willis, T. 193
Wilson, G.M. 191
Wiskott–Aldrich syndrome 283
Witebsky, Ernest 178–179, 187, 188, 189, 190
Witebsky's criteria 199
Wolfe, H. 149
Woodville, William 4, 9
Wright, Almroth E. 45, 46, 289, 305, 307

X-linked agammaglobulinemia 273, 281–283
xenograft 258

Yalow, Rosalyn Sussman 292, 293
yellow fever vaccine 270, 276
Yersin, Alexandre 18

Zinkernagel, Rolf 156, 157, 238, 239
Zinsser, Hans 127, 138–139